Infection Prevention and Safe Practice

POCKET GUIDE TO

Infection Prevention and Safe Practice

SUSAN D. SCHAFFER, PhD, FNP

Associate Professor, School of Nursing
Family Nurse Practitioner, Old Dominion University
Norfolk, Virginia

LAUREL S. GARZON, DNSc, RN

Assistant Professor of Perinatal Nursing
Director, Perinatal Clinical Specialist Program and
Neonatal Nurse Practitioner Program
Old Dominion University
Norfolk, Virginia

DORRI L. HEROUX, RN, BSN, MSHS, CIC

Infection Control Coordinator
Group Health Cooperative of Puget Sound
Tacoma, Washington

DENISE M. KORNIEWICZ, DNSc, RN, FAAN

Associate Dean for Academic Affairs
Associate Professor, Georgetown University
Washington, D.C.

with **43** *illustrations*

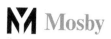

Mosby

St. Louis Baltimore Boston Carlsbad Chicago Naples New York
Philadelphia Portland London Madrid Mexico City Singapore
Sydney Tokyo Toronto Wiesbaden

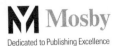

Mosby

Dedicated to Publishing Excellence

A Times Mirror Company

Publisher: Nancy Coon
Editor: Barry Bowlus
Senior Developmental Editor: Nancy C. Baker
Project Manager: Patricia Tannian
Senior Production Editor: Suzanne C. Fannin
Book Design Manager: Gail Morey Hudson
Manufacturing Supervisor: Linda Ierardi
Editing and Production: Graphic World Publishing Services
Cover Designer: Teresa Breckwoldt

Printed in the United States of America
Composition by: Graphic World, Inc.
Printing/binding by: R. R. Donnelley & Sons Company

Mosby–Year Book, Inc.
11830 Westline Industrial Drive
St. Louis, Missouri 63146

Library of Congress Cataloging in Publication Data

Pocket guide to infection prevention and safe practice / Susan D. Schaffer . . . [et al.]
    p.   cm.
   Includes bibliographical references and index.
   ISBN 0-8151-7593-0
   1. Hospitals—Sanitation—Handbooks, manuals, etc. 2. Nosocomial infections—Prevention—Handbooks, manuals, etc. 3. Cross infection—Prevention—Handbooks, manuals, etc. I. Schaffer, Susan D.
   [DNLM: 1. Cross Infection—prevention & control—handbooks. 2. Infection Control—methods—handbooks. 3. Nursing Care—standards—handbooks. WC 39 P7385 1996]
RA969.P63 1996
614.4′4—dc20
DNLM/DLC
for Library of Congress
                              95-32784
                              CIP

95 96 97 98 99 / 9 8 7 6 5 4 3 2 1

Contributors

CAROLINE BAGLEY BURNETT, RN, ScD
Assistant Professor
School of Nursing and Lombardi Cancer Center
Georgetown University
Washington, D.C.

PENNY E. CRAWFORD, RN, MSN, FNP
Family Nurse Practitioner, Certified Wound, Ostomy,
Continence Nurse
Great Neck Family Practice
Virginia Beach, Virginia

JOANNE R. DUFFY, DNSc, RN, CCRN
Administrator, Cardiac Care and Transplant Services
Fairfax Hospital
Falls Church, Virginia

DORRIE K. FONTAINE, RN, DNSc
Clinical Associate Professor
School of Nursing
Georgetown University
Washington, D.C.

MARYANNE F. LACHAT, RNC, PhD
Clinical Assistant Professor
School of Nursing
Georgetown University
Washington, D.C.

SANDRA W. McCLESKEY, RN, PhD
Assistant Professor
School of Nursing and Department of Pharmacology
Georgetown University
Washington, D.C.

JENNIFER McMURRAY, RN, NNP, MSN
Director of Neonatal Outreach Network
Childrens Hospital of the King's Daughters
Norfolk, Virginia

KATHLEEN M. NEILL, RN, DNSc
Assistant Professor
School of Nursing
Georgetown University
Washington, D.C.

PATRICIA C. SEIFERT, RN, MSN, CRNFA, CNOR
Operating Room Coordinator, Cardiac Surgery
Department of Surgery
The Arlington Hospital
Arlington, Virginia

LAURA SESSIONS, RN, MSN
University of Maryland Medical Systems
Baltimore, Maryland

SHEILA M. SPARKS, DNSc, RN, CS
Assistant Professor
School of Nursing
Georgetown University
Washington, D.C.

Preface

It is an increasing challenge for nurses and other health care professionals in the 1990s to prevent and manage infection in patients and health care workers (HCWs), to meet the budgetary constraints of the health care organization, and to comply with the latest directives from accrediting and regulatory agencies. HCWs require current infection control information to meet this challenge.

Nosocomial (hospital-acquired) infections are increasing in the United States, affecting 5% to 7% of people who are admitted to an acute-care hospital. Factors contributing to this increase are the increasingly debilitated patients who are admitted to hospitals and the increasing use of invasive, high-risk technology. HCWs must understand body defense mechanisms and how they are threatened by patient treatments and procedures to apply isolation precautions and prevent nosocomial infections.

Although hepatitis B is now vaccine preventable, human immunodeficiency virus (HIV) and hepatitis C continue to pose risks for HCWs who experience needle stick or other contaminated sharp instrument exposures. Implementation of the 1991 Blood-borne Pathogens Standard foreshadows the increasing influence of the Occupational Safety and Health Administration (OSHA) on HCW protection. HCWs require knowledge of regulatory trends and national organizational recommendations to minimize their risks of occupational infection.

Pocket Guide to Infection Prevention and Safe Practice summarizes and reinforces information needed to promote safety of patients and HCWs related to infection and communicable disease. The emphasis is on infection control (preventing infection) rather than management of infection. "Stop and Think" figures featured in many of the chapters summarize infection control strategies used to break the chain of infection in specific situations. Unit I describes the role of regulatory, accreditation, and professional agencies in infection prevention and management, identifies reportable diseases, and identifies infection control resources. An overview of the roles of the Joint Commission for the Accreditation of Healthcare Organizations (JCAHO), the Centers for Disease Control and Prevention (CDC), and OSHA related to infection control is provided along with current initiatives of these organizations.

Unit II presents concepts of immunity and the chain of infection. Patient risks for infection and signs and symptoms of patient infections are reviewed. This unit includes the CDC 1994 Draft Guidelines for Isolation Precautions in Hospitals that supersede previous recommendations for patient protection and that incorporate aspects of universal precautions, body substance isolation, and the 1983 CDC isolation precautions. An extensive chapter on HCW safety reviews HCW immunization, work exclusion for workers with infections, and the management of blood and body fluid exposures. Strategies for disinfection, sterilization, and surgical asepsis are included.

Unit III focuses on the prevention of patient infection during specific procedures. Sections in these chapters on home care acknowledge the importance of this health care trend. Although most of these chapters focus on procedures that are applicable for all patients, chapters on the neonatal procedures and obstetrical procedures reflect specialty approaches. A chapter on the immunocompromised patient acknowledges special approaches that are needed for the patient whose immune system is reduced.

This book is addressed to all HCWs who are interested in preventing infection in their patients and in themselves.

Susan D. Schaffer, PhD, FNP

Contents

UNIT I Trends and Regulations in Infection Control

1 Trends in Health Care: Implications for Infection Control Practice, 3

2 The Role of Regulatory, Accreditation, and Professional Agencies, 7

3 Reportable Diseases, 19

4 Infection Control Resources, 50

UNIT II Infection Control Strategies

5 The Infectious Process: Body Defenses and Chain of Infection, 57

6 Hand Washing: The Most Important Method of Prevention and Control, 74

7 Isolation Precautions, 81

8 Preventing and Managing Infections in Health Care Workers, 116

9 Cleaning, Disinfecting, and Sterilizing, 139

10 Surgical Asepsis, 162

UNIT III Infection Control and Nursing Procedures

11 Collecting Blood and Body Fluid Specimens, 181

12   The Immunocompromised Patient, 202

13   Surgical Procedures, 224

14   Catheterization, 241

15   Wound and Ostomy Management, 273

16   Burn Care, 292

17   Intravenous Techniques, 304

18   Gastrointestinal Procedures, 342

19   Dialysis, 351

20   Respiratory Care 363

21   Obstetrical Procedures 387

22   Neonatal Procedures, 396

23   Postmortem Care, 409

POCKET GUIDE TO

Infection Prevention and Safe Practice

TRENDS AND REGULATIONS IN INFECTION CONTROL

I

Trends in Health Care: Implications for Infection Control Practice

1

Trends in Infectious Diseases

Recent developments in the health care environment have stimulated interest in infection control practices in traditional and nontraditional health care settings. These developments relate to trends in infectious diseases and their human and monetary costs. The increase in infectious diseases that cannot be readily controlled by antibiotics or are resistant to antibiotics has renewed the interest of health care workers, health care administrators, regulatory agencies, and accrediting agencies, in infection control policies and practices. Concerns about occupational transmission of human immunodeficiency virus (HIV) and hepatitis B virus have generated an increased focus on infection control practices, especially universal precautions. These occupational concerns are translated into regulations in the form of the Occupational Safety and Health Administration (OSHA) Bloodborne Pathogens Standard.[1] Methicillin-resistant *Staphylococcus aureus,* vancomycin-resistant *Enterococcus faecium,* and multidrug-resistant tuberculosis currently challenge the efforts of infection control specialists in hospitals, long-term care facilities, ambulatory care centers, and home health settings. Efforts to define the most effective strategies to prevent and contain infection continue.

Cost Issues

In the context of increasing interest in cost-effective health care, the presence and costs of nosocomial infections are now closely scrutinized by providers, by third-party payers, and by patients. By their nature, nosocomial infections generate concern about the quality and efficacy of health care services.[2] There is increasing reluctance on the part of third-party payers to pay for this adverse outcome of treatment.[2]

Many patients who were formerly kept in the hospital are now being discharged to long-term care and home health care settings. This trend is certainly driven by cost considerations. However, it is also influenced by trends in supportive care for the dying and by physicians' perceptions that home care limits the risk of patient exposure to organisms from other patients. Infection control measures are needed in ambulatory care and home settings because these patients may be immunocompromised, may have communicable diseases, or may have invasive devices. Methods for preventing the spread of infection must be adapted because patients must be protected from acquiring new infection. Family caregivers must be protected and taught infection prevention practices, such as hand washing, and strategies for disposal of contaminated needles and other potentially infectious items.

Ethical and Legal Principles Related to Infectious Diseases

The Code for Nurses holds that nurses provide service to all persons without regard for socioeconomic status or the nature of health problems. The code also states that information of a confidential nature must be protected.[3] These principles support the ethical obligation of nurses to care for persons with infectious disease unless the care involves the risk of significant personal harm to the nurse.[4] The Employment at Will Doctrine provides legal support for the right of employers to discharge employees for refusal to care for assigned patients.[5]

However, the HIV epidemic has challenged our thinking about fundamental ethical and legal issues, such as the right of privacy, informed consent, and confidentiality. Although the chances of occupational transmission are remote, the discovery that HIV can be transmitted to health care workers has led to a reassessment of the balance between the duty to provide health care and the privacy interests of patients and providers.

Widespread HIV screening of patients or providers has been

generally dismissed as inefficient; however, recent legal decisions uphold the right of employers to know the HIV status of employees who provide services that are considered to be invasive or that present an opportunity for an exchange of body fluids.[6] Employees who experience exposure to a patient's blood or body fluids may have a right to know the HIV status of the patient. These rights have generally been codified into state laws. Employers who know of their employee's positive HIV status are required to keep this information confidential, just as employees must maintain patient confidentiality.

The Americans with Disabilities Act of 1990 includes HIV infection, and suspicion of HIV infection, as a condition that is categorized as a handicap. Employers must make reasonable accommodations for employees with handicaps who are otherwise qualified for their positions.[7] A hospital was recently cited under this act for transferring a nurse infected with HIV from an intensive care unit to a secretarial position. The nurse was reinstated because it was found that he followed universal precautions and performed no invasive procedures.[8] Health care providers must remain attentive to the evolving legal environment related to infection while remembering their duty to provide care for all patients and protection for their employees.

Research and Infection Control

Given the high cost of many infection control and isolation procedures and the risks to patients and providers if these procedures are ineffective, it is unfortunate that there are few rigorous studies documenting the efficacy and cost effectiveness of isolation precautions.[9] Although the various protocols currently in use for infection control all have advocates, research is needed before any conclusions are drawn about their relative efficacy and cost effectiveness. Universal precautions are now legally enforceable through the implementation of the OSHA Bloodborne Pathogens Standard, but they have not been shown to prevent contaminated-needle injuries, which account for 80% of occupationally acquired HIV.[10] The engineering controls being marketed to prevent needle stick injuries lack rigorous evaluation of efficacy.

Continuing questions about infection control protocols and the evolution of variant organisms mandate that health care workers participate in and remain abreast of research. The most effective systems for infection control will be those that are easy to use correctly, are cost effective, and are shown to be safe.

References

1. U.S. Department of Labor/OSHA. Occupational exposure to blood-borne pathogens: final rule, *Federal Register* 56(235):64004, 1991.
2. Wakefield DS: Understanding the costs of nosocomial infections. In Wenzel RP, editor: *Prevention and control of nosocomial infections,* (ed 2), Baltimore, 1993, Williams & Wilkins.
3. American Nurses Association. *Code for nurses with interpretive statements,* Kansas City, Mo, 1985, American Nurses Association.
4. American Nurses Association. *Ethics in nursing: position statements and guidelines,* Kansas City, Mo, 1988, American Nurses Association.
5. Greve PA: Medical, ethical, and legal issues associated with HIV, *J Intravenous Nurs* 14(suppl):S-30, 1991.
6. *Leckelt v. Board of Commissioners of Hospital District No. 1,* 714 F. Supp. 1377 (D.C. La. 1989).
7. *The Americans with Disabilities Act of 1990.* 1990. U.S. Code. Vol. 42, sec. 12101 *et seq.*
8. Pugliese G: Court rules on applicability of OSHA's bloodborne pathogen rule on dental practice, home healthcare settings, and temporary staffing, *Infect Control Hosp Epidemiol* 14(4):235, 1993.
9. Garner JS, Hierholzer WJ: Controversies in isolation policies and practices. In Wenzel RP, editor: *Prevention and control of nosocomial infections,* (ed 2), Baltimore, 1993, Williams & Wilkins.
10. American Nurses Association: Needlesticks put RNs at risk, *Am Nurs* 2, Dec 1990.

The Role of Regulatory, Accreditation, and Professional Agencies

2

Understanding the roles of national agencies in the prevention and management of infection requires an understanding of the underlying purpose and enforcement capabilities of those agencies. Organizations discussed in this chapter include the Joint Commission for the Accreditation of Healthcare Organizations (JCAHO), the Occupational Safety and Health Administration (OSHA), and Centers for Disease Control and Prevention (CDC). An overview of each agency is presented, and the remainder of the chapter focuses on current initiatives of each agency related to infection control.

Joint Commission on Accreditation of Healthcare Organizations

JCAHO is a national organization that accredits health care organizations that demonstrate compliance with JCAHO published standards. JCAHO implemented the first formal hospital infection control requirements when it published infection control standards in 1976 as a requirement for hospital accreditation. These standards are revised and published annually, reflecting changes in infection control practice to protect patients and health care workers.

Although JCAHO accreditation is voluntary, it is viewed as critical by most hospitals because 43 states recognize this accreditation in licensure decisions and 13 states accept accreditation in place of state licensure inspection. Accreditation of a health care facility by JCAHO is also required for Medicare and Medicaid participation.[1]

JCAHO Infection Control Standards

JCAHO infection control standards published in 1994 (1995 guidelines) require documentation of an effective, hospitalwide program for the surveillance, prevention, and control of infection, with oversight of infection control activities provided by a multidisciplinary committee. The 1995 guidelines provide examples of evidence of performance for the surveillance, prevention, and control of infection.[2] The box on p. 9 outlines three broad standards related to infection control that hospitals are expected to achieve for accreditation.

Responsibility for the infection control program must be assigned to a person with training in infection surveillance, prevention, and control functions. This person must be knowledgeable in epidemiologic principles, infectious disease, and either adult education principles or patient care practices. Patient care support services must be available to assist in the prevention and control of infections, and these services must have adequate direction, staffing, and facilities to perform required infection surveillance, prevention, and control functions.[2]

In 1986 JCAHO began a major initiative to reshape the nature of accreditation based on a goal of continual improvement in the quality of care. This initiative, the Agenda for Change, shifts the focus of evaluation from an organization's capacity to provide good care (process indicators) to its actual performance (outcome indicators). An essential component of the Agenda for Change is the development of useful performance measures and the establishment of an interactive reference database by which organizations can both monitor and compare their performance with other organizations.[3]

An Infection Control Expert Task Force was convened by JCAHO in 1990 to begin infection control indicator development. After face validity (reasonableness) and the collectibility of initial indicators were determined, a second 2-year round of testing was initiated in 1992. This second phase of testing evaluated (1) the capacity of a wide variety of hospitals to collect and transmit indicator data, (2) the capacity of JCAHO to receive and analyze indicator data and transform the data into comparative reports, (3) the reliability and validity of the data for identifying opportunities for improvement, and (4) the cost and usefulness of the indicators.[4]

Testing on infection control indicators was completed in August 1994. Hospitals seeking accreditation that voluntarily enroll in the Indicator Measurement System will begin using these finalized

---

1995 JCAHO Standards for Surveillance, Prevention, and Control of Infection

IC.1   The organization has a functioning coordinated process in place to reduce the risks of endemic and epidemic nosocomial infections in patients and health care workers.

- The process is managed by an individual who is qualified by virtue of education, training, certification, and/or licensure.

IC.2   In patient care and employee health activities there are mechanisms or processes designed to reduce the risks of endemic and epidemic nosocomial infections. These mechanisms include:

- Case findings and identification of nosocomial infections, as appropriate to demographics, to provide surveillance data for the organizations.
- Reporting of information about infections, as appropriate, to the organization and to public health agencies.
- Implementation of strategies to reduce risks for and/or to prevent nosocomial infections in patients, employees, and visitors.
- Implementation of strategies to control outbreaks of nosocomial infections when such are identified.

IC.3   An objective of the nosocomial infection risk reduction process is improvement in the risks of, trends in, and, where appropriate, rates of epidemiologically significant infections.

- Appropriate management systems support the nosocomial infection risk reduction process to ensure adequate data analysis, interpretation, and presentation of findings.

From Joint Commission on Accreditation of Healthcare Organizations: Surveillance, prevention, and control of infection, *1995 Accreditation manual for hospitals,* 1994, Joint Commission on Accreditation of Healthcare Organizations.

1996 JCAHO Infection Control Indicators

Indicator 1
Numerator: Selected inpatient and outpatient surgical
  procedures complicated by a surgical site infection
Denominator: Number of selected inpatient and
  outpatient surgical procedures

Indicator 2
Numerator: Ventilated patients who develop pneumonia
Denominator: Inpatient (ICU/non-ICU) ventilator days

Indicator 3
Numerator: Inpatients with a central or umbilical line
  who develop primary blood stream infection.
Denominator: Inpatient (ICU/non-ICU) central or
  umbilical line days

From Joint Commission on Accreditation of Healthcare Organizations: The indicator measurement system, *1996 Draft medication use/infection control indicators,* 1995, Joint Commission on Accreditation of Healthcare Organizations.

indicators in 1996.[5] These are listed in the box above. It is anticipated that use of the infection control indicators will assist hospitals in monitoring and improving patient care. JCAHO may initiate an inquiry of institutions with unusually high rates of infection compared with peer institutions. Of primary interest will be how the institution responded to the high rates.[4]

Occupational Safety and Health Administration

The Occupational Safety and Health Act of 1970 (PL 91-596, 1970) was passed by a bipartisan congress in response to escalating rates of job-related accidents, worker-related disabilities, and new cases of occupational diseases. This act established OSHA, a branch of the U.S. Department of Labor that is charged with conducting research, developing safety standards, monitoring job-related illness, and inspecting workplaces. OSHA standards are legally enforceable and employers violating standards are subject to fines. Section 18 of the act permits any state to develop and enforce its own occupational safety and health standards, but these must be equivalent to or higher than OSHA standards. Although the general duty clause of the act requires all employers to maintain working environments safe from hazards, promulgation of the 1991 Bloodborne Pathogens Standard marked the first OSHA regulation directed specifically at the 7 million health care workers in the United States.

OSHA: Bloodborne Pathogens Standard

In 1986 to 1987, following the first documented reports of occupationally acquired HIV in health care workers (HCWs),[6] several unions representing HCWs and the American Nurses Association[7] petitioned OSHA to promulgate an emergency infection control standard. Although OSHA believed an emergency standard was not justified, congressional hearings in 1987 led to a decision by OSHA to enforce the CDC universal precautions guidelines while OSHA's standard rulemaking procedure was pursued.[8] The final standard was published in December 1991 with an effective date of March 1992. The applicability of the standard to dentists, temporary medical personnel, and home health employers was recently upheld by a federal appeals court.[9] An overview of the Bloodborne Pathogens Standard is presented in the box on pp. 12-13.

OSHA: Guidelines for Preventing the Transmission of Tuberculosis in Health Care Facilities

On October 8, 1993, OSHA issued guidelines to enforce the protection of exposed HCWs against *Mycobacterium tuberculosis* *(TB)*. This OSHA HCW initiative was prompted by an escalating rate of new cases of active TB in the general public, by the emergence of multidrug-resistant strains of *M. tuberculosis,* and by outbreaks of TB in hospitals across the United States.[10] OSHA's enforcement guidelines are based on the 1990 CDC[11] guidelines except that high-efficiency particulate air (HEPA) respirators are specified as the minimum level of respiratory protection when employees perform high-risk procedures such as sputum induction, bronchoscopy, or administration of aerosolized pentamidine. HCWs must also wear HEPA filtered masks to enter isolation rooms housing persons who may have TB or to transport such persons in a closed vehicle. OSHA determined that the dust mist respirators used by many hospitals are not adequate protection against the

1991 OSHA Bloodborne Pathogens Standard: An Overview

Scope and Application

The Standard on Occupational Exposure to Bloodborne Pathogens applies to all workers with occupational exposures to blood or other potentially infectious material (OPIM).

Exposure Control Plan

Every employer with an employee who may be reasonably anticipated to have occupational exposure to bloodborne pathogens must have a written exposure control plan designed to eliminate or minimize employee exposure. The plan must contain (1) a documented exposure determination, (2) a schedule and method for implementing the exposure control plan, and (3) a procedure for evaluating exposure incidents.

Methods of Compliance

Universal Precautions: Universal precautions must be used to prevent exposure to all blood or OPIM. If it is difficult to differentiate the type of body fluid or tissue, it should be handled as if it were infectious.

Engineering Controls: Engineering controls refer to methods of isolating or removing a hazard from the workplace. These include needle disposal containers and mechanical devices to reduce handling of contaminated needles.

Work Practice Controls: Work practice controls are techniques that reduce the likelihood of exposure by changing the way a task is performed. Examples are hand washing, avoidance of needle recapping or needle breaking, and the use of a mechanical device to disassemble needle-bearing devices. Eating, drinking, smoking, and applying lip balm or contact lenses are prohibited in areas of likely exposure. Food and beverages may not be kept where blood or OPIM are kept. Blood or tissue specimens must be transported in labeled impenetrable containers.

Personal Protective Equipment: The employer must provide gloves, gowns, shoe covers, goggles, masks, and resuscitation bags. Personal protective equipment (PPE)

1991 OSHA Bloodborne Pathogens Standard: An Overview—cont'd

must be used whenever contact with blood or OPIM is anticipated, except under rare and temporary circumstances when the employee believes it would prevent the delivery of health care or would impose a greater hazard to the employee. The employer is responsible for the maintenance of PPE.

Orientation and Training: Initial and annual training related to the standard must be provided to each potentially exposed employee during working hours, and at no cost to the employee (annual training must be provided within 12 months of initial training). Records must be kept of training sessions.

Labels and Signs: Biohazard warning labels must be placed on all substances containing blood or OPIM.

Regulated Waste: Waste containing liquid blood or OPIM must be placed in special labeled containers and disposed of properly. Contaminated needles must be placed in closeable, labeled, puncture-resistant containers. Contaminated laundry must be labeled and contained in leakproof containers.

Housekeeping: Contaminated work areas must be decontaminated appropriately. Products used for decontamination must be effective against tuberculosis and HIV.

Hepatitis B Vaccination: Hepatitis B vaccination must be offered to all potentially exposed employees within 10 days of employment. Records related to this vaccination must be maintained. Employees who decline vaccination must sign a standardized declination form.

Post-exposure Plans: All employees experiencing an occupational exposure incident must report it immediately. All medical procedures and prophylaxis related to an occupational exposure incident must be provided by the employer. Confidential medical records must be kept related to the exposure.

From U.S. Department of Labor/OSHA: Occupational exposure to bloodborne pathogens: final rule, *Federal Register* 56(235):64004, 1991; U.S. Department of Labor/OSHA: *Enforcement standards for the occupational exposure to bloodborne pathogens standard,* Washington, DC, 1992, U.S. Office of Health Compliance Assistance.

infectious droplet nuclei of TB because these masks do not reach full filtering efficiency until they are loaded with dust (a condition unlikely in health care facilities).[9]

OSHA's enforcement guidelines also specify that warnings must be placed outside a respiratory isolation room and that employee medical records related to TB exposure, skin testing, and infection must be handled in accordance with OSHA requirements. All positive TB skin tests in HCWs are presumed to be employment related and must be recorded on the organization's OSHA 200 log.[12]

Centers For Disease Control and Prevention

The CDC is the Public Health Service agency responsible for providing direction and leadership in the prevention and control of diseases and other preventable conditions. The CDC is concerned with the protection of both HCWs and patients who may be exposed to infection. Although the CDC cannot enforce regulation related to hospital infection control practice, its guidelines and recommendations have become standards for governmental regulations and legislation.

CDC Guidelines for Preventing the Transmission of Tuberculosis in Health Care Facilities

In October 1994 the CDC published updated guidelines for preventing transmission of tuberculosis in health care settings. These guidelines replace the 1990 CDC guidelines. The new guidelines emphasize the importance of (1) the hierarchy of control measures, including administrative controls and personal respiratory equipment, (2) health care facility risk assessment and development of a written TB control plan, (3) early identification and management of persons with TB, (4) purified protein derivative skin testing programs, and (5) HCW education.[13] Components of an optimal TB control program are listed in the box on pp. 15-17. CDC recommendations for frequency of TB risk assessment and repeat skin testing for employees can be found in Chapter 8.

CDC Guidelines for Infection Control in Hospital Personnel

The search for practices that are efficient, safe, and economical in protecting patients and HCWs from infection has generated much

Optimum Tuberculosis Control Program for All Health Care Facilities

I. Initial and periodic risk assessment
  A. Evaluate health care worker's (HCW's) purified protein derivative (PPD) test conversion data
  B. Determine tuberculosis (TB) prevalence among patients
  C. Reassess risk each PPD testing period
II. Written TB infection control plan
  A. Document all aspects of TB control
  B. Identify individual(s) responsible for TB control program
  C. Explain and emphasize hierarchy of controls
III. Implementation
  A. Assignment of responsibility
    1. Assign responsibility for TB control program to individual(s)
    2. Ensure that persons with expertise in infection control, occupational health, and engineering are identified and included
  B. Risk assessment and periodic reassessment of program
    1. Select initial risk protocols
    2. Observe HCW's infection control practices
    3. Repeat risk assessment at appropriate intervals
  C. Early detection of patients with TB
    1. Symptom screen for each patient
      a) On initial encounter in emergency room or ambulatory care setting
      b) Before or at admission
    2. Radiologic and bacteriologic screening for patients with symptoms of TB
  D. Management of outpatients with possible infectious TB
    1. Promptly initiate TB precautions
    2. Place patients in separate waiting areas of TB isolation rooms
    3. Give patients mask and box of tissues; instruct to cover mouth while coughing

From Centers for Disease Control and Prevention: Guidelines for preventing the transmission of mycobacterium tuberculosis in healthcare facilities, 1994, *Federal Register* 59(208):54242, 1994.

Continued.

Optimum Tuberculosis Control Program for All Health Care Facilities—cont'd

E. Isolation for infectious TB patients
  1. Prompt isolation and initiation of treatment for patients with suspected or known infectious TB
  2. Monitoring of response to treatment
  3. Appropriate criteria for discontinuation of isolation

F. Engineering recommendations
  1. Local exhaust and general ventilation should be designed in collaboration with persons with expertise in ventilation engineering
  2. In areas where infectious TB patients receive care, use single-pass system or recirculation after high-efficiency particulate air (HEPA) filtration
  3. Use additional measures, if needed, in areas where TB patients may receive care
  4. Health care facilities should be designed to achieve the best possible ventilation air flows
  5. Regularly monitor and maintain engineering controls
  6. Monitor and maintain TB isolation room negative pressure daily while in use relative to hallway and all surrounding areas
  7. Exhaust TB isolation room air to outside or, if unavoidable, recirculate within room after HEPA filtration

G. Respiratory protection
  1. Devices should meet recommended performance criteria
  2. Devices should be worn by persons in settings where administrative and engineering controls are not likely to provide adequate protection (e.g., TB isolation rooms, treatment rooms, and other high-risk areas)
  3. A respiratory protection program is required where respiratory protection is used

Optimum Tuberculosis Control Program for All Health Care Facilities—cont'd

  H. Cough-inducing procedures
   1. Should not be performed on TB patients unless absolutely necessary
   2. Should be performed using local exhaust, in a HEPA filtered booth, or in individual TB isolation room
   3. After completion, TB patients should remain in booth or enclosure until cough subsides
  I. HCW TB education
   1. All HCWs should receive periodic education appropriate to their job
   2. Should include epidemiology of TB in the facility
   3. Should emphasize concepts of pathogenesis and occupational risk
   4. Should describe practices that reduce TB transmission
  J. HCW counseling and screening
   1. Counsel all HCWs regarding TB and TB infection
   2. Counsel all HCWs about increased risk if immunocompromised
   3. PPD test all HCWs on employment and repeat at periodic intervals
   4. Screen asymptomatic HCWs for active TB
  K. Evaluate HCW PPD test conversion and possible nosocomial TB transmission
  L. Coordinate efforts with public health department

controversy. The controversy increased when OSHA's Bloodborne Pathogens Standard mandated the application of blood and body fluid precautions to all persons. The debate continues with 1994 CDC draft guidelines for isolation precautions. (See Chapter 7.)

References

1. McDonald LL, Pugliese G: Regulatory, accreditation, and professional agencies influencing infection control programs. In Wenzel RP (editor):

Prevention and control of nosocomial infections, (ed 2), Baltimore, 1993, Williams & Wilkins.

2. Joint Commission on Accreditation of Healthcare Organizations: Surveillance, prevention, and control of infection, *1995 Accreditation manual for hospitals,* 1994, Joint Commission on Accreditation of Healthcare Organizations.

3. Joint Commission on Accreditation of Healthcare Organizations: The Joint Commission's agenda for change, *Accreditation standards for education and training* (appendix), 1990, Joint Commission on Accreditation of Healthcare Organizations.

4. Kazlauskas KL, Nadzam, DM: The agenda for change: development of the joint commission infection control indicators, *Infect Control Hosp Epidemiol* 13(6):331, 1992.

5. Joint Commission on Accreditation of Healthcare Organizations: The indicator measurement system, *1996 Draft medication use/infection control indicators.* Personal communication, April 1995.

6. Bowers E: Worker protection under OSHA's bloodborne pathogens standard, *Job Safety Health Q* 3(4):14, 1992.

7. Miramontes H: Progress in establishing safety protocols based on CDC and OSHA recommendations, *Infect Control Hosp Epidemiol* 11(10):561, 1990.

8. Fleming SH: OSHA's bloodborne pathogens team: a common goal—worker protection, *Job Safety Health Q* 3(4):16, 1992.

9. Pugliese G: Hospital may lose federal funding for discriminating against HIV-positive healthcare worker, *Infect Control Hosp Epidemiol* 14(3):177, 1993.

10. Clark RA: OSHA enforcement policy and procedures for occupational exposure to tuberculosis, *Infect Control Hosp Epidemiol* 14(12):694, 1993.

11. Dooley SW et al: Guidelines for preventing the transmission of tuberculosis in health-care settings, with special focus on HIV-related issues, *MMWR* 39(RR-17): 1, 1990.

12. Decker MD: OSHA enforcement policy for occupational exposure to tuberculosis, *Infect Control Hosp Epidemiol* 14(12):689, 1993.

13. Centers for Disease Control and Prevention: Guidelines for preventing the transmission of mycobacterium tuberculosis in health-care facilties, 1994, *Federal Register* 59(208):54242, 1994.

Reportable Diseases

3

Prompt and accurate reporting of infectious diseases provides a basis for future investigations and strategies for control of these diseases. In the United States the Centers for Disease Control and Prevention (CDC) is responsible for infectious disease surveillance. The CDC recommends that selected infectious diseases be reported to its National Notifiable Diseases Surveillance System (NNDSS), a national reporting system that collects, compiles, and publishes data on infectious diseases from each state.[1]

However, individual practitioners do not report infectious diseases directly to the CDC. Instead, each state reports to the CDC through a state department with authority derived from state legislature. State regulations specify which diseases are notifiable (in addition to those that are on the NNDSS list), who is responsible for reporting the disease, what information is required to define each case, the speed with which diseases must be reported, and to whom the information is reported. Many states require patient demographic data, presenting symptoms, laboratory results, physician's name, and treatment given.

Within hospitals and other health care organizations responsibility for identifying reportable diseases and notifying appropriate authorities lies with the clinician who diagnoses the case, although state statutes frequently require reporting by hospitals. Oversight of this function within hospitals is frequently a responsibility of the Infection Control Practitioner.

It is helpful for nurses and other health care workers to be familiar with nationally reportable diseases and the criteria for confirming disease cases so that they can participate in the process of diagnosis and reporting. Knowledgeable health care workers may serve a valuable role in reminding clinicians that certain diseases are reportable. Accurate reporting requires that suspicious cases of infectious disease be confirmed using uniform standards before they are reported to state health departments and to the CDC.

Infectious Diseases that Are Reportable in Some States

Animal bites
Blastomycosis
Campylobacteriosis
Chickenpox/herpes zoster
    (varicella-zoster virus)
Chlamydia trachomatis
Coccidioidomycosis
Conjunctivitis
Dengue fever
Diarrhea caused by ecoli
    (especially 0157:h7)
Food-associated illness
Gastroenteritis
Giardiasis
Guillain-Barré syndrome
Hantavirus
Herpes simplex
Histoplasmosis
Human immunodeficiency
    virus
Impetigo

Influenza
Kawasaki syndrome
Listeriosis
Mycobacteria (atypical)
Nonspecific urethritis
Nosocomial infection
Opthalmia neonatorum
Pelvic inflammatory
    disease
Q fever
Relapsing fever
Reye's syndrome
Scarlet fever
Staphylococcal disease
Streptococcal disease
Toxic shock syndrome
Toxoplasmosis
Trachoma
Typhus
Vibriosis
Water-borne infection

From Chorba TL et al: Mandatory reporting of infectious diseases by clinicians, *JAMA* 262(21):3018, 1989.

Case definitions have been published by the CDC[1,2] in order to promote accuracy. Some diseases require laboratory confirmation for diagnosis, others are confirmed by clinical symptomatology alone. Diseases included in the NNDSS and criteria for case definitions are listed in Table 3-1. Probable cases are reportable to the NNDSS pending appropriate laboratory confirmation.

In addition, familiarity is needed with infectious diseases that are reportable within one's own state, although some of these diseases may not be nationally notifiable. The box above lists infectious diseases that are reportable in some states only. Because no uniform standards for case definitions or reporting have been developed for diseases that are not nationally reportable, diseases that may be reportable by states are listed without additional data.

Table 3-1 Case definitions for diseases reportable by state health departments to the notifiable diseases surveillance system of the CDC

Disease	Clinical Description	Laboratory Criteria for Diagnosis	Case Classification	Comments
AIDS	Life threatening condition resulting from progressive impairment of immune response; characterized by opportunistic infections and cancers	CD4+ T-lymphocyte count (≤200) or CD4+ T-lymphocyte percentage (<14% of total lymphocytes) or one of 26 clinical conditions in the presence of documented HIV infection	Laboratory confirmation of CD4+ status of HIV infection plus one of 26 clinical conditions listed below[*]	Many states require reporting of HIV infection, not just clinical AIDS

From Centers for Disease Control: Case definitions for public health surveillance, *MMWR* 39(RR-13):1,1990; Centers for Disease Control: Surveillance for occupational acquired HIV infection, *MMWR* 41:823, 1992.

CDC, Centers for Disease Control and Prevention; *AIDS*, acquired immunodeficiency syndrome; *HIV*, human immunodeficiency virus; *ELISA*, enzyme-linked immunosorbent assay; *HAV*, hepatitis A virus; *HBsAg*, Hepatitis B surface antigen; *IgM*, immunoglobulin M; *HBcAg*, hepatitis B core antigen; *HCV*, hepatitis C virus; *RIBA*, recombinant immunoblotting assay; *HDV*, hepatitis delta virus; *IF*, immunofluorescence; *CSF*, cerebrospinal fluid; *VDRL*, Venereal Disease Research Laboratory test; *RPR*, rapid plasma reagin test; *BUN*, blood urea nitrogen; *SGOT*, serum glutamate oxaloacetate transaminase; *DNA*, deoxyribonucleic acid.

[*]Clinical conditions associated with AIDS include the following: candidiasis of bronchi, trachea, esophagus, or lungs; invasive cervical cancer; extrapulmonary coccidioidomycosis (disseminated or extrapulmonary); cryptococcosis; cryptosporidiosis; cytomegalovirus disease (other than spleen, liver, and nodes) or cytomegalovirus retinitis; encephalopathy; (HIV-related) herpes simplex virus (chronic ulcers, esophagitis, or bronchitis); histoplasmosis; isosporiasis; Kaposi's sarcoma; lymphoma (Burkitt's, immunoblastic, or primary); *Mycobacterium tuberculosis* (any site); *Mycobacterium avium*-complex; *Microbacterium kansasii* or other species (disseminated or extrapulmonary); *Pneumocystis carinii* pneumonia; any recurrent pneumonia; progressive multifocal leukoencephalopathy; salmonella septicemia (recurrent); toxoplasmosis of brain; or wasting syndrome due to HIV.

Continued.

Table 3-1   Case definitions for diseases reportable by state health departments to the notifiable diseases surveillance system of the CDC—cont'd

Disease	Clinical Description	Laboratory Criteria for Diagnosis	Case Classification	Comments
Amebiasis	Infection of large intestine or other organ by *Entamoeba histolytica*	Cysts of trophozoites in stool or trophozoites in biopsy/culture	Laboratory confirmation or demonstration of antibody in the case of symptomatic persons with extraintestinal disease	Asymptomatic carriage is not reportable
Anthrax	Acute bacterial illness that may be cutaneous, respiratory, intestinal, or oropharyngeal	Positive culture or immunofluorescence, or 4× rise between acute and convalescent titer 2 weeks apart, or ELISA titer ≥64	Clinically compatible illness that is laboratory confirmed	
Aseptic meningitis	Acute illness with meningeal symptoms, fever, and cerebrospinal fluid pleocytosis	No evidence of bacterial or fungal meningitis	Clinically compatible illness with no laboratory evidence of bacteria or fungus	Most commonly caused by a viral agent

Botulism, foodborne	Acute illness with symmetric paralysis	Botulinal toxin in serum, stool, food, or isolation of organism in stool	Clinically compatible illness that is laboratory confirmed or that occurs among persons who ate same food as persons with lab confirmation	May be diagnosed without lab confirmation if clinical and epidemiologic evidence is overwhelming
Botulism, infant	Illness characterized by constipation, and poor feeding that may be followed by weakness and impaired respiration	Detection of botulinal toxin in stool or isolation of organism in stool	Clinically compatible illness occurring in child under age 1	
Botulism, wound	Wound infection with *Clostridium botulinum*	Detection of botulinal toxin in serum or isolation of organism in wound	Clinically compatible illness that is laboratory confirmed in patients with no food exposure and a fresh contaminated wound within 2 weeks	

Continued.

Table 3-1 Case definitions for diseases reportable by state health departments to the notifiable diseases surveillance system of the CDC—cont'd

Disease	Clinical Description	Laboratory Criteria for Diagnosis	Case Classification	Comments
Botulism, other	Illness compatible with botulism	Detection of botulinal toxin or organism in clinical specimen	Clinically compatible illness without ingestion of suspect food or wounds	
Brucellosis	Illness characterized by fever, night sweats, anorexia, fatigue, weight loss, and arthralgia	Detection of *Brucella* sp. by culture or immunofluorescence, 4× rise between acute and convalescent titer 2 weeks apart	Probable: Clinically compatible case that is linked to a confirmed case or that has supportive serology (one titer ≥160) Confirmed: Laboratory confirmation	

Chancroid	Painful genital ulceration and inguinal adenopathy	Isolation of *Haemophilus decreyi* from clinical specimen	Probable: Clinically compatible case with no evidence of syphilis or herpes Confirmed: Laboratory confirmation
Cholera†	Illness characterized by vomiting and diarrhea	Isolation of toxigenic *Vibrio cholerae* 01 from stool or vomitus, significant rise in acute/convalescent titer, or significant fall in antibodies in early and late convalescent sera in those not recently vaccinated	Clinically compatible illness that is laboratory confirmed	Only confirmed cases of strain 01 should be reported

†Case report universally required by international health regulations (reporting by telephone or other rapid means is mandated).

Continued.

Table 3-1 Case definitions for diseases reportable by state health departments to the notifiable diseases surveillance system of the CDC—cont'd

Disease	Clinical Description	Laboratory Criteria for Diagnosis	Case Classification	Comments
Diphtheria	Upper respiratory infection characterized by adherent pharyngeal membrane	Isolation of *Corynebacterium diphtheriae* from clinical specimen	Probable: Meets clinical case definition Confirmed: Meets clinical case definition and either laboratory confirmed or linked to a laboratory-confirmed case	
Encephalitis (primary)	Illness in which encephalitis is the major presentation		Confirmed: Clinically compatible illness diagnosed by a physician as primary encephalitis	Excludes postinfectious encephalitis

Encephalitis (postinfectious)	Encephalitis that follows or occurs with other viral illnesses that are not central nervous system illnesses		Confirmed: Clinically compatible illness diagnosed by a physician as postinfectious encephalitis	Includes encephalitis, which occurs after chickenpox and after mumps
Gonorrhea	A sexually transmitted infection characterized by urethritis, cervicitis, or salpingitis; may be asymptomatic	Isolation of *Neisseria gonorrhoeae* from a clinical specimen or gramnegative intracellular diplococci in a male urethral smear	Probable: Gramnegative diplococci in a female endocervical smear or a written report by a physician Confirmed: Laboratory confirmation	
Granuloma inguinale	Painless or minimally painful granulomatous lesions in the anogenital region	Intracytoplasmic Donovan bodies in smears or biopsies	Confirmed: Clinically compatible case with laboratory confirmation	

Continued.

Table 3-1 Case definitions for diseases reportable by state health departments to the notifiable diseases surveillance system of the CDC——cont'd

Disease	Clinical Description	Laboratory Criteria for Diagnosis	Case Classification	Comments
Haemophilus influenzae (invasive disease)	Meningitis, bacteremia, epiglottitis, or pneumonia	Isolation of *Haemophilus influenzae* from a normally sterile site	Probable: Clinically compatible illness with detection of *H. influenzae* type b antigen in cerebrospinal fluid Confirmed: Clinically compatible illness that is culture confirmed	
Hepatitis A	Viral infection characterized by discrete onset of symptoms and jaundice	IgM anti-HAV positive	Case meets clinical case definition and is laboratory confirmed	
Hepatitis B	Viral infection characterized by discrete onset of symptoms and jaundice	HBsAg positive or IgM HBcAg positive	Case meets clinical case definition and is laboratory confirmed	

Hepatitis C Note: Although Hepatitis C is now recognized as a specific entity, it is reported to the CDC as non-A, non-B Hepatitis	Viral infection characterized by discrete onset of symptoms and jaundice	Anti-HCV positive and positive RIBA (supplemental assay) or IgM anti-HAV negative and HBsAg negative and serum aminotransferase levels $>2\frac{1}{2} \times$ normal	Case meets clinical case definition and is laboratory confirmed	Specific test for Hepatitis C requires 6 months between onset of disease and detectable antibody; hence non-A, non-B hepatitis should be reported
Hepatitis delta	Viral infection characterized by discrete onset of symptoms and jaundice	HBsAg or IgM anti-HBcAg positive and anti-HDV positive	Case meets clinical case definition and is laboratory confirmed	Virus exists only in the presence of hepatitis B virus infection

Continued.

Table 3-1 Case definitions for diseases reportable by state health departments to the notifiable diseases surveillance system of the CDC—cont'd

Disease	Clinical Description	Laboratory Criteria for Diagnosis	Case Classification	Comments
Legionellosis (Legionnaires' disease)	Illness with acute onset, fever, cough, and x-ray confirmed pneumonia	Isolation of *legionella* from normally sterile site, or 4× or greater rise in reciprocal IF titer to ≥128 against *Legionella pneumophila* serogroup 1, or demonstration by direct fluorescent antibody testing or urine radioimmunoassay	Probable: Clinically compatible disease with antibody titer ≥256 from a single convalescent phase serum titer Confirmed: Laboratory confirmation	

Leprosy (Hansen's disease)	Disease of skin, peripheral nerves, and mucosa of upper airway	Demonstration of acid-fast *bacilli* in skin or dermal nerve obtained from full thickness skin biopsy of a lesion	Clinically compatible case that is laboratory confirmed
Leptospirosis	Illness with fever, headache, chills, myalgia, conjunctival suffusion	Isolation of *Leptospira* from a clinical specimen or 4× titer increase in acute and convalescent phase specimens taken 2 weeks apart and studied at the same laboratory, or demonstration by immunofluoresence	Probable: Clinically compatible case with supportive serology (titer ≥200) Confirmed: Clinically compatible case that is laboratory confirmed

Continued.

Table 3-1 Case definitions for diseases reportable by state health departments to the notifiable diseases surveillance system of the CDC—cont'd

Disease	Clinical Description	Laboratory Criteria for Diagnosis	Case Classification	Comments
Lyme disease	Systemic disease with dermatologic, rheumatologic, neurologic, and cardiac abnormalities. Clinical case is defined by *erythema migrans* or at least one late manifestation	Isolation of *Borrelia burgdorferi*, or antibodies in serum or cerebrospinal fluid, or significant change in antibody response in acute/convalescent phase serum samples	Confirmed: A case that meets one of the clinical case definitions	Characteristic skin lesion (*erythema migrans*) occurs in 60%-80% of patients

Lymphogran-uloma venereum	Genital lesions, suppurative regional lymphadenopathy, or hemorrhagic proctitis	Isolation of *Chlamydia trachomatis*, serotypes L1-L3 or inclusion bodies by immunofluorescence, or positive serologic test	Probable: Clinically compatible case with one or more tender fluctuant inguinal lymph nodes with a single *Chlamydia trachomatis* titer >64
			Confirmed: Laboratory confirmation
Malaria	Chills followed by fever and sweating	Demonstration of malaria parasites in blood films	Confirmed: A person's first attack of laboratory-confirmed malaria that occurs in the United States
			A subsequent attack in one person caused by a different *Plasmodium* sp. is counted as an additional case

Continued.

Table 3-1   Case definitions for diseases reportable by state health departments to the notifiable diseases surveillance system of the CDC—cont'd

Disease	Clinical Description	Laboratory Criteria for Diagnosis	Case Classification	Comments
Measles (red) (rubeola)	Rash lasting ≥3 days with temperature ≥38.3° C and cough, coryza, or conjunctivitis	Isolation of measles virus from clinical specimen or significant rise in antibody level, or positive serologic test for measles IgM antibody	Probable: Meets clinical case definition without links to another case Confirmed: Case that is laboratory confirmed or that meets clinical case definition and is linked to a probable or confirmed case	Two probable cases that are linked are considered confirmed

Meningococcal disease	Meningitis or meningococcemia	Isolation of *Neisseria meningitides* from a normally sterile site	Probable: Positive antigen test in CSF or clinical purpura fulminans in absence of positive blood culture. Confirmed: Clinically compatible case that is culture confirmed	Antigen tests in urine or serum are unreliable for diagnosis
Mumps	Unilateral or bilateral tender, self-limited swelling of parotid or other salivary gland, lasting ≥2 days without other cause	Isolation of virus from clinical specimen or significant rise in mumps antibody level, or positive serologic test for mumps IgM antibody	Probable: Meets clinical case definition. Confirmed: Laboratory confirmation or meets clinical case definition and is linked to a confirmed or probable case	Two cases that are linked would be considered confirmed even in the absence of laboratory confirmation

Continued.

Table 3-1   Case definitions for diseases reportable by state health departments to the notifiable diseases surveillance system of the CDC—cont'd

Disease	Clinical Description	Laboratory Criteria for Diagnosis	Case Classification	Comments
Pertussis	Cough lasting at least 2 weeks with paroxysms of coughing or inspiratory "whoop," or posttussive vomiting and without other causes	Isolation of *Bordetella pertussis* from clinical specimen	Probable: Meets clinical case definition. Confirmed: Clinically compatible case that is laboratory confirmed or linked to a laboratory confirmed case	Direct fluorescent antibody testing of nasopharyngeal secretions is not considered laboratory confirmation
Plague†	Fever and leukocytosis presenting as regional lymphadenitis, septicemia, pneumonia, or pharyngitis	Isolation of *Yersinia pestis* from a clinical specimen or 4× change in serum antibody to *Y. pestis*	Probable: Clinically compatible illness with supportive laboratory results. Confirmed: Laboratory confirmation	

Poliomyelitis, paralytic	Acute onset of flaccid paralysis of one or more limbs without other cause without sensory or cognitive losses		Probable: Case that meets clinical case definition Confirmed: Case that meets clinical case definition and patient has neurologic deficit 60 days later, who died or whose status is unknown	All suspected cases are reviewed by an expert panel before final classification
Psittacosis	Illness with fever, chills, headache, photophobia, respiratory disease and myalgia	Isolation of *Chlamydia psittaci* from clinical specimen or 4× rise in antibody-titer between two serum specimens obtained 2 weeks apart and studied at the same laboratory	Probable: Clinically compatible illness that is linked to a confirmed case with supportive serology (titer ≥32) Confirmed: Laboratory confirmation	Serologic findings may also occur with *Chlamydia trachomatis* or *Chlamydia pneumoniae*

Continued.

Table 3-1 Case definitions for diseases reportable by state health departments to the notifiable diseases surveillance system of the CDC—cont'd

Disease	Clinical Description	Laboratory Criteria for Diagnosis	Case Classification	Comments
Rabies, animal		Positive direct fluorescent antibody test or isolation of rabies virus	Confirmed: Laboratory confirmation	
Rabies, human	Acute encephalomyelitis that usually progresses to coma or death within 10 days	Direct fluorescent antibody of viral antigens in clinical specimen or isolation of rabies virus or identification of a rabies neutralizing antibody titer ≥5 in serum of CSF of unvaccinated person	Clinically compatible case with laboratory confirmation	Laboratory confirmation by all of noted methods is recommended

Rheumatic fever	Inflammatory illness with carditis, polyarthritis, chorea, subcutaneous nodules, and *erythema marginatum* (major criteria)	No specific laboratory test exists	Confirmed: Illness with two major criteria or one major and two minor criteria with supporting evidence of preceding group A streptococcal infection	Minor criteria include previous rheumatic fever, arthralgia, fever, elevated erythrocyte sedimentation rate, positive C-reactive protein, and prolonged PR interval
Rocky Mountain spotted fever	Illness of acute onset and fever, usually with myalgia, headache, and petechial rash	Rise of 4× in antibody titer or a single titer ≥64 by immunofluorescent antibody test or ≥16 by complement fixation	Probable: Clinically compatible case with supportive serology Confirmed: Laboatory confirmation	Petechial rash appears on palms and soles in two-thirds of cases

Continued.

Table 3-1   Case definitions for diseases reportable by state health departments to the notifiable diseases surveillance system of the CDC—cont'd

Disease	Clinical Description	Laboratory Criteria for Diagnosis	Case Classification	Comments
Rubella (3-day measles)	Acute illness with generalized maculopapular rash, temperature 37.2° C, and arthralgia, arthritis, lymphadenopathy, or conjunctivitis	Isolation of rubella virus or significant rise in rubella antibody or positive serologic test for rubella IgM antibody	Suspect: Any generalized rash illness of acute onset Probable: Case that meets case definition Confirmed: Case that is laboratory confirmed or that meets clinical case definition and is linked to a laboratory-confirmed case	Congenital Rubella syndrome also reportable

Salmonellosis	Diarrhea, abdominal pain, nausea, and sometimes vomiting	Isolation of *Salmonella* from a clinical specimen	Probable: Clinically compatible illness that is linked to a confirmed case Confirmed: Laboratory confirmation
Shigellosis	Diarrhea, fever, nausea, cramps, and tenesmus	Isolation of *shigella* from a clinical specimen	Probable: Clinically compatible case linked to a confirmed case Confirmed: Laboratory confirmation
Syphilis (primary)	Infection characterized by chancre	Demonstration of *Treponema pallidum* in clinical specimen by darkfield, fluorescent antibody, or equivalent microscopic method	Probable: Clinically compatible case with one or more ulcers (chancres) and a reactive serologic test Confirmed: Clinically compatible case that is laboratory confirmed	Clinical illness is not required for reporting

Continued.

Table 3-1 Case definitions for diseases reportable by state health departments to the notifiable diseases surveillance system of the CDC—cont'd

Disease	Clinical Description	Laboratory Criteria for Diagnosis	Case Classification	Comments
Syphilis (secondary)	State of infection characterized by localized or diffuse mucocutaneous lesions and generalized adenopathy	Demonstration of *Treponema pallidum* in clinical specimens by darkfield, fluorescent antibody, or equivalent microscopic methods	Probable: Clinically compatible case with a reactive nontreponemal test titer of ≥4 Confirmed: A clinically compatible case that is laboratory confirmed	
Syphilis (latent)	Stage of infection in which organism persists without symptoms or signs		Presumptive: No past diagnosis of syphilis and a reactive nontreponemal test and a reactive treponemal assay for antibody to *Treponema pallidum*	VDRL and RPR are nontreponemal tests

| Neurosyphilis | Evidence of central nervous system infection with *Treponema pallidum* | Reactive serologic test for syphilis and reactive VDRL in CSF | Presumptive: Syphilis of any stage, a negative VDRL in CSF, and both elevated CSF protein without other cause and clinical symptoms without other known cause
Confirmed: Meets laboratory criteria for neurosyphilis |

Continued.

Table 3-1 Case definitions for diseases reportable by state health departments to the notifiable diseases surveillance system of the CDC—cont'd

Disease	Clinical Description	Laboratory Criteria for Diagnosis	Case Classification	Comments
Syphilis (congenital)	Wide spectrum of defects present at birth due to *Treponema pallidum*	Demonstration of *Treponema pallidum* by dark-field microscopy or other specific stains in specimens from lesions, placenta, umbilical cord, or other material	Presumptive: Infant whose mother had untreated or inadequately treated syphilis at delivery or infant who has reactive treponemal test for syphilis and evidence on x-ray or exam, reactive CSF VDRL or elevated CSF cell count, or a reactive antibody test Confirmed: Laboratory confirmation	Reporting criteria includes syphilitic stillborns

Tetanus	Acute onset of hypertonia and generalized muscle spasm without other apparent medical cause	Confirmed: A case that meets the clinical case definition	
Toxic shock syndrome	Temperature ≥38.9° C, diffuse macular erythroderma, desquamation 1-2 weeks after onset, hypotension and 3 or more indicators of multisystem involvement with negative blood, throat, or cerebrospinal fluid cultures and negative titers for Rocky Mountain spotted fever, leptospirosis, or measles	Probable: A case with 5 of 6 clinical indicators Confirmed: A case with all 6 clinical findings including desquamation unless patient dies before desquamation could occur	Multisystem involvement indicators include vomiting or diarrhea, myalgia, mucous membrane hyperemia, 2× normal BUN or creatinine, 2× normal SGOT, platelets <100,000 mm^3, or altered consciousness

Continued.

Table 3-1 Case definitions for diseases reportable by state health departments to the notifiable diseases surveillance system of the CDC—cont'd

Disease	Clinical Description	Laboratory Criteria for Diagnosis	Case Classification	Comments
Trichinosis	Eosinophilia, fever, myalgia, and periorbital edema	Demonstration of larvae or cysts of *Trichinella spiralis* on muscle biopsy or positive serology	Confirmed: Clinically compatible case that is laboratory confirmed	
Tuberculosis	Chronic bacterial infection characterized by formation of granulomas; lung is most common site, but others may be involved	Isolation of *Mycobacterium tuberculosis* from clinical specimen, demonstration of organism by DNA probe, or demonstration of acid-fast *bacilli* in clinical specimen	Confirmed: Case that is laboratory confirmed or that meets clinical case definition	Clinical case definition: Positive tuberculin skin test, other compatible signs and symptoms such as chest x-ray, treatment with 2 or more antituberculous medications, or completed diagnostic evaluation

Tularemia	An illness which may take a variety of forms	Isolation of *Francisella tularensis* from a clinical specimen or demonstration by immunofluorescence of a 4× rise in acute and convalescent specimens taken ≥2 weeks apart, analyzed at the same time and in the same lab	Probable: Clinically compatible disease with supportive serology Confirmed: Laboratory confirmation	Clinical evidence is supported by history of tick or deerfly bite, exposure to infected tissue, or infected water
Typhoid fever	Sustained fever, headache, malaise, relative bradycardia, GI symptoms, and nonproductive cough	Isolation of *Salmonella typhi* from clinical specimen	Probable: Clinically compatible case linked to a confirmed case Confirmed: Laboratory confirmation	

Continued.

Table 3-1   Case definitions for diseases reportable by state health departments to the notifiable diseases surveillance system of the CDC—cont'd

Disease	Clinical Description	Laboratory Criteria for Diagnosis	Case Classification	Comments
Yellow fever	Mosquito-borne disease characterized by constitutional symptoms followed by a brief remission and recurrence of fever, hepatitis, and albuminuria	A rise of 4× or greater in yellow fever antibody titer without recent immunization	Probable: Clinically compatible illness with supportive serology Confirmed: Laboratory confirmation	

References

1. Centers for Disease Control: Case definitions for public health surveillance, *MMWR* 39(RR-13):1, 1990.
2. Centers for Disease Control: Surveillance for occupational acquired HIV infection, *MMWR*, 41:823, 1992.

Infection Control Resources

4

There are many information resources available to health care providers to protect patients and health care workers from infections and diseases. Chapter 2 discussed and described the regulatory and professional agencies involved in the regulation and oversight of infection control practices. These agencies also provide consultation to health care providers during outbreaks of nosocomial or community-acquired infections and answer specific infection control procedural or policy questions. In hospital and long-term care facilities (LTCFs) formal infection control programs are mandated. Formal committees provide oversight for the programs that are administered by infection control practitioners. Other settings such as ambulatory care and home health care settings may not have a formal program but are still required to meet infection control standards. The purpose of this chapter is to discuss available resources and how health care providers may access them.

Infection Control Practitioner

Infection control practitioners (ICPs) are normally nurses or microbiologists with specific education in infection control, research, and epidemiology. Many ICPs are nationally certified by the Association for Practitioners in Infection Control and Epidemiology (APIC) using the initials C.I.C. to designate their certification. Additional courses of study are provided by the APIC and the Centers for Disease Control and Prevention (CDC) to prepare and update ICPs for certification. Hospital and LTCF administrators give an ICP the authority to take direct and immediate action in situations requiring intervention to stem outbreaks of infection. ICPs use principles of epidemiology, statistics, and microbiology to identify and control nosocomial infections and communicable diseases within the health care setting.[1,2]

The ICP develops plans for the surveillance, prevention, and control of infection and educates health care providers about infection prevention. Using national standards for cleaning, sanitation, disinfection, and sterilization practices, the ICP provides guidance for health care providers to meet infection control practice standards, protecting patients and themselves from the harm of cross infection. The monitoring of overall infection rates, particularly the percentage of antibiotic-resistant infections and clusters of infection, are important parts of an ICP's role. Device-related infections, surgical site infections, and infections in neonates are particular areas of concern.

In hospital and LTCF settings suspected nosocomial or community-acquired infections are reported to the ICP, who recommends specific actions and determines if infections must be reported to the local health authority. (Reportable diseases are listed in Chapter 3.) Formal surveillance methods performed by the ICP are the primary method of detection for nosocomial infections. If there is a discernible pattern of infection in a unit, the ICP reviews infection prevention measures to identify breaches of technique, for example, shared equipment between patients or improper disinfection practices. If there is an outbreak of an infection, the ICP manages the epidemiological investigation and recommends specific infection control practices to stem the outbreak. If an airborne infection is identified, the ICP determines if others were exposed to the infection before isolation was initiated and takes action to evaluate, recommend treatment, and follow up with involved patients, staff, and visitors.[1-3]

Although all health care settings will not have an ICP, a telephone call to the local hospital provides access to a highly informed infection control professional who will readily offer assistance and guidance.

Association for Practitioners in Infection Control and Epidemiology

The APIC is a national association located in Washington, D.C., for those who work in or are interested in infection control. It sponsors certification programs, annual conventions, educational courses, and resource materials and publishes scientific journals. The APIC works closely with the CDC to research and publish guidelines recognized as national standards of infection control practice. In addition, there are local or regional chapters comprised of the ICPs in the area. Both the national and local chapters are excellent resources for those in ambulatory care and home health care.

Centers for Disease Control and Prevention

As stated in Chapter 2, the CDC, located in Atlanta, provides direction, leadership, and investigation in the prevention and control of diseases and other preventable conditions. Scientists and researchers are available to anyone who calls for assistance in epidemic or outbreak investigations or with specific questions about cleaning, disinfection, sterilization, and waste disposal practices. They recommend infection control and medical interventions for people who are exposed to diseases and may actually come to the area involved to assist in the investigation. CDC employees may be located full time in state departments of health.

State and Local Departments of Health

State and local departments of health are excellent resources for information and assistance with disease and waste management interventions. The local departments of health are readily available for questions and support. The Communicable Disease division and the tuberculosis division assist with or lead exposure investigations. The Waste Management division assists with interpretation of local or regional ordinances to manage infectious or biomedical waste.

Written Resources

The following resources are relevant and helpful as references in all health care settings.

Subject	Resource
Reference books on communicable diseases	■ Benenson AS, editor: *Control of communicable diseases in man,* ed 15, Washington, DC, 1990, American Public Health Association.
	■ American Academy of Pediatrics Infectious Disease

Subject	Resource
	Committee: *The report of the committee on infectious diseases: the red book,* ed 22, Elk Grove Village, Ill, 1991, American Academy of Pediatrics Infectious Disease Committee.
All aspects of infection control practices and procedures	■ Association for Professionals in Infection Control and Epidemiology, *APIC infection control and applied epidemiology: Principles and practice,* St Louis, 1996, Mosby.
Hand washing	■ Larson E: APIC guideline for the use of topical antimicrobials, *Am J Infect Control* 16:253, 1988.
Disinfection	■ Rutala WA: APIC guideline for selection and use of disinfectants, *Am J Infect Control* 18:99, 1990. ■ Block SS, editor: *Disinfection, sterilization, and preservation,* ed 4, Philadelphia, 1991, Lea & Febiger.
Sterilization	■ Reichert M, Young J, editors: *Sterilization technology for the health care facility,* Gaithersburg, Md, 1993, Aspen. ■ Block SS, editor: *Disinfection, sterilizaton, and preservation,* ed 4, Philadelphia, 1991, Lea & Febiger.
Endoscopes	■ Martin MA, Reichelderfer M: APIC guidelines for infection prevention and control in flexible endoscopy, *Am J Infect Control* 22: 19, 1994.

References

1. Soule, B, editor: *The APIC curriculum for infection control practice,* vol 1-2, Dubuque, Iowa, 1983, Kendall/Hunt.
2. Joint Commission on Accreditation of Healthcare Organizations: Surveillance, prevention, and control of infection, *1995 Accreditation manual for hospitals,* Chicago, 1994, Joint Commission on Accreditation of Healthcare Organizations.
3. Association for Professionals in Infection Control and Epidemiology, *APIC infection control and applied epidemiology: principles and practice,* St Louis, 1996, Mosby.

INFECTION CONTROL STRATEGIES

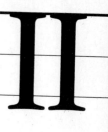

II

The Infectious Process: Body Defenses and Chain of Infection

5

Patients in heath care settings are at risk for development of infection from endogenous and exogenous sources. Hospital and long-term care facility patients are already susceptible hosts, that is, they are frequently elderly and poorly nourished. In addition, underlying medical disorders (e.g., malignancies, diabetes, renal failure, human immunodeficiency virus, and cirrhosis) decrease T- and B-cell–mediated immune function. Breaches of body integrity such as urinary catheters and IV devices impair the body's defense mechanisms, decreasing the ability of the integumentary, gastrointestinal (GI), genitourinary (GU), and respiratory systems to resist invasion by endogenous and exogenous microorganisms.[1]

Patient treatments also impair the immune defenses of the body. Stool softeners, GI stimulants, and enemas are demonstrated as independent risk factors for *Clostridium difficile* diarrhea.[2] Treatment with broad-spectrum antibiotics increases the risk of *C. difficile* infection in the 5% of persons who normally carry this bacteria in their GI systems. Immunosuppressive agents and oral corticosteroids decrease the ability of the body to resist infection.

Exogenous infection risks for patients and health care providers result from inadequate or absent hand washing or other breaches of aseptic technique. These breaches result in the spread of microorganisms from health care workers to patients and between patients. Contamination of the surfaces of equipment such as ventilators, electronic thermometer probe covers, bronchoscopes, and sigmoidoscopes can cause infections with *Pseudomonas, C. difficile,* and *mycobacteria.*[2] Failure to diagnose contagious respiratory infections results in inadequate or absent isolation techniques or incorrect isolation techniques (leaving doors to isolation rooms open or not using masks). Patients are also at risk from organisms with increased virulence. Antibiotic overusage in hospitals and long-term care facilities fosters the development of antibiotic-resistant bacteria that may cause epidemics resulting from breaches of hand washing and aseptic techniques.[3] The spread of vancomycin-resistant *Enterococcus faecium* and methicillin-resistant *Staphylococcus aureus* are examples of this phenomenon. Multidrug-resistant tuberculosis (MDR TB) occurs when patients start and stop their medication. MDR TB is then passed from person to person.

The key to controlling or preventing infection lies with a clear understanding of how the body defends itself and how pathogenic organisms that cause infections or diseases bypass these defenses. Knowledge of the microbiology of pathogenic organisms gives us more data to make decisions for infection control strategies or practices. The chain of infection concept captures the cycle of infection and demonstrates how to prevent or control infections. This chapter is the basis for all the infection control and prevention strategies in the following chapters.

Body Defense Mechanisms

In humans, defense against infectious agents (viruses, bacteria, *rickettsiae, fungi,* and parasites) includes three components, mechanical, biological, and chemical. Mechanical defense mechanisms work to exclude microorganisms from the body, either by preventing their entry or by eliminating or ejecting them through body orifices once they enter. Biological mechanisms isolate, disable, or engulf invading microorganisms once they gain entry into tissues. Chemical defenses refer to endogenous body secretions, lysozymes, immunoglobulins that fight invading agents, and such exogenous chemical prophylaxis as immunizations and antibiotics. Working together, the three components provide health and well-being to the host. If the components are not working well, are absent, or are bypassed, the host becomes susceptible to infection.

Mechanical Defense Mechanisms

The body's mechanical defense mechanisms, or barriers, exclude or eject invading microorganisms. These defenses are very effective and constitute the body's primary defenses against invasion. If the defenses are broken, entry of pathogenic microorganisms may cause infection or disease. Whether an infection results from breach of defenses depends on the virulence of the organism, the size of the inoculum, and the susceptibility of the host.[4,5]

The skin, the body's largest organ, is the first line of mechanical defense and protects the body from constant bombardment of pathogenic and nonpathogenic organisms, dirt, and grime. When the skin is invaded with devices, such as intravenous catheters, or is burned or surgically cut, the patient becomes a susceptible host. Endogenous and exogenous organisms find this once highly resistant path and migrate into the body causing infection. Endogenous refers to the patient's own normal flora, and exogenous refers to organisms from outside the patient. Exogenous examples are unwashed hands or contaminated equipment and solutions. Normal flora provide protection by producing antibiotic substances and by competing for essential nutrients. If the normal flora are upset, such as with the use of antibiotic therapy, subsequent contamination by pathogenic organisms can lead to infection.

Other mechanical defenses are actions the body takes to rid itself of such irritants as microorganisms, dirt, dust, and waste products. Examples of these actions are coughing, sneezing, tearing, sweating, shedding dead skin, excreting urine and feces, and the actions of the mucous membranes and cilia that wash and push irritants up or out of the body. Table 5-1 lists the body's mechanical defenses and their actions.

Biological Defense Mechanisms

The body's normal immune response plays a large role in deterring a microorganism's ability to cause infection. In response to invasion by microorganisms, antigen-presenting cells of the immune system recognize specific antigens of the invader. The antigens are then attacked by lymphocytes programmed to recognize them. Two types of lymphocytes are involved in this process: B-lymphocytes (plasma cells), which produce specific antibodies that bind to the invaders, or cytotoxic T-lymphocytes, which kill the invaders. Once the antibodies or the cytotoxic T-lymphocytes come in contact with the invading microorganism, a full-fledged immune response occurs using the complement cascade and additional immune cells from the lymph nodes and bone marrow. The complement cascade is a series of proteolytic

Table 5-1   Mechanical body defense mechanisms and actions

Defense Mechanisms	Actions
Gastrointestinal system	Saliva and stomach acidity break down enteric organisms
	Excretes waste products
	Produces and secretes immunoglobulins (antibodies)
	Secretes enzymes and bile
Genitourinary system	Mucosa blocks bacterial adherence to bladder
	Excretes waste products
Integumentary system (skin)	Prevents penetration
	Contains secretions with antibacterial actions
	Normal skin flora provides antibacterial activity
	Sheds dead skin cells containing bacteria
Lymphatic system	Tears provide antibacterial action and mechanically remove entrapped organisms
	Sweat rids skin of irritants
Respiratory system	Expulsion by sneezing and coughing
	Secretes lysozymes and immunoglobulins
	Upper tract: mucus entraps organisms and blocks adherence to mucosa, cilia remove organisms, nasal hairs trap organisms
	Lower tract: secretions and macrophages ingest organisms and carry them to the lymph nodes for excretion

enzymes each activating the next member of the cascade. The function of activated complement proteins from several levels of the cascade is to assist the immune cells by coating microorganisms so they can be more easily phagocytized (consumed), and to participate in bacterial cell lysis. In some cases the invading organisms are eliminated from the body. Sometimes the inflammation produced by the immune response walls off the microorganism by forming, for example, a tubercle or cyst that protects the rest of the body from infection.[6,7]

Chemical Defense Mechanisms

Endogenous and exogenous chemicals assist the body in evading infection. Secretions found on body surfaces contain chemicals that destroy unwanted pathogens. Hydrochloric acid in the stomach breaks down food that contains pathogens and mucus swallowed from the respiratory tract. Lysozymes are enzymes that destroy bacteria by removing cell walls; they are found in body secretions such as tears, mucus, and saliva. Exogenous chemicals include antibiotic therapy, immune serum globulin, and immunizations. All of these chemicals work in concert to provide protection against or to stop infection and disease.

Bypassing Body Defense Mechanisms

Health care providers may have little effect on the biological and the chemical body defense mechanisms of their susceptible hosts. However, they have a profound effect on the mechanical defense mechanisms. For example, a 60-year-old female with severe chronic obstructive pulmonary disease (COPD) is admitted to the intensive care unit postoperatively. Her surgical procedure was a gastric resection. She is intubated and on the ventilator. She has an arterial line to monitor her blood gases. She has a subclavian intravenous injection for total parenteral nutrition (TPN). She has a nasogastric (NG) tube for bowel decompression and a urinary catheter.

A review of Table 5-1 demonstrates how many of this patient's normal body defense mechanisms are bypassed and why she is now more susceptible to a nosocomial infection. Penetration of the skin occurred by surgical incision and two invasive devices entered directly into her bloodstream. The respiratory mechanisms are bypassed because of intubation. This knocks out the expulsion mechanism and the mucous membrane and cilia activities and provides an open path into the lungs that is further invaded by suctioning procedures. Her respiratory system is already compromised because of the COPD. The NG tube interferes with saliva and stomach acid activities, especially if antacids are used to protect against stress ulcers. Peristalsis, tears, and saliva production are decreased because of the anesthetic agents used during surgery. The urinary catheter provides a direct path to the sterile bladder and bypasses normal mucosal activity. Urine now flows into the catheter bag and becomes a medium for the growth of microorganisms that migrate up into the bladder. The patient is now extremely susceptible for at least four nosocomial infections, bacteremia, pneumonia, urinary tract infection (UTI), and wound infection, any of which could severely impair her chances for recovery.

Understanding the body's defense mechanisms and how easily they are bypassed in health care settings is integral to protecting patients from infections. Figure 5-1 lists the affected defense mechanisms of the patient discussed in the preceding paragraph. When health care providers stop and think about this aspect of the infection process, they understand why infection control strategies work when they are practiced. The next step is to add knowledge of the chain of infection to fully understand how infections and diseases spread from patient to patient, patient to health care provider, and health care provider to patient.

Defining Infections

An infection is defined as a process by which a susceptible host is invaded by a pathogenic (or infectious) agent that grows and multiplies, causing harm to the host. The principal infectious agents are viruses, bacteria, *rickettsiae, fungi,* and parasites. It is important to distinguish between colonization and infection. Colonization occurs when a microorganism invades a host, grows, and multiplies but does not cause infection. The missing word in the colonization definition is the word *susceptible*. Patients or health care providers can be colonized with pathogens but not exhibit symptoms of infection. If they become susceptible, infection can occur. For instance, many people are colonized with *Staphylococcus aureus* without being ill; these people are known as carriers. Carriers can pass on the organism to others who are susceptible and who then become infected.

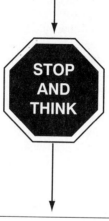

Example:
The postoperative gastric resection patient with chronic obstructive pulmonary disease arrives in the intensive care unit

STOP AND THINK

Altered defense mechanisms:

Integumentary system: surgical incision, foreign body (central and peripheral lines, nasogastric tube, urinary catheter) invasion sites

Respiratory system: mucous membranes, cilia, secretions, cough and sneeze reflexes, foreign body (suction tube) invasion

Gastrointestinal system: peristalsis, gag reflex, secretions, excretions, saliva, stomach acidity, foreign body (nasogastric tube) invasion

Genitourinary system: mucous membranes, excretion, foreign body (catheter) invasion

Figure 5-1.
Examples of altered body defense mechanisms affecting a postoperative gastric resection patient with chronic obstructive pulmonary disease.

There are three other factors that must be present for infection to occur: pathogenicity, virulence, and dose. Pathogenicity is the organisms' ability to invade tissue and cause infection or disease. Virulence is a measure of the severity of the infection or disease. Dose is the amount of organisms available to cause infection or disease. These factors and susceptibility of the host must be present to cause infection or disease.[4,5]

A communicable or infectious disease is one in which a specific disease is transferred from one person to another either directly or indirectly. For example, endocarditis is an infection, but is not communicable to others. TB is a communicable disease because it is spread to other humans by means of respiratory droplets. Not all TB patients are infectious, that is, able to communicate or transfer the disease to others. Many are infected with the organism, but only about 10% of those infected progress to active disease. They can then become infectious, or able to transmit the disease, to others.[4,5]

A nosocomial infection is an infection that was not incubating or apparent at the time of a patient's admission to the health care setting.[8] Nosocomial infections can be caused by the patient's endogenous flora or by microorganisms found in the facility's environment. Nosocomial infections can result in increased health care costs, prolonged recovery time, disability, and death of the patient. About 25% of nosocomial infections are considered preventable.[9] The most prevalent nosocomial infections are surgical wound infections, UTIs, primary bacteremias, and lower respiratory infections such as pneumonia.

Infections are categorized as local or general. Localized infections are accompanied by inflammation, namely, pain, heat, redness, swelling, and loss of function. Local infections include those that are site-specific and that manifest inflammation, purulence, or dysuria. Generalized infections are those that include general body dysfunction and may exhibit systemic symptoms such as fever, chills, tachycardia, hypotension, or confusion. Individuals who present signs and symptoms of infection may need antibiotic therapy or other treatments to ward off the invading agent.[6]

Chain of Infection

The chain of infection is a classic concept of infection control. If all the links of the chain are present, infection will spread from person to person. If one link is eliminated or broken, the spread of

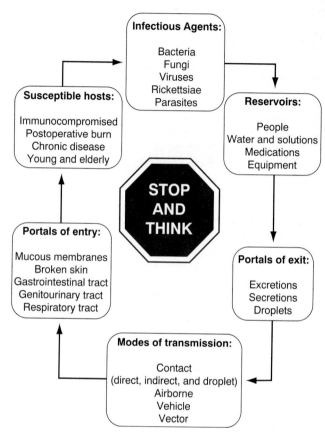

Figure 5-2.
The six components of the chain of infection.

infection can be prevented or stopped. Figure 5-2 displays the six components necessary for a pathogen to be transmitted from one individual to another.[4,5]

Infectious agents refer to biological, physical, or chemical entities capable of causing infection or disease. In humans, agents include viruses, bacteria, *rickettsiae, fungi,* and parasites.

Reservoirs are places in which an infectious agent can survive, grow, multiply, and await transfer to a susceptible host. Common reservoirs are humans and animals (hosts), plants, soil, water, and organic matter on inanimate objects (fomites). In healthy individuals the normal mucosa of the skin, intestine, or vagina act as human reservoirs. Common reservoirs associated with nosocomial infections include patients, health care workers, equipment, and the environment. Two types of human reservoirs are those with acute disease and those who are asymptomatic disease carriers. A carrier is an infected person without discernible clinical disease or symptoms. Humans can transmit disease in either situation.

Portals of exit are paths by which an infectious agent may leave the reservoir. Portals of exit include the respiratory tract, GU and GI tracts, skin and mucous membranes, transplacenta, and blood. Any body fluid is likely to contain viruses or bacteria. Examples are excretions, secretions, and droplets.

Modes of transmission are the mechanisms used to transport the infectious agent from the reservoir to a susceptible host. These modes have four main categories: (1) contact, (2) airborne, (3) vehicle, and (4) vector. The contact mode has three subcategories: (1) direct, (2) indirect, and (3) droplet. Table 5-2 describes and defines the modes of transmission. The examples in the table demonstrate that infectious agents may have more than one mode of transmission. For example, TB is listed in both the droplet contact and airborne categories and hepatitis B is listed in the direct contact, indirect contact, and vehicle categories.[4,5,7]

The mode of transmission is the most susceptible link of the chain and is the easiest to break.[4,5,7] It is also the most important link for health care providers to understand. Many times, there is little that health care providers can actively do about the infectious agent or the susceptible host, but they can interrupt the mode of transmission by practicing infection control strategies. These strategies are based heavily on the body's defense mechanisms and the chain of infection, specifically the modes of transmission.

Portals of entry are paths by which an infectious agent enters the susceptible host. These portals are the respiratory tract, GU and GI tracts, broken skin, mucous membranes, and placenta. Examples are surgical wounds and intravenous sites.

Susceptible hosts do not possess sufficient resistance against exposure to an infectious agent and prevention of infection or disease. Specific characteristics influencing susceptibility are age, chronic or active disease history, nutritional status, immune status, medication, and burns, trauma, or surgery. Sex, ethnicity, socio-

Table 5-2 Definitions and examples of the modes of transmission

Mode	Definitions and Examples	Infectious Agent Examples
Contact	Transference of the infectious agent by touching or manipulating reservoirs	
	Examples: infected hosts, contaminated fomites, contact with droplets	
Direct	Person-to-person transmission	RSV, HIV, hepatitis A and B, *staphylococcus, streptococcus*, gonorrhea, *Pseudomonas,* chickenpox, *Escherichia coli*
	Examples: touching, kissing, sexual intercourse, fecal and oral contact	
Indirect	Fomites maintain the life of the agent	RSV, hepatitis B, *staphylococcus, Pseudomonas, Klebsiella, E. coli,* CMV
	Examples: surgical instruments, urinary catheter bags, contaminated needles, dressings, toys, handkerchiefs, bedding, objects transferred mouth to mouth	
Droplet	Large, heavy droplet particles, forcibly expelled from the infected host; it is considered contact because it involves close association between hosts (3 feet or less)	Chickenpox, influenza, TB, mumps, measles, rubella, *streptococcus*, pertussis, *Haemophilus influenzae,* meningitis
	Examples: coughing, sneezing, singing	

Continued.

Modified from Benenson AS, editor: *Control of communicable diseases in man*, ed 15, Washington, DC, 1990, American Public Health Association.

RSV, respiratory syncytial virus; *HIV*, human immunodeficiency virus; *CMV*, cytomegalovirus; *TB* tuberculosis.

Table 5-2 Definitions and examples of the modes of transmission—cont'd

Mode	Definitions and Examples	Infectious Agent Examples
Airborne	Easily confused with droplet contact; however, these are small, light bacteria and viruses contained in droplet nuclei or dust particles which are carried on air currents and can stay in the air for long periods	Measles, TB, *aspergillus*, *Legionella*
Vehicle	Substances that maintain the life of the agent until it is ingested or inoculated into the susceptible host Examples: water, blood, serum, plasma, medications, food, feces	Food: *salmonella*, *Staphylococcus aureus* Blood: HIV, hepatitis B and C, CMV Water: hepatitis A, cholera, *shigella*, polio, typhoid, *Legionella*, *E. coli*, *Giardia*
Vector	Arthropods or other invertebrates transmit the agent by biting the susceptible host or by depositing the agent on skin or food; the vector may be infected itself (mosquito) or act as a carrier of the agent (flies) Examples: mosquitoes, ticks, flies, rodents	Malaria, Rocky Mountain spotted fever, yellow fever, plague, rabies

economic status, lifestyle, heredity, and occupation are also factors that may contribute to susceptibility.[5,10]

Recognizing Patient Infections

All patients should be surveyed for signs and symptoms of infection in acute care, ambulatory care, and home health care settings. Patient characteristics, such as underlying diseases and country of origin, should be identified. These characteristics may place them at high risk for certain infections or diseases. Document and report symptoms of infection. Chapter 3 lists diseases that must be reported to state or local departments of health. The patient's medical provider must be notified to initiate appropriate therapy, although nurses may take initial steps to place patients on respiratory precautions or in isolation if airborne or droplet contact is the suspected mode of transmission.

Signs and Symptoms

Questions about throat pain or dysphagia, cough and sputum production, nausea, vomiting, diarrhea, dysuria or flank pain, joint swelling or erythema, headache or neck stiffness, genital, pelvic or anorectal pain, or pruritus help identify infections. Subjective symptoms such as nausea, pain, or fatigue may also be clues. For patients with a persistent cough for longer than 3 weeks, bloody sputum, weight loss, anorexia, or fever, consider TB and take appropriate respiratory precautions; that is, the patient should be masked, placed in a room with negative pressure ventilation, and taught to cover his or her mouth when coughing.[11]

The cardinal sign of infection is fever. Temperatures between 98.6° and 100.4° F or 37° and 38° C are considered within normal range. A localized infection presents inflammation (increased redness, tenderness, swelling, and warmth) and possible fever. However, it should be realized that elderly or severely immuno-suppressed patients have a blunted response to infection and may not develop fever. It is important to observe the patient for enlarged or tender lymph nodes, skin rashes, wounds, bites, needle marks, discharge or pruritus of eyes, ears, or nose, and abnormal breath sounds such as rales. Additionally, chills, tachycardia, hypotension, or confusion may be signs of infection.[4]

Laboratory and Radiology Studies

Leukocytes are white blood cells (WBCs) that defend the body against infectious agents. The average adult has 5000 to 10,000 leukocytes per millimeter of blood. Examination of the total WBC count and WBC differential identifies patients at risk for infection; for example, decreased WBC counts of less than 4000 indicate leukopenia and elevated WBC counts of greater than 10,000 indicate leukocytosis. In bacterial infections the age of polymorphonuclear neutrophils (PMNs) is assessed. A left shift means that more than 20% of the PMN are immature, suggesting bacterial infection. In virtually all viral infections, lymphocytes are increased (adult normal is 34% of the total leukocyte count). Radiology studies assess patients with cough, shortness of breath, and fever to identify infiltrates representing pneumonia.[3]

Prevention and Control Strategies

The development of infection depends on a complex interaction of host susceptibility, infectious agents, and modes of transmission. Patient and health care factors interact to produce significant infection risks. Identification of infection risks, of those already infected, and of recommended infection control strategies minimize the incidence and serious consequences of infections in patients and in health care workers. Prevention and control methods focus on three areas: (1) increasing host resistance, (2) inactivating the infectious agent, and (3) breaking the modes of transmission.

Host resistance is increased by using vaccines and toxoids for active immunization or immunoglobulins (antibodies) for passive immunization. General health, adequate nutrition, and exercise also add to the host's resistance.[4]

Inactivation of the infectious agent is accomplished by physical and chemical methods. Physical methods include heat (pasteurization and sterilization) and adequate cooking for foods. Chemical methods include water chlorination, equipment and environmental disinfection, and antibiotics.[4,5]

As stated earlier, the mode of transmission is the easiest link to break in the chain. Breaking the mode of transmission is accomplished by isolation of infectious patients; chemoprophylaxis of their contacts after exposure; using hand washing and aseptic techniques in the management of excretions, secretions, and blood;

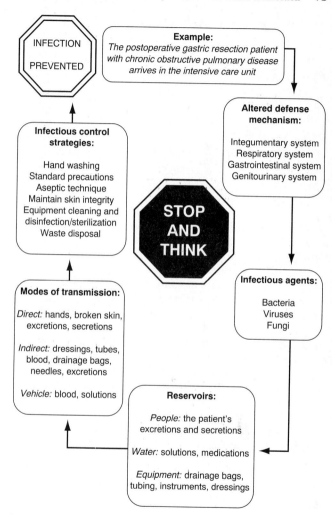

Figure 5-3.
Examples of using and understanding altered body defense mechanisms and factors in the chain of infection to select correct strategies.

and managing contaminated instruments, equipment, and medical waste.

Summary

Understanding the infection process is crucial to protect patients and health care providers from nosocomial infections and communicable diseases. Using the previous patient example, Figure 5-3 illustrates the interrelationship of altered body defense mechanisms, the chain of infection, and the strategies to prevent a nosocomial infection in this situation. The illustration combines all three concepts into one circle that is broken at the end by the use of infection prevention strategies.

The remainder of Part II of this guide book describes recommended infection control strategies for infection prevention and control including hand washing, universal precautions, environmental controls, and surgical aseptic techniques.

Part III incorporates the general strategies from Part II into specific recommendations for infection prevention and control for common procedures or with specific patient groups. Specific body defense mechanisms, chain of infection factors, and prevention strategies are illustrated at the end of each chapter to assist in understanding these important concepts. When health care providers stop and think about the aspects of the infection process, selection of the correct infection control strategies for safe nursing practice becomes clear.

References

1. Weber DJ, Rutala WA: Environmental issues and nosocomial infections. In Wenzel RP, editor: *Prevention and control of nosocomial infections,* ed 2, Baltimore, 1993, Williams & Wilkins.

2. Pannuti CS: Hospital environment for high-risk patients. In Wenzel RP, editor: *Prevention and control of nosocomial infections,* ed 2, Baltimore, 1993, Williams & Wilkins

3. Neu HC: Antimicrobial agents: role in the prevention and control of nosocomial infections. In Wenzel RP, editor: *Prevention and control of nosocomial infections,* ed 2, Baltimore, 1993, Williams & Wilkins.

4. Soule B, editor: *The APIC curriculum for infection control practice,* vol 1-2, Dubuque, Iowa, 1983, Kendall/Hunt.

5. Benenson AS, editor: *Control of communicable diseases in man,* ed 15, Washington, DC, 1990, American Public Health Association.

6. Benhaim R, Hunt TK: Natural resistance to infection: leukocyte functions, *J Burn Care Rehabil* 13(2):289, 1992.
7. Mentzer SJ, Burakoff SJ, Faller DV: Adhesion of T lymphocytes to human endothelial cells is regulated by the LFA-1 membrane molecule, *J Cell Physiol* 126:285, 1986.
8. Garner JS et al: CDC definitions for nosocomial infections, *Am J Infect Control* 16:128, 1988.
9. Gurevic I: *Infectious diseases in critical care nursing: prevention and precautions,* Rockville, Md, 1989, Aspen.
10. Klein RS: Universal precautions for preventing occupational exposures to human immunodeficiency virus type I, *Am J Med* 90:141, 1991.
11. Centers for Disease Control and Prevention: Guidelines for preventing the transmission of mycobacterium tuberculosis in healthcare facilities, 1994. *Federal Register* 59(208):54242, 1994.

Hand Washing: The Most Important Method of Prevention and Control

6

As stated in Chapter 5, the easiest link to break in the chain of infection is the mode of transmission. In health care settings, hands are one of the most efficient modes of transmission for nosocomial infections. Therefore, hand washing becomes the most important method of control and prevention. The purpose of hand washing is to decrease the bioburden (number of organisms) on the hands and to prevent their spread to noncontaminated areas, such as patients, health care workers (HCWs), and equipment.[1-4]

The lack of proper hand washing places both patients and health care providers at risk for infections or diseases. Inadequate HCW hand washing transfers organisms such as *staphylococcus, Escherichia coli, Pseudomonas,* and *Klebsiella* directly to susceptible hosts, thereby causing nosocomial infections and epidemics in all types of patient settings. At the same time, inadequate hand washing places the HCW at risk for such viral diseases as hepatitis A, B, C, and D; human immunodeficiency virus; chickenpox; and bacterial infections such as *staphylococcus, streptococcus, and E. coli.*[1,2,5,6]

Resident and Transient Organisms

The two types of organisms found on the skin are resident and transient. Resident organisms can be an individual's normal (or colonizing) flora. They live on the skin, growing and multiplying, but rarely cause infections except when introduced into the body through invasive procedures. They are not easily removed by scrubbing, can be cultured from the skin, and are usually aerobic, gram-positive organisms. Aerobic means that the organism needs oxygen to survive. *Staphylococcus aureus* is an excellent example of a resident organism. Many HCWs carry *S. aureus* without sequelae but are able to shed organisms into nonintact skin areas of susceptible hosts, causing infection. Other examples of aerobic, gram-positive organisms are *streptococci* and *Corynebacterium.*[4,5,7]

Transient organisms are much the opposite of resident organisms. They survive less than 24 hours on the skin, can be easily removed by washing or scrubbing, and are usually anaerobic, gram-negative organisms. Anaerobic means that the organism cannot survive for long in the presence of oxygen. They use the hands as a short-lived mode of transmission while looking for a susceptible host or a reservoir where they can survive. Transient organisms readily cause infection once they enter a susceptible host. Examples are *Pseudomonas, E. coli, salmonella,* and *shigella.* These types of organisms become the focus of hand washing because they can be readily transmitted on hands unless removed by mechanical friction and soap and water washing.[4,7]

Types of Hand Washing Soaps

Both plain soaps and antimicrobial soaps are available in the health care setting. Using mechanical friction, **plain soap** physically removes dirt and transient organisms from the skin. It has no bactericidal activity. Plain soap comes in many forms (bar, liquid, leaflet, and powder), all of which are acceptable for use. (If bar soap is used, it is prudent to use small bars that can be changed frequently and soap racks that promote drainage.) **Antimicrobial soaps** contain chemicals that kill transient and some resident organisms, not just remove them from the skin. Antimicrobials provide persistent chemical activity, which means that the chemical stays on the skin to continue to kill organisms. The choice of using an antimicrobial soap or a plain soap should be based on the need to reduce and maintain minimal counts of resident organisms and to remove mechanically transient organisms.[7] In this way it is possible to identify high-risk situations in which patients are compromised and a maximum reduction in bacterial counts is desirable. Such

Table 6-1 Agents for hand washing before nonsurgical and surgical procedures

	Hand Washing Agent	Procedure Description	Examples
General Patient Care Procedures			
	Plain soap	Contact with intact skin and mucous membranes or with equipment (in addition, gloves should be used when in contact with blood and body fluids)	Patient bathing, taking vital signs, emptying bedpans and drainage bags, collecting urine or stool specimens
Nonsurgical Procedures			
	Plain soap	Instruments come in contact with intact mucous membranes	Bronchoscopy, GI endoscopy, tracheal suction, cystoscopy, urinary catheterization
	Plain soap or antimicrobial soap	Insertion of peripheral IV or arterial cannula; insertion and prompt removal of a sterile needle in deep tissues or body fluids, usually to obtain specimens or instill therapeutic agents	IV therapy, arterial pressure monitoring; spinal tap, thoracentesis, abdominal paracentesis

Antimicrobial soap	Percutaneous insertion of a central catheter or wire	Hyperalimentation, CVP and wedge pressure monitoring, angiography, cardiac pacemaker insertion
Surgical Procedures		
Plain soap	Minor skin surgery	Skin biopsy, suturing of small cuts, lancing boils, mole removal
Antimicrobial soap	Insertion of a sterile tube or device through tissue into a normally sterile tissue or fluid; other procedures (major and minor surgery) that enter tissue below the skin	Chest tube insertion, culdoscopy, laparoscopy, peritoneal catheter insertion; hysterectomy, cholecystectomy, herniorrhaphy

Modified from Soule B, editor: *The APIC curriculum for infection control practice*, vol 1-2, Dubuque, Iowa, 1983, Kendall/Hunt; Larson E: APIC guidelines for the use of topical antimicrobials, *Am J Infect Control* 16:253, 1988.
GI, gastrointestinal; *IV*, intravenous; *CVP*, central venous pressure.

high-risk situations are invasive procedures such as surgery or the presence of invasive devices (intravenous [IV] and urinary catheters) and immune deficits from such events as alterations in humoral or cellular immunity, skin damage (burns, decubital ulcers, wounds), and extremities of age.[7] Guidelines for the soap to use in a specific procedure are listed in Table 6-1.

Indications for Hand Washing

Hands are one of the most implicated vehicles for transmission of pathogenic microorganisms to patients. Hand washing reduces the transfer of microbes to patients and inhibits the growth of microorganisms on the nails, hands, and forearms. Indications for hand washing are:

1. Before and after each patient contact or procedure, such as handling used dressings, used sputum containers, secretions, excretions, drainage, or blood
2. Before and after handling in-use patient devices, for example, IV catheters, urinary catheters, urine drainage bags, and respiratory equipment
3. After using the restroom and after blowing or wiping the nose
4. Before and after eating
5. Before and after collecting specimens
6. When hands are obviously soiled
7. When coming on duty and when going off duty

Hand washing facilities must be readily available to assist the HCW in performing this critical procedure. If they are not readily available, waterless antiseptic hand rinses should be available to use until the HCW can get to a sink, for example, in home care settings, ambulatory care settings, or ambulances.[3,4,6-8]

Hand Washing Procedure

The two methods of hand washing are the routine and the surgical hand scrubs. Chapter 10 contains the procedure for the surgical hand scrub. The procedure below describes the routine hand washing required for all other times and settings. The three components for hand washing are soap, water, and friction. Vigorous mechanical friction is the most important aspect; it removes the transient organisms. The procedure should take at least 10 to 15 seconds.

1. Wet hands with running water
2. Apply soap in the middle of the wet hands
3. Lather well
4. Use vigorous friction by rubbing the hands together; pay attention to nail beds and the webs between the fingers and thumbs
5. Rinse hands thoroughly with water and leave water running
6. Pat hands dry with a paper towel
7. Turn water off with a paper towel[1-4,8]

Home Care Considerations

Patients with infections or communicable diseases who are discharged from the hospital must be taught proper hand washing techniques and be knowledgeable about the applicable modes of transmission. It is best to include family members or caregivers when teaching patients about these techniques.

Home HCWs need to be aware of the patient's condition and use proper hand washing techniques and appropriate precautions within the home environment. If water is not available, rinseless antiseptic hand products or antiseptic hand wipes can be used to clean the hands until the HCW can reach a sink.[4,9]

Summary

The importance of hand washing cannot be overemphasized because infectious agents are easily and readily transmitted via the hands and everything the hands touch. Hand washing is absolutely essential to prevent and control nosocomial infections. There is no better substitute. It is one of the oldest, simplest, and most consistent methods available to prevent the spread of infectious agents from one person to another. It is a safety practice that protects patients, heath care personnel, families, and visitors.[2-4,7]

References

1. Butz A: *Personal cleanliness: the importance of cleanliness and infection prevention.* Proceedings of the sixth annual symposium of the soap and detergent association, NY, 1989.

2. Larson E: Evaluating handwashing techniques, *J Adv Nur* 10:547, 1985.

3. Palmer M: *Infection control: a policy and procedure manual,* Philadelphia, 1984, WB Saunders.

4. Soule B, editor: *The APIC curriculum for infection control practice,* vol 1-2, Dubuque, Iowa, 1983, Kendall/Hunt.

5. Benenson A, editor: *Control of communicable diseases in man,* ed 15, Washington, DC, 1990, American Public Health Association.

6. U.S. Department of Labor/OSHA: Occupational exposure to bloodborne pathogens: final rule, *Fed Reg* 56(235):64004,1991.

7. Larson E: APIC guidelines for the use of topical antimicrobials, *Am J Infect Control* 16, 1988.

8. Centers for Disease Control: *Guideline for handwashing and hospital environmental control,* Atlanta, 1985, Centers for Disease Control, Public Health Service, U.S. Department of Health and Human Services.

9. Macheca MK: Medical patient care. In Potter PA, Perry AG, editors: *Fundamentals of nursing: concepts and practice,* ed 3, St Louis, 1993, Mosby.

Isolation Precautions

Routes of infection transmission have been understood for many years. This knowledge has been the basis for the development of policies and practices to prevent the spread of infection. This chapter reviews the evolution of isolation practices in U.S. hospitals and provides the background for the Centers for Disease Control and Prevention (CDC) 1994 draft recommendations that follow. Guidelines are provided for the use of personal protective equipment (PPE) and for adapting isolation techniques to home care.

Evolution of Isolation Practices

In 1983 the CDC endorsed two systems of isolation precautions. Category-specific isolation precautions grouped infectious diseases based on modes of transmission and epidemiology; isolation procedures were then based on these broad categories. Disease-specific isolation precautions were individualized based on known transmission routes and epidemiology of diseases.[1]

These systems were endorsed by many hospitals although they both proved to have drawbacks. Category-specific isolation overisolated some patients (some infections within a category may actually require fewer precautions than others in the same category). Disease-specific isolation required higher levels of training for personnel and increased the potential for mistakes.[2] A flaw of both systems is that they were not applied until an infectious disease was actually diagnosed, resulting in the potential for spread of infection before diagnosis.

Universal Precautions

In 1985 the CDC published recommendations for preventing occupational bloodborne pathogen transmission in health care settings. The strategies outlined in the universal precautions protocol marked a shift in infection control practices in the United States.

Updated in 1987 and 1988, these recommendations, known as universal precautions (UP), protect health care workers (HCWs) by emphasizing the need to regard all patients as potentially infected with bloodborne pathogens. HCWs are advised to use appropriate PPE such as gloves, gowns, and protective facewear when contact with blood or blood-based body fluids of a patient is anticipated. Appropriate handling and disposal of used needles and other sharp instruments are also emphasized. The box on p. 83 gives an overview.

Many features of UP were subsequently codified in the Bloodborne Pathogens Standard promulgated by the Occupational Safety and Health Administration (OSHA, 1991). (See Chapter 2.) Although use of UP for all patients eliminates the need for additional precautions to prevent bloodborne pathogens, it does not eliminate the need for additional precautions for patients known or suspected to be infected with organisms transmitted by direct, airborne, or droplet contact routes of transmission.[2]

Body Substance Isolation

A system called body substance isolation (BSI) was developed between 1984 and 1990 as an alternative to diagnosis and category-driven isolation systems. The purpose of BSI is to protect patients from cross-transmission of microorganisms from hands of HCWs.[3,4] Like UP, BSI holds that all patients are potentially infectious. This system focuses on the isolation from patients of all moist and potentially infectious body substances (urine, blood, feces, sputum, saliva, wound drainage, and other body fluids) primarily through the use of gloves. BSI proponents hold that wearing fresh gloves before contact with any moist body substances will adequately prevent transmission of all infections except those transmitted by airborne or droplet contact routes. In BSI, signs are placed on the doors of patients with airborne infection; anyone wishing to enter the room is referred to the floor nurse for further instructions.[3]

Although many components of UP and BSI are similar, a major difference between them is that BSI emphasizes the application of fresh examination gloves just before contact with all moist body substances[4] and BSI does not emphasize hand washing after removal of gloves unless hands are visibly soiled because of glove punctures.[2] However, as with UP, BSI does not eliminate the need

Universal Blood and Body Fluid Precautions: An Overview

Universal precautions are intended to supplement rather than replace recommendations for routine infection control such as washing hands and using gloves to prevent gross microbiological contamination of hands.

- All health care workers should routinely use appropriate barrier precautions to prevent skin and mucous membrane exposure when contact is anticipated with blood, semen, vaginal secretions, cerebrospinal fluid, synovial fluid, pleural fluid, peritoneal fluid, pericardial fluid, amniotic fluid, or any body fluid containing visible blood. Barrier protection should also be used for handling items or surfaces soiled with blood or other specified body fluids. Gloves should be worn for venipuncture, and for touching blood and body fluids, mucous membranes, or nonintact skin. Masks, gowns, and protective eyewear should be worn for procedures likely to generate droplets, splashes, or sprays of blood or other listed body fluids.

- Gloves should be changed after contact with each patient and should not be washed or reused. Hands should be washed immediately after gloves are removed.

- Precautions should be taken to prevent injuries when using needles, scalpels, and other sharp instruments or devices; when handling sharp instruments after procedures; when cleaning used instruments; and when disposing of used instruments.

- Needles, used disposable syringes, scalpel blades, and other sharp items should be placed in puncture-resistant containers for disposal. Containers should be located as close to the area of use as is practical. Reusable sharps should be placed in puncture-resistant containers for transport to the reprocessing area.

- Resuscitation bags should be available in areas where the need for resuscitation is predictable to avoid mouth-to-mouth contact.

- Health care workers with open lesions should refrain from direct patient care and from handling patient-care equipment.

Modified from Centers for Disease Control: Recommendations for prevention of HIV transmission in health-care settings, *MMWR* 36(2-s), 3s, 1987; Centers for Disease Control: Update: universal precautions for prevention of transmission of human immunodeficiency virus, hepatitis B virus, and other bloodborne pathogens in health care settings, *MMWR* 37(24):377, 1988.

for additional precautions with patients known or suspected to have infections transmitted by contact with environmental fomites or through airborne or droplet particles.

CDC 1994 Draft Guidelines for Isolation Precautions in Hospitals

The CDC 1994 Draft Guidelines for Isolation Precautions in Hospitals incorporates recommendations by the Hospital Infection Control Practices Advisory Committee (HICPAC) and the CDC National Center for Infectious Diseases. These guidelines are intended to supersede previous CDC recommendations for isolation precautions for use in hospitals, although hospitals are encouraged to adapt these guidelines to meet their own needs. Development of these guidelines was driven by the following objectives: (1) to maintain epidemiological soundness; (2) to recognize the importance of all body fluids, secretions, and excretions in the transmission of nosocomial pathogens; (3) to contain adequate precautions for infections transmitted by the airborne, droplet, and contact routes of transmission; (4) to be as simple and user-friendly as possible; and (5) to provide new terms to avoid confusion with existing systems.[5]

Standard Precautions

The revised guidelines contain two tiers of precautions. The first tier contains standard precautions that are designed for the care of all patients in hospitals regardless of their diagnosis or presumed infection status. Standard precautions synthesize the major features of UP and BSI. Standard precautions apply to blood, all body fluids, secretions, excretions (regardless of whether or not they contain visible blood), nonintact skin, and mucous membranes. The box on pp. 85-87 lists these guidelines. Hospitals are directed to develop a system to ensure that patients, personnel, and visitors are educated about the use of precautions and their responsibility for adherence to them. Hospitals are also directed to evaluate adherence to precautions and to use findings to direct improvements.

Transmission-Based Precautions

The second tier of precautions, transmission-based precautions, is designed as a supplement to standard precautions and for use with patients documented or suspected to be infected or colonized with highly transmissible or epidemiologically important pathogens. There are three types of transmission-based precautions—airborne, droplet, and contact precautions. The box on pp. 88-91 outlines the implementation standards for these precautions. For definitions of airborne, droplet, and contact transmission, see Chapter 5.

Temporary Clinical Syndrome Precautions

Recognizing that patients are admitted before definitive diagnoses, the CDC published additional guidelines addressing the issue of undiagnosed communicable patients. These guidelines relate to clinical syndromes or symptoms of the patient. Until a diagnosis is made and infection or disease is ruled out, these temporary precautions will decrease nosocomial transfer. Table 7-1 lists those symptom-specific situations that are highly suspicious for transmissible infections.

Text continued on p. 95.

Standard Precautions: An Overview

Standard precautions should be used for the care of all hospitalized patients.

Hand washing
Wash hands after touching blood, body fluids, secretions, excretions, and contaminated items, whether or not gloves are worn. Wash hands immediately after gloves are removed and between patient contacts.

Gloves
Wear gloves when touching blood, body fluids, secretions, excretions, and contaminated items. Put on clean gloves just before touching mucous membranes and nonintact skin. Remove gloves promptly after use, before touching noncontaminated items and environmental surfaces, and before going to another patient. Wash hands immediately to avoid transfer of microorganisms to other patients or environments.

Modified from Centers for Disease Control and Prevention: Draft guidelines for isolation precautions in hospitals, *Federal Register* 59(214):55552, 1994.

Continued.

Standard Precautions—cont'd

Mask, eye protection, face shield
Wear a mask and eye protection or a face shield to protect mucous membranes of the eyes, nose, and mouth during procedures and patient-care activities that are likely to generate splashes or sprays of blood, body fluids, secretions, and excretions.

Gown
Wear a clean gown to protect skin and prevent soiling of clothing during procedures and patient-care activities that are likely to generate splashes or sprays of blood, body fluids, secretions, or excretions or to cause soiling of clothing. Remove a soiled gown as promptly as possible and wash hands to avoid transfer of microorganisms to other patients or environments.

Patient-care equipment
Handle used patient-care equipment soiled with blood, body fluids, secretions, or excretions in a manner that prevents skin and mucous membrane exposure, contamination of clothing, and transfer of microorganisms to other patients and environments. Reusable equipment must be processed appropriately before it is used for the care of another patient. Single-use items must be appropriately discarded.

Linen
Handle, transport, and process used linen soiled with blood, body fluids, secretions, and excretions in a manner that prevents skin and mucous membrane exposure and contamination of clothing.

Standard Precautions—cont'd

Needle disposal

Take care to prevent injuries when using needles, scalpels, and other sharp instruments or devices; when handling sharp instruments after procedures; when cleaning used instruments; and when disposing of used needles. Never recap used needles or manipulate them with any other technique that involves directing the point of a needle toward any part of the body. A one-handed scoop technique or a mechanical device for holding the needle sheath may be used. Do not remove used needles from disposable syringes by hand, and do not bend, break, or manipulate used needles by hand. Place used disposable syringes and needles, scalpel blades, and other sharp items in appropriate puncture-resistant containers located as close as practical to the area in which the items were used. Place reusable syringes and needles in a puncture-resistant container for transport to the reprocessing area.

Resuscitation equipment

Use mouthpieces, resuscitation bags, or other ventilation devices as an alternative to mouth-to-mouth resuscitation in areas where the need for resuscitation is predictable.

Patient placement

Place a patient who contaminates the environment or who does not assist in maintaining appropriate environmental control in a private room. If a private room is not available, consult with infection control professionals regarding patient placement or other alternatives.

Transmission-Based Precautions

1. Airborne precautions should be used in addition to standard precautions for patients known or suspected to be infected with microorganisms transmitted by airborne droplet nuclei (5 microns or smaller).

   A. **Patient placement**
   Place the patient in a private room that has (1) monitored negative air pressure in relation to surrounding areas, (2) a minimum of six air changes per hour, and (3) appropriate discharge of air outdoors or, if this is not possible in retrofitted isolation rooms, use monitored high-efficiency filtration of room air before the air is circulated to other areas in the hospital. Keep the room door closed and the patient in the room. When a private room is not available, place the patient in a room with a patient who has active infection with the same microorganism but no other infection unless otherwise recommended. When a private room is not available and cohorting is not desirable, consult with infection control professionals.

   B. **Respiratory protection**
   Wear respirator protection when entering the room of a patient with known or suspected infectious tuberculosis. Do not enter the room of patients known or suspected to have measles or *varicella* if susceptible to these infections.

   C. **Patient transport**
   Limit the movement and transport of the patient to essential purposes only. If transport or movement is necessary, minimize patient dispersal of droplet nuclei by placing a surgical mask on the patient.

   D. Some examples of infections or diseases requiring airborne precautions are tuberculosis, measles, and *varicella* (including disseminated zoster).

Modified from Centers of Disease Control and Prevention: Draft guidelines for isolation precautions in hospitals, *Federal Register* 59(214):55552, 1994.

Transmission-Based Precautions—cont'd

2. Droplet precautions should be used in addition to standard precautions for a patient known or suspected to be infected with microorganisms transmitted by droplets larger than 5 microns that can be transmitted by coughing, sneezing, talking, or by the performance of procedures such as suctioning.
   A. **Patient placement**
      Place the patient in a private room or in a room with a patient who has active infection with the same microorganism but no other infection. When a private room is not available and cohorting is not possible, maintain a separation of at least 3 feet between the infected patient and other patients and visitors.
   B. **Masking**
      Wear a mask when working within 3 feet of a patient.
   C. **Patient transport**
      Limit the movement and transport of the patient to essential purposes only. If transport or movement is necessary, minimize patient dispersal of droplets by placing a surgical mask on the patient.
   D. Some examples of infections or diseases requiring droplet precautions are *Neisseria meningitidis,* multidrug-resistant *Streptococcus pneumonia,* pertussis, *Streptococcal pharyngitis,* influenza, mumps, and rubella.
3. Contact precautions should be used in addition to standard precautions for a patient known or suspected to be infected or colonized with epidemiologically important microorganisms that can be transmitted by hand or skin-to-skin contact or indirect contact with environmental surfaces or patient-care items in the patient's room.

Continued.

Transmission-Based Precautions—cont'd

A. **Patient placement**
   Place the patient in a private room or in a room with a patient who has active infection with the same organisms but no other infection. When a private room is not available and cohorting is not possible, consult with infection control professionals.

B. **Gloves and hand washing**
   Wear gloves when entering the patient's room. Remove gloves before leaving the patient's room and scrub hands with an antimicrobial agent. After glove removal and hand washing, ensure that hands do not touch potentially contaminated environmental surfaces.

C. **Gowns**
   Wear a gown when entering the patient's room if you anticipate that your clothing will have substantial contact with the patient, environmental surfaces, or items in the patient's room or if the patient is incontinent or has diarrhea, an ileostomy, or wound drainage not contained by a dressing. Remove the gown before leaving the patient's environment. After gown removal, ensure that clothing does not contact potentially contaminated environmental surfaces.

D. **Patient transport**
   Limit the movement and transport of the patient to essential purposes only. If the patient is transported out of the room, ensure that precautions are maintained.

Transmission-Based Precautions—cont'd

E. **Environmental control**

Ensure that patient care items, bedside equipment, and frequently touched surfaces receive daily cleaning.

F. **Patient care equipment**

When possible, dedicate the use of noncritical patient-care equipment and items such as stethoscopes, sphygmomanometers, bedside commodes, or electronic rectal thermometers to a single patient (or cohorted patients) to avoid sharing between patients. If use of common equipment is unavoidable, items must be adequately cleaned and disinfected before use with another patient.

G. **Additional precautions for preventing the spread of vancomycin-resistance**

Consult the Hospital Infection Control Practices Advisory Committee report on preventing the spread of vancomycin-resistance. (*Federal Register* 59(94): 25758, 1994.)

H. Some examples of infections or diseases requiring contact precautions are uncontained major abscesses or decubitus ulcers, scabies, pediculosis, staphylococcal skin infections, *impetigo,* enteric infections (*Clostridium difficile, Escherichia coli*) 0157:H7, respiratory syncytial virus.

Table 7-1 Clinical syndromes or conditions warranting additional empiric precautions to prevent transmission of epidemiologically important pathogens pending confirmation of diagnosis*

Clinical Syndrome or Condition†	Potential Pathogens‡	Empiric Precautions
Diarrhea		
Acute diarrhea with likely infectious cause in incontinent or diapered patient	Enteric pathogens§	Contact
Diarrhea in adult with history of broad spectrum or long-term antibiotics	*Clostridium difficile*	Contact
Meningitis	*Neisseria meningitidis*	Droplet
Generalized Rashes of Unknown Etiology		
Petechial or ecchymotic with fever	*Neisseria meningitidis*	Droplet
Vesicular	*Varicella*	Airborne and contact
Maculopapular with rhinitis and fever	Rubeola (measles)	Airborne
Respiratory Infections		
Cough, fever, or upper lobe pulmonary infiltrate in HIV-negative patient	*Mycobacterium tuberculosis*	Airborne

Cough, fever, pulmonary infiltrate in any lung location in HIV-positive patient	*Mycobacterium tuberculosis*	Airborne
Paroxysmal or severe persistent cough during periods of pertussis activity	*Bordetella pertussis*	Droplet
Respiratory infections, particularly bronchiolitis and croup in infants and young children	Respiratory syncytial or parainfluenza virus	Contact

Modified from Centers for Disease Control and Prevention: Draft guidelines for isolation precautions in hospitals, *Federal Register* 59(214):55552, 1994.

HIV, human immunodeficiency virus.

*Infection control professionals are encouraged to modify or adapt this table according to local conditions. To ensure that appropriate empiric precautions are always implemented, hospitals must have systems in place to routinely evaluate patients according to these criteria as part of their preadmission and admission care.

†Patients with the syndromes or conditions listed may have atypical signs or symptoms; for example, pertussis in neonates or adults may not have paroxysmal or severe cough. The clinician's index of suspicion should be guided by the prevalence of specific conditions in the community as well as clinical judgment.

‡The organisms listed are not intended to represent the complete or even most likely diagnoses, but rather possible etiologic agents that require additional precautions beyond standard precautions until they can be ruled out.

§These pathogens include entero-hemorrhagic *Escherichia coli* 0157:H7, *shigella*, hepatitis A, and rotavirus.

Continued.

Table 7-1 Clinical syndromes or conditions warranting additional empiric precautions to prevent transmission of epidemiologically important pathogens pending confirmation of diagnosis*

Clinical Syndrome or Condition†	Potential Pathogens‡	Empiric Precautions
Risk of Multidrug-Resistant Microorganisms		
History of infection or colonization with multidrug-resistant organisms‖	Resistant bacteria	Contact
Skin, wound, or urinary tract infection in patient with recent hospital or nursing home stay in facility where multidrug-resistant organisms are prevalent	Resistant bacteria	Contact
Skin or Wound Infection		
Abscess or draining wound that cannot be covered	*Staphylococcus aureus*, group A streptococcus	Contact

‖Resistant bacteria judged by the infection control program, based on current state, regional, or national recommendations, to be of special clinical or epidemiological significance.

Precautions for Selected Infections and Conditions

In an appendix to the guidelines, the CDC lists diseases and infections and the types and duration of precautions needed. When the diagnosis is known, users can refer to this part of the guidelines to select the appropriate types of precautions and to find out how long the precautions need to be kept in place. This information is presented in its entirety in Table 7-2.

Guidelines for Use of Personal Protective Equipment

PPE for nonsurgical settings consists of gowns, gloves, masks, eyewear, and face shields. Examples of appropriate use of PPE are presented in the following section.

Gowns

Wear gowns during procedures that are likely to generate splashes of blood or other body fluids that may contaminate clothes or uniforms. Examples of patient care activities requiring gowns are wound cleansing and irrigating procedures, handling drainage, pouring contaminated fluids into hoppers (or toilets), and during major dressing changes.

Gloves

Wear a clean pair of gloves for all procedures involving mucous membranes, nonintact skin, and moist body substances (feces, urine, sputum, saliva, and wound drainage). Wear gloves to touch items or surfaces soiled with blood or body fluids, to perform venipuncture, to collect blood gases, or to access other vascular sites. Remove gloves and wash hands after each patient. Do not wash hands while wearing gloves because glove integrity cannot be assured.[6] See the box on p. 113 for specific glove guidelines.

Face Protection: Masks, Eyewear, Face Shields

Use masks alone when there is a risk of respiratory (airborne or droplet) transmission of an infectious agent (rubella, mumps, tuberculosis). Masks (in conjunction with eyewear) provide full face protection from splashes of blood or body fluids and protect against exposure of oral and nasal mucous membranes.

Text continued on p. 113.

Table 7-2 Type and duration of precautions needed for selected infections and conditions

Infection/Condition	Precautions Type[a]	Precautions Duration[b]
Abscess		
Draining, major[c]	C	DI
Draining, minor or limited[d]	S	
Acquired immunodeficiency syndrome (AIDS)[e]	S	
Actinomycosis	D, C	DI
Adenovirus infection, in infants and young children	S	
Amebiasis	S	
Anthrax		
Cutaneous	S	
Pulmonary	S	
Antibiotic-associated colitis (see *Clostridium difficile*)		
Arthropodborne viral encephalitides (eastern, western, Venezuelan equine encephalomyelitis; St. Louis, California encephalitis)	S[f]	
Arthropodborne viral fevers (dengue fever, yellow fever, Colorado tick fever)	S[f]	
Ascariasis	S	
Aspergillosis	S	
Babesiosis	S	
Blastomycosis (North American, cutaneous, or pulmonary)	S	
Botulism	S	

Bronchiolitis (see respiratory infections in infants and young children)

Condition		
Brucellosis (undulant, Malta, Mediterranean fever)	S	
Campylobacter gastroenteritis (see gastroenteritis)		
Candidiasis, all forms including mucocutaneous	S	
Catscratch fever (benign innoculation lymphoreticulosis)	S	
Cellulitis, uncontrolled drainage	C	DI
Chancroid (soft chancre)	S	
Chickenpox (varicella)	A, C	F[g]
Chlamydia trachomatis		
Conjunctivitis	S	
Genital	S	
Respiratory	S	
Cholera (see gastroenteritis)		

Modified from Centers for Disease Control and Prevention: Draft guidelines for isolated precautions in hospitals, *Federal Register* 59(214):555631, 1994.

[a] A, airborne; C, contact; D, droplet; S, standard; when A, C, and D are specified, also use S.

[b] CN, until off antibiotics and culture negative; DH, duration of hospitalization; DI, duration of illness (with wound lesions, DI means until they stop draining); U, until time specified in hours (hrs) after initiation of effective therapy; F, see footnote.

[c] No dressing or dressing does not adequately contain drainage.

[d] Dressing covers and adequately contains drainage.

[e] Also see syndromes or conditions listed in Table 7-1.

[f] Install screens in windows and doors in endemic areas.

[g] Maintain precautions until all lesions are crusted. Use varicella-zoster immune globulin (VZIG) when appropriate, and discharge exposed susceptible patients before the tenth day after the exposure, if possible. Place remaining exposed susceptible patients on precautions beginning 10 days after exposure and continue until 21 days after last exposure (up to 28 days if VZIG has been given). Susceptible persons should stay out of the rooms of patients on precautions.

Continued.

Table 7-2 Type and duration of precautions needed for selected infections and conditions—cont'd

Infection/Condition	Precautions	
	Type[a]	Duration[b]
Closed-cavity infection		
Draining, limited or minor	S	
Not draining	S	DI
Clostridium		
C. botulinum	S	
C. difficile	C	
C. perfringens		
Food poisoning	S	
Gas gangrene	S	
Coccidioidomycosis (valley fever)		
Draining lesions	S	
Pneumonia	S	
Colorado tick fever	S	
Congenital rubella	C	F[h]
Conjunctivitis		
Acute bacterial	S	
Chlamydia	S	
Gonococcal	S	
Acute viral (acute hemorrhagic)	C	DI

Coxsackie virus (see enteroviral infection)

Creutzfeldt-Jakob disease	S[i]	
Croup (see respiratory infections in infants and young children)		
Cryptococcosis	S	
Cryptosporidiosis (see gastroenteritis)		
Cysticercosis	S	
Cytomegalovirus infection, neonatal or immunosuppressed	S	
Decubitus ulcer, infected		
Major[e]	C	DI
Minor or limited[d]	S	
Dengue	S[f]	
Diarrhea, acute-infective etiology suspected (see gastroenteritis)		
Diphtheria		
Cutaneous	C	CN[j]
Pharyngeal	D	CN[j]
Echinococcosis (hydatidosis)	S	
Echovirus (see enteroviral infection)		
Encephalitis or encephalomyelitis (see specific etiologic agents)		
Endometritis	S	
Enterobiasis (pinworm disease, oxyuriasis)	S	

[h]Place infant on precautions during any admission until 1 year of age unless nasopharyngeal and urine cultures are negative for virus after age 3 months.
[i]Additional special precautions are necessary for handling and decontamination of blood, body fluids, and tissues, and contaminated items from patients with confirmed or suspected disease. See latest College of American Pathologists (Northfield, Ill) guidelines or other references.
[j]Until two cultures taken at least 24 hours apart are negative.

Continued.

Table 7-2 Type and duration of precautions needed for selected infections and conditions—cont'd

Infection/Condition	Precautions	
	Type[a]	Duration[b]
Enterococcus sp. (see multidrug-resistant organisms if epidemiologically significant or vancomycin resistant)		
Enterocolitis, *Clostridium difficile*.........	C	DH
Enteroviral infections		
Adults.........	S	
Infants and children.........	C	DI
Epiglottitis, due to *Haemophilus influenzae*.........	D	U[24 hrs]
Epstein-Barr virus infection, including infectious mononucleosis.........	S	
Erythema infectiosum (also see Parvovirus B19).........	S	
Escherichia coli gastroenteritis (see gastroenteritis)		
Food poisoning		
Botulism.........	S	
Clostridium pefringens or *welchii*.........	S	
Staphylococcal.........	S	
Furunculosis—staphylococcal		
Infants and young children.........	C	DI
Gangrene (gas gangrene).........	S	
Gastroenteritis		

Campylobacter sp.	S[k]	
Cholera	S[k]	
Clostridium difficile	C	DI
Cryptosporidium sp.	S[k]	
Escherichia coli		
Enterohemorrhagic 0157:H7	S[k]	
Diapered or incontinent	C	DI
Other species	S[k]	
Giardia lamblia	S[k]	
Rotavirus	S	
Diapered or incontinent	C	DI
Salmonella sp. (including *S. typhi*)	S[k]	
Shigella sp.	S[k]	
Diapered or incontinent	C	DI
Vibrio parahaemolyticus	S[k]	
Viral (if not covered elsewhere)	S[k]	
Yersinia enterocolitica	S[k]	
German measles (rubella)	D	DI
Giardiasis (see gastroenteritis)		
Gonococcal ophthalmia neonatorum (gonorrheal ophthalmia, acute conjunctivitis of newborn)	S	

Continued.

[k]Use contact precautions for diapered or incontinent children <6 years of age for duration of illness.

Table 7-2 Type and duration of precautions needed for selected infections and conditions—cont'd

Infection/Condition	Precautions	
	Type[a]	Duration[b]
Gonorrhea.	S	
Granuloma inguinale (donovanosis, granuloma venereum).	S	
Guillain-Barré syndrome.	S	
Hand, foot, and mouth disease (see enteroviral infection)		
Hemorrhagic fevers (for example, Lassa fever)[l]	C	DI
Hepatitis, viral		
Type A.	S	
Diapered or incontinent patients.	C	F[m]
Type B (HB$_s$Ag positive).	S	
Type C and other unspecified non-A, non-B.	S	
Type E.	S	
Herpangina (see enteroviral infection)		
Herpes simplex (*Herpesvirus hominis*)		
Encephalitis.	S	
Neonatal[n].	C	DI
Mucocutaneous, disseminated or primary, severe.	C	DI
Mucocutaneous, recurrent (skin, oral, genital).	S	
Herpes zoster (varicella-zoster)		

Localized in immunocompromised patient, or disseminated	A, C	DI
Localized in normal patient	S	
Histoplasmosis	S	
Hookworm disease (ancylostomiasis, uncinariasis)	S	
Human immunodeficiency virus (HIV) infection[e]	S	
Impetigo	C	U[24 hrs]
Infectious mononucleosis	S	
Influenza	D°	DI
Kawasaki syndrome	S	
Lassa fever[l]	C	DI
Legionnaires' disease	S	
Leprosy	S	
Leptospirosis	S	
Listeriosis	S	
Lyme disease	S	

[l]Call state health department and CDC for advice about management of a suspected case.

[m]Maintain precautions in infants and children <3 years of age for duration of hospitalization; in children 3 to 14 years of age, until 2 weeks after onset of symptoms; and in others, until 1 week after onset of symptoms.

[n]For infants delivered vaginally or by C-section and if mother has active infection and membranes have been ruptured for more than 4 to 6 hours.

[o]This recommendation is made recognizing the logistic difficulties and physical plant limitations that may face hospitals admitting multiple patients with suspected influenza during community outbreaks. If sufficient private rooms are unavailable, consider cohorting patients, or at the very least, avoid room sharing with high risk patients.

Continued.

Table 7-2 Type and duration of precautions needed for selected infections and conditions—cont'd

Infection/Condition	Precautions Type[a]	Precautions Duration[b]
Lymphocytic choriomeningitis.	S	
Lymphogranuloma venereum.	S	
Malaria.	S	
Marburg virus disease[1]	C	DI
Measles (rubeola), all presentations.	A	DI
Melioidosis, all forms.	S	
Meningitis		
Aseptic (nonbacterial or viral meningitis).	S	
Bacterial, gram-negative enteric, in neonates.	S	
Fungal.	S	
Haemophilus influenzae, known or suspected.	D	U[24 hrs]
Listeria monocytogenes.	S	
Neisseria meningitidis (meningococcal) known or suspected.	D	U[24 hrs]
Pneumococcal.	S	
Tuberculosis[P].	S	
Other diagnosed bacterial.	S	
Meningococcal pneumonia.	D	U[24 hrs]
Meningococcemia (meningococcal sepsis).	D	U[24 hrs]

Molluscum contagiosum	S	
Mucormycosis	S	
Multidrug-resistant organisms, infection or colonization[q]		
Gastrointestinal	C	CN
Respiratory	C	CN
Pneumococcal	D	CN
Skin, wound, or burn	C	CN
Mumps (infectious parotitis)	D	F[r]
Mycobacteria, nontuberculosis (atypical)		
Pulmonary	S	
Wound	S	
Mycoplasma pneumonia	D	DI
Necrotizing enterocolitis	S	
Nacardiosis, draining lesions or other presentations	S	
Norwalk agent gastroenteritis (see viral gastroenteritis)		
Orf	S	
Parinfluenza virus infection, respiratory in infants and young children	C	DI

[p]Patient should be examined for evidence of current (active) pulmonary tuberculosis. If evidence exists additional precautions are necessary (see tuberculosis).

[q]Resistant bacteria judged by the infection control program, based on current state, regional, or national recommendations, to be of special clinical and epidemiologic significance.

[r]For 9 days after onset of swelling.

Continued.

Table 7-2 Type and duration of precautions needed for selected infections and conditions—cont'd

Infection/Condition	Precautions	
	Type[a]	Duration[b]
Parvovirus B19	D	F[s]
Pediculosis	C	U[24 hrs]
Pertussis (whooping cough)	D	F[t]
Pinworm infection	S	
Plague		
Bubonic	S	
Pneumonic	D	U[72 hrs]
Pleurodynia (see enteroviral infection)		
Pneumonia		
Adenovirus	D, C	DI
Bacterial not listed elsewhere (including gram-negative bacterial)	S	
Chlamydia	S	
Fungal	S	
Haemophilus influenzae		
Adults	S	
Infants and children (any age)	D	U[24 hrs]
Legionella	S	

Meningococcal..	D	U$^{24\ hrs}$
Multidrug-resistant bacterial (see multidrug-resistant organisms)		
Mycoplasma (primary atypical pneumonia)...	D	DI
Pneumococcal...	S	
Multidrug-resistant (see multidrug-resistant organisms)		
Pneumocystis carinii..	S[u]	
Pseudomonas cepacia in cystic fibrosis (CF) patients, including respiratory tract colonization....	C[v]	DH
Staphylococcus aureus..	S	
Streptococcus, Group A		
Adults..	S	
Infants and young children..	D	U$^{24\ hrs}$
Viral		
Adults..	S	
Infants and young children (see respiratory infectious disease, acute)......	S	
Poliomyelitis...	S	
Psittacosis (ornithosis)...	S	
Q fever...	S	
Rabies..	S	

[s]Maintain precautions for duration of hospitalization when chronic disease occurs in an immunodeficient patient. For patients with transient aplastic crisis or red cell crisis, maintain precautions for 7 days.

[t]Maintain precautions until 5 days after patient is placed on effective therapy.

[u]Avoid placement in the same room with an immunocompromised patient.

[v]Avoid cohorting or placement in the same room with a cystic fibrosis patient who is not infected or colonized with *P. cepacia*.

Continued.

Table 7-2 Type and duration of precautions needed for selected infections and conditions—cont'd

Infection/Condition	Precautions Type[a]	Duration[b]
Rat-bite fever (*Streptobacillus moniliformis* disease, *Spirillum minus* disease)	S	
Relapsing fever	S	
Resistant bacterial infection or colonization (see multidrug-resistant organisms)		
Respiratory infectious disease, acute (if not covered elsewhere)		
Adults	S	
Infants and young children[e]	C	DI
Respiratory syncytial virus infection, in infants and young children, and immunocompromised adults.	C	DI
Reye's syndrome	S	
Rheumatic fever	S	
Rickettsial fevers, tickborne (Rocky Mountain spotted fever, tickborne typhus fever)	S	
Rickettsialpox (vesicular rickettsiosis)	S	
Ringworm (dermatophytosis, dermatomycosis, tinea)	S	
Ritter's disease (staphylococcal scalded skin syndrome)	C[w]	DI
Rocky Mountain spotted fever	S	
Roseola infantum (exanthem subitum)	S	
Rotavirus infection (see gastroenteritis)		
Rubella (German measles) (also congenital rubella)	D	F[x]
Salmonellosis (see gastroenteritis)		

Scabies	C	U$^{24\ hrs}$
Scalded skin syndrome, staphylococcal (Ritter's disease)	C^w	DI
Schistosomiasis (bilharziasis)	S	
Shigellosis (see gastroenteritis)		
Sporotrichosis	S	
Spirillum minus disease (rat-bite fever)	S	
Staphylococcal disease (*S. aureus*)		
Skin, wound, or burn:		
Major^c	C	DI
Minor or limited^d	S	
Enterocolitis	S	
Multidrug-resistant (see multidrug-resistant organism)		
Pneumonia	S	
Scalded skin syndrome	C	DI
Toxic shock syndrome	S	
Streptobacillus moniliformis disease (rat-bite fever)	S	
Streptococcal disease (group A *Streptococcus*)		
Skin, wound, or burn		
Major^c	C	U$^{24\ hrs}$
Minor or limited^d	S	

^{w}Blistering is due to the hematogenous dissemination of toxin, not to presence of organisms in the blisters. However, such patients may be heavily colonized with staphylococci because of their skin problems; thus, contact precautions are recommended.

^{x}Until 7 days after onset of rash.

Continued.

Table 7-2 Type and duration of precautions needed for selected infections and conditions—cont'd

Infection/Condition	Precautions	
	Type[a]	Duration[b]
Endometritis (puerperal sepsis)	S	
Pharyngitis in infants and young children	D	U[24 hrs]
Pneumonia in infants and young children	D	U[24 hrs]
Scarlet fever in infants and young children	D	U[24 hrs]
Streptococcal disease (group B *Streptococcus*), neonatal	S	
Streptococcal disease (not group A or B), unless covered elsewhere	S	
Multidrug-resistant (see multidrug-resistant organisms)		
Strongyloidiasis	S	
Syphilis		
Skin and mucous membrane, including congenital, primary, secondary	S	
Latent (tertiary) and seropositivity without lesions	S	
Tapeworm disease		
Hymenolepis nana	S	
Taenia solium (pork)	S	
Other	S	
Tetanus	S	
Tinea (fungus infection dermatophytosis, dermatomycosis, ringworm)	S	
Toxoplasmosis	S	

Continued.

Toxic shock syndrome (staphylococcal disease)	S	
Trachoma, acute	S	
Trench mouth (Vincent's angina)	S	
Trichinosis	S	
Trichomoniasis	S	
Trichuriasis (whipworm disease)	S	
Tuberculosis		
Extrapulmonary, draining lesion (including scrofula)	S	
Extrapulmonary, meningitis[D]	S	
Pulmonary, confirmed or suspected or laryngeal disease	A	F[y]
Skin test positive with no evidence of current pulmonary disease	S	
Tularemia		
Draining lesion	S	
Pulmonary	S	
Typhoid (*Salmonella typhi*) fever (see gastroenteritis)	S	
Typhus, endemic and epidemic	S	
Urinary tract infection (including pyelonephritis), with or without urinary catheter	S	
Varicella (chickenpox)	A, C	F[g]
Vibrio parahaemolyticus (see gastroenteritis)	S	
Vincent's angina (trench mouth)	S	

[y] Discontinue precautions only when tuberculosis (TB) patient is on effective therapy, is improving clinically, and has three consecutive negative sputum smears collected on different days, or TB is ruled out.

Table 7-2 Type and duration of precautions needed for selected infections and conditions—cont'd

Infection/Condition	Precautions	
	Type[a]	Duration[b]
Viral diseases		
Respiratory (if not covered elsewhere)		
Adults..	S	
Infants and young children (see respiratory infectious disease, acute)		
Whooping cough (pertussis)..	D	F[t]
Wound infections		
Major[c]	C	DI
Minor or limited[d]	S	
Yersinia enterocolitica gastroenteritis (see gastroenteritis)		
Zoster (varicella-zoster)		
Localized in immunocompromised patient, disseminated.......	A, C	F[g]
Localized in normal patient..	S	
Zygomycosis (phycomycosis, mucormycosis).....................	S	

Guidelines for Use of Gloves

1. Wear gloves on both hands whenever contact with blood and body fluid is anticipated.
2. Choose appropriate gloves for the job (e.g., examination gloves for patient contact; utility gloves for cleanup).
3. Wash hands before applying gloves.
4. Never reuse gloves.
5. Change gloves if you notice gross defects.
6. Keep fingernails short to avoid punctures.
7. Do not wear rings, bracelets, or other jewelry that might tear gloves.
8. Remove gloves by inversion (turn them inside out).
9. Discard gloves in appropriate receptacle.
10. Wash hands immediately following removal.

Modified from Korniewicz D: Effectiveness of glove barriers used in clinical settings, *Medsurg Nurs* 1(1):29 Sept 1992; Korniewicz D, Kirwin M, Larson E: Do your gloves fit the task? *Am J Nurs* 91(6):38, 1991; U.S. Environmental Protection Agency: *Guide for infectious waste management,* pub no 530-SW-86-014, Washington, DC, May 1986, U.S. Environmental Protection Agency.

Masks and eyewear should be used when assisting with procedures or when performing procedures such as wound cleaning, dressing, tubing, catheter changes, or instrument decontamination.[7] Masks may be used without eyewear (e.g., around active tuberculosis patients), but eyewear should not be used without masks.

Patient Concerns Related to Personal Protective Equipment

Discuss any psychosocial concerns expressed by the patient or family about the use of protective attire. A clear explanation about the rationale for use of PPE helps patients and their families accept the use of PPE that may subject the patient to social isolation.

Homecare Considerations

Families who care for patients at home need education about common ways that germs are spread. They need to be educated about strategies to avoid contact with body fluids and fomites such as needles, bandages, or bedpans. If patients require respiratory precautions at home, they and their families will need to be

Infection Control Practices Adapted for Home Care

Hand washing procedure: Hand washing should always occur before handling dressings, tubes, or medications; after using the bathroom; after handling any items that may be contaminated with body fluids (dressings); after removing gloves; after handling or caring for pets; and before eating.

Gloves: Latex or vinyl gloves should be worn if you think you might have contact with blood or other body fluids; before touching cut or scraped skin or mucous membranes (eyes, nose, mouth); and before handling soiled linen or clothing. Gloves should be removed immediately after use and disposed of properly. They must not be reused. Gloves do not need to be worn for casual contact such as bathing of unbroken skin, feeding a person, or assisting with walking.

Spills: Blood and other body fluid spills should be cleaned up by following these steps: (1) put on gloves, (2) wipe up spill with paper towels, (3) clean spill area with disinfectant (bleach, alcohol, cleanser, Lysol, or hydrogen peroxide), (4) dispose of cleanup materials and gloves in a plastic bag, and (5) wash hands.

Waste disposal: Bodily waste (stool, urine, blood) can be safely flushed down the toilet. Care should be taken to avoid splashing during disposal. Soiled dressings or bandages, used gloves, disposable equipment, or other contaminated medical waste should be placed in tied plastic bags. Needles, syringes, lancets, and other sharp objects should be handled with care. Never recap, bend, or break needles after use. Needles and other used sharp instruments may be placed in a hard plastic soda bottle. Put tape over the closed bottle cap when the bottle is full. Contact the waste disposal company to determine if the medical waste bag or filled bottle may be placed in the garbage can.

Laundry: Linen and clothing soiled with blood or body fluids can be washed in the washer using detergent and hot water. Dry in the family dryer on the hot cycle. One cup of household bleach may be added to each load of laundry.

Modified from Group Health Cooperative of Puget Sound: *Protect yourself when you take care of others: infection control practices for home care,* Seattle, 1993, Group Health Cooperative of Puget Sound.

educated about the importance of covering the mouth with tissues while coughing, disposing of tissues appropriately, and the use of masks by the patient and by care providers. For patients with bloodborne infection, family members need to be educated about washing hands, wearing gloves, cleaning spills, disposing of wastes, and doing laundry. Families will often need assistance in identifying sources for appropriate PPE. HCWs who provide health care in the home will need to remember to bring PPE with them to the home.[8] See the box on p. 114 for infection control practices adapted for families providing home care.

Summary

Although there has been conflict over the efficacy of various isolation techniques in the prevention of nosocomial infections, it is anticipated that the synthesis of universal precautions and body substance isolation described as standard precautions will help eliminate confusion and compensate for the inadequacies of previous systems of isolation precautions. However, it is important for HCWs to remember that isolation precautions can protect only if they are used consistently and appropriately.

References

1. Garner JS, Simmons BP: *CDC guideline for isolation precautions in hospitals,* 1983, U.S. Department of Health and Human Services.
2. Garner JS, Hierholzer WJ: Controversies in isolation policies and practices. In Wenzel RP, editor: *Prevention and control of nosocomial infections,* ed 2, Baltimore, 1993, Williams & Wilkins.
3. Lynch P et al: Rethinking the role of isolation precautions in the prevention of nosocomial infections, *Ann Intern Med* 107:243, 1987.
4. Jackson MM, Lynch P: An attempt to make an issue less murky: a comparison of four systems for infection precautions, *Infect Control Hosp Epidemiol* 12(7):448, 1991.
5. Centers for Disease Control and Prevention: Draft guidelines for isolation precautions in hospitals, *Fed Reg* 59(214):55552, 1994.
6. Korniewicz D: Effectiveness of glove barriers used in clinical settings, *Medsurg Nurs* 1(1):29, 1992.
7. Centers for Disease Control: Update: universal precautions for prevention of transmission of human immunodeficiency virus, hepatitis b virus, and other bloodborne pathogens in health care settings, *MMWR* 37(24):377, 1988.
8. American Hospital Association: *Infection control in hospitals,* ed 5, Chicago, 1991, American Hospital Association.

Preventing and Managing Infections in Health Care Workers

8

In 1991 and 1994 the Occupational Safety and Health Administration (OSHA) mandated health care worker (HCW) disease protection using Centers for Disease Control and Prevention (CDC) guidelines. This chapter describes these requirements for protection against bloodborne diseases and tuberculosis and also addresses the management of other infectious disease risks for HCWs.

The prevention of HCW infection (and possible subsequent patient infection) in all health care settings requires that HCWs use appropriate infection control and isolation practices. Published standards explicate both required (OSHA) and recommended (CDC) infection control standards.

OSHA requires that HCWs be skin tested routinely for tuberculosis and have access to engineering controls, work practice controls, and hepatitis B virus (HBV) immunization. OSHA also requires that HCWs who are exposed to blood or body fluids be assessed for bloodborne infection, receive medical intervention as indicated, and receive counseling about the possible implications of their exposure.

The CDC recommends that HCWs be immunized for common vaccine-preventable diseases (in addition to HBV). HCWs with transmissible infections must be identified quickly and be excluded from the workplace or from direct patient contact until they are no longer infectious.

Work Practice Controls

Work practice controls are policies and procedures that employers are required to document, implement, and enforce. It is the employer's responsibility to provide and to enforce the controls; however, it is the HCW's responsibility to practice and use the controls. The purpose of work practice controls is to protect employees from exposure to infections and diseases. Work practice controls must address such issues as hand washing, decontamination, disinfection and sterilization, environmental cleaning schedules, sharps handling, biomedical waste disposal, the use of engineering controls, and the use of appropriate personal protective equipment (PPE). At a minimum PPE includes vinyl or latex gloves, gowns, and protective eye and face wear. (See Chapter 7.)

Engineering Controls

Careful application of universal precautions as mandated by the OSHA Bloodborne Pathogens Act (1991) minimizes blood and body fluid exposure from splashes and aerosols, but these precautions—such as handwashing and wearing gloves and goggles—do not prevent needlesticks.[1] The use of engineering controls such as conveniently placed nonpenetrable needle disposal containers and work practice controls such as prohibition of needle recapping and manual handling of needles have brought about a reduction in needlestick injuries but have not eliminated them.[2,3] The significance of the problem is demonstrated by the 39 occupational human immunodeficiency virus (HIV) seroconversions documented by the CDC.[4]

Needles are necessary devices for penetrating a patient's skin (examples are those used in starting intravenous (IV) infusions or giving direct injections). However, devices have been developed to eliminate exposed needles when skin penetration is not required (e.g., needleless IV connectors). Other devices make it possible to protect HCWs' hands from necessary needles (e.g., devices with self-sheathing or retractable needles and devices with needles that are recessed behind protective covers).

Reports now document the efficacy of these devices in reducing needlesticks without compromising patient safety.[5] Some even document cost savings when the cost of postexposure follow up is factored in.[6,7] These devices are safer for the HCW who uses them initially, and they reduce injury to housekeepers and other persons who handle the medical trash. However, some health care organizations are slow to adopt these devices, citing such factors as significantly increased costs (approximately 3 to 4 times the cost of standard devices) and questionable efficacy.

In the bloodborne pathogens standard, OSHA emphasizes engineering and work practice controls as the first line of defense against contaminated sharps injuries and states that "personal protective equipment shall be used when occupational exposure remains after institution of these controls." [8] OSHA also refers specifically to resheathing or retracting syringe devices, estimating that use of these devices could reduce needlesticks by more than 50%. The Food and Drug Administration (FDA) took OSHA standards a step further when it issued an FDA safety alert in April 1992. This alert states that because IV tubing–needle assemblies have a higher risk of needlestick injury than any other needled devices, "the use of exposed needles on IV administration sets or the use of needled syringes to access IV administration ports or injection sites are unnecessary and should be avoided." [9]

Despite the apparent intent of OSHA and the FDA to encourage the use of safety-engineered devices to prevent needlestick injuries in health care settings, risk managers, health and safety committees, and HCWs still need to learn about these devices, and ongoing evaluation of device efficacy is necessary.

Health Care Worker Immunity: Vaccine Use and Tuberculosis Testing

In 1987 and 1989 the CDC issued immunization recommendations for HCWs.[10,11] These recommendations encourage health care facilities to develop comprehensive policies for HCW immunization against influenza; HBV; measles, mumps, and rubella (the measles-mumps-rubella [MMR] vaccine); and poliomyelitis. Although the CDC does not specifically recommend the tetanus/diphtheria vaccine for HCWs, it is generally recommended for general health maintenance. In 1991 OSHA strengthened the CDC recommendations by requiring that employers offer HBV vaccine within 10 days of employment at no charge to HCWs who have occupational exposure to blood or other potentially infected material.[8]

Administrative Requirements for Vaccine Administration

Health care providers who administer HBV vaccines, diphtheria/ tetanus vaccines, polio vaccines, and MMR vaccines (or their components) are required to record and maintain a permanent record of the provider's name, address, type of vaccine, manufacturer's lot number, and date of administration. This record keeping is also advised for all other vaccines. Since 1988 the National Vaccine Inquiry Compensation Program has required that adverse vaccine reactions be reported to the U.S. Department of Health and Human Services. Adults who are given vaccines must be advised about the benefits and risks of vaccination and should have the opportunity to ask questions. The CDC has developed information statements related to vaccines, which may be used to educate vaccine recipients.

Tips for Vaccine Use

Indications, side effects, tips for administration, and contraindications to vaccine use are listed in Table 8-1. In general, inactivated vaccines may be given simultaneously at different sites with no decrease in antibody response and no increase in side effects.[12] Most inactivated and live vaccines may also be administered together, but live vaccines must be given either together or separated by at least 4 weeks because the antibody response to the second live virus vaccine might be reduced if given earlier. Live virus vaccines can also interfere with tuberculin test results unless the tuberculin test is administered simultaneously or 4 to 6 weeks later.[12]

Immune globulin does not interfere with inactivated vaccines, but it will interfere with live virus replication and should be given either two weeks after live virus vaccine or 6 weeks to 3 months before live virus vaccine.[12] HCWs who are immunosuppressed as a result of disease or therapy should not receive live virus vaccines.

Tuberculin Testing

HCW exposure to active tuberculosis (TB) is a growing problem in health care facilities, with 1% to 2% of HCWs converting to

Table 8-1 Adult health care worker preventive vaccine recommendations

Vaccine	Indication	Use/Dose	Side Effects	Contraindications
Tetanus/Diphtheria toxoid	Recommended every 10 years after primary series as routine adult health care (not critical as condition of employment)	Use Td ≥ age 7 /0.5 ml IM	Local/minor	Anaphylactic or neurologic reaction to previous dose
Polio (IPV & E-IPV) (inactivated vaccines)	Adults who have not completed primary series	OPV (Live vaccine) should not be used in adults, or in children if a household member is immunosuppressed/unit dose	Poliomyelitis in patients and contacts possible with OPV	Avoid in pregnancy

Influenza	Workers who care for persons with chronic illness or those ≥ 65, and workers who have chronic illness (chronic obstructive pulmonary disease, cardiac disease)	Administer annually prior to flu season (between mid-October and mid-November)/ 0.5 ml IM	Primarily local/minor	Hypersensitivity to eggs, defer until 2nd trimester of pregnancy if possible
Hepatitis B	Must be provided for all HCWs with potential exposure to blood or serum-based body fluids	3 doses at 0, 1, and 6 months; must be given in deltoid. Routine boosters not recommended/ 1.0 ml IM	Local/minor	Hypersensitivity to yeasts

Continued.

Modified from Fedson DE, Immunizations for health-care workers and patients in hospitals. In Wenzel RP, editor: *Prevention and control of nosocomial infections*, ed 2, Baltimore, 1993, Williams & Wilkins.

Td, tetanus diptheria; *IM*, intramuscular; *OPV*, oral polio virus; *HCW*, health care worker; *subQ*, subcutaneous.

Table 8-1 Adult health care worker preventive vaccine recommendations—cont'd

Vaccine	Indication	Use/Dose	Side Effects	Contraindications
Measles/mumps/rubella	All HCWs entering employment in medical facilities unless two doses of active vaccine or immune by titer*	/0.5 ml subQ	Local/minor	Hypersensitivity to eggs or neomycin, immunocompromise, pregnancy or within 3 months of conception

*Physician documented history of measles acceptable as evidence of immunity in those born before 1957. (Modified from Krause PJ et al: Quality standard for assurance of measles immunity among health care workers. *Infect Control Hosp Epidemiol*, 15(3):193, 1994.)

positive purified protein derivative (PPD) skin tests each year.[13] Increasing numbers of active TB cases with multiple antibiotic resistance highlight the ongoing threat of this infection to HCWs and have prompted the CDC and OSHA to take a new look at guidelines for transmission prevention. (See Chapter 2.)

Initial Employee Screening and Testing

The 1994 CDC Tuberculosis Guidelines recommend that all new employees undergo two-step testing with five tuberculin units of PPD injected just under the surface of the skin of the volar or ventral surface of the arm. (New employees with documentation of a negative PPD within the past year are not required to undergo boosted testing.[14]) PPD tests should be read by designated, trained personnel (not by the employee) between 48 and 72 hours after injection. The second PPD test should be given 3 weeks later to look for a possible boosted reaction.[15] Persons with known HIV infection should be tested for anergy with *Candida* antigen and tetanus toxoid when they have their PPD test.[14]

Interval PPD Screening

The CDC guidelines recommend that the frequency of skin testing for ongoing employees be based on the most recent TB risk assessment conducted for the facility, specific unit, or occupational group of the facility. This protocol is summarized in Table 8-2.

PPD Follow Up

A positive PPD indicates infection, not active disease, which explains why further medical screening is necessary. Persons with a positive PPD without further signs of active disease need not be excluded from work. Interpretation of PPD skin tests is presented in the box on pp. 126-127.

Persons with newly positive tuberculin tests or conversions within 2 years should be evaluated with a chest x-ray scan, history, and physical examination to rule out active disease. If the chest x-ray scan is negative, preventive therapy with isoniazid (INH) may be offered to prevent a latent infection from progressing to active TB. The decision to offer INH is based on many factors, including age, preexisting medical conditions, and household contacts with active TB. The usual preventive therapy of oral INH is 300 mg daily for 6 to 12 months (12 months for persons with HIV infection or

Table 8-2 CDC standard for frequency of tuberculosis risk assessment and repeat skin testing

Very Low Risk (Variable PPD and Risk Assessments) †	Low Risk (Annual PPD and Risk Assessments)	Intermediate Risk (PPDs and Risk Assessments every 6 Months)	High Risk (PPD and Risk Assessments every 3 Months)
PPD test conversion rate is not higher than areas without occupational exposure to TB patients or not higher than previous rates	PPD test conversion rate is not higher than areas without occupational exposure to TB patients or not higher than previous rates	PPD test conversion rate is not higher than areas without occupational exposure to TB patients or not higher than previous rates	PPD test conversion rate *is* significantly higher than areas without occupational exposure to TB patients or than previous rates *or*
No evidence of patient-to-patient transmission	No clusters of PPD test conversions	No clusters of PPD test conversions	There *is* a cluster of PPD test conversions *or*
	No evidence of patient-to-patient transmission	No evidence of patient-to-patient transmission	There is evidence of patient-to-patient transmission

No TB patients admitted as inpatients to facility during preceding year and plan to refer confirmed TB patients for inpatient care	< 6 TB patients hospitalized/year‡	≥ 6 TB patients hospitalized/year‡

From Centers for Disease Control: Guidelines for preventing the transmission of tuberculosis in health-care facilities, 1994, *Federal Register* 59(208):54242, 1994.

PPD, purified protein derivative; *TB,* tuberculosis.

*Risk assessment includes analysis of employee PPD conversion data, number of TB cases, presence of clusters, evidence of patient-to-patient transmission, and evaluation of ventilation system. Negative pressure of isolation rooms should be evaluated daily for all risk levels.

†This category generally applies only to an entire facility. Health care workers who are involved in the initial assessment and diagnostic evaluation of patients in ambulatory care, emergency, and admitting departments may need routine PPD screening and may need to be involved in a respiratory protection program.

‡Refers to an area or unit.

Note: Facilities determined to be at *minimal risk* (no TB patients in community or facility during previous year) do not need to maintain an ongoing PPD skin-testing program. However, baseline PPD testing may be advisable so that if exposure occurs, conversions can be identified.

Summary of Interpretation of Tuberculosis Skin Test

A. A reaction of ≥ 5 mm is classified as positive in the following persons:
   1. Persons with HIV infection or risk factors for HIV infection with unknown HIV status
   2. Persons who have had recent close contact with persons with active TB*
   3. Persons who have fibrotic chest radiographs consistent with old healed TB
B. A reaction of ≥ 10 mm is classified as positive in all persons who do not meet any of the preceding criteria but who have other risk factors for TB, including the following:
   1. High risk groups
      a. Intravenous drug users known to be HIV seronegative
      b. Persons with other medical conditions reported to increase the risk of progressing from latent TB infection to active TB, including silicosis, gastrectomy, jejunoileal bypass surgery, being 10% or more below ideal body weight, chronic renal failure, diabetes, high-dose corticosteroid and other immunosuppressive therapy, some hematologic disorders (e.g., leukemia) and other malignancies
   2. High prevalence groups
      a. Foreign-born persons from high prevalence countries in Asia, Africa, the Caribbean, and Latin America
      b. Persons from medically underserved, low income populations
      c. Residents of long-term care facilities (prisons, nursing homes)
      d. Persons from high risk populations in their communities as determined by local public health authorities

From Centers for Disease Control: Guidelines for preventing the transmission of tuberculosis in health-care facilities, 1994, *Federal Register* 59(208):54242, 1994. *HIV*, human immunodeficiency virus; *TB*, tuberculosis.
*Recent close contact implies household contact or unprotected occupational exposure similar in intensity and duration to household contact.

Summary of Interpretation of Tuberculosis Skin Test—cont'd

C. Induration of ≥ 15 mm is classified as positive for persons who do not meet any of the above criteria.

D. Recent converters are defined on the basis of both induration and age.

1. ≥ 10 mm increase within a 2-year period is classified as positive for persons < 35 years

2. ≥ 15 mm increase within a 2-year period is classified as positive for persons ≥ 35 years

3. ≥ 5 mm increases under certain circumstances (see A, p. 126)

---

chest x-ray scans showing old healed TB).[15] The addition of Pyridoxine 100 mg daily with INH prevents peripheral neuritis.[15]

Because fatal hepatitis has occasionally been reported as a consequence of INH, persons taking this drug are monitored monthly for symptoms of hepatitis. Because INH-associated hepatitis occurs more frequently in persons older than 35, a transaminase measurement should be obtained from persons in this age group before initiation of therapy and then monthly until treatment is completed. Persons with daily alcohol use or chronic liver disease or persons who inject drugs also have an increased risk of hepatitis associated with INH and should have more frequent clinical and laboratory monitoring.[14] Persons with positive PPD conversions and negative chest x-ray scans do not need additional screening (interval PPDs or chest x-ray scans) unless they become symptomatic.[14]

Employee Work Exclusions

It is often difficult to determine when HCWs with common health conditions should be at work and when they should be excluded. Work restriction guidelines for each institution should always be consulted. Table 8-3 offers guidelines.

Text continued on p. 132.

Table 8-3 Work exclusions for health care workers

Health Condition	Mode of Transmission*/ Incubation Period	Work Exclusion?	Work Return-Restrictions/Notes
Chickenpox (varicella-zoster)	Direct contact, droplet contact, airborne/2-3 weeks	Yes	Until lesions are crusted/Isolate nonimmune, exposed workers from patient care from days 10-21 after exposure
Conjunctivitis (acute, bacterial)	Direct contact/24-72 hours	No	/No direct patient contact until discharge gone
Diarrhea	Direct contact with feces	Yes	When symptoms resolve and salmonella ruled out (see Chapter 7)
Draining wounds/lesions	Direct contact	Yes	When no longer draining
Hepatitis A	Direct and indirect contact with feces and contaminated food/15-50 days	Yes	7 days after onset of jaundice
Hepatitis B	Direct and indirect contact with semen or blood, perinatal/45-180 days	No	/Use universal precautions. Institutional policy may prohibit invasive procedures

Herpes zoster/shingles	Direct contact with lesions, vesicle fluid may be airborne/2-3 weeks	No	/Lesions must be covered; should not care for nonimmune or immunosuppressed patients
Human immunodeficiency virus	Direct and indirect contact with semen or blood/2 months-10 years	No	/Use universal precautions. Institutional policy may prohibit invasive procedures
Herpes simplex (type 1)	Direct contact with saliva/2-12 days	No	/Should not care for newborns, children with eczema or burns, or immunosuppressed patients
Influenza	Direct, droplet, airborne/1-5 days	Yes	3-5 days from onset of symptoms
Lice/scabies	Direct contact/2-6 weeks	Yes	Until treated

Epidemiologic data from Benenson AS, editor: Control of communicable diseases in man, ed 15, Washington, DC, 1990, American Public Health Association.

*For further discussion and definitions of modes of transmission see Chapter 5.

Continued.

Table 8-3 Work exclusions for health care workers—cont'd

Health Condition	Mode of Transmission*/ Incubation Period	Work Exclusion?	Work Return-Restrictions/Notes
Measles (rubeola)	Airborne and droplet contact/ 1-3 weeks	Yes	From 5-21 days after exposure or until 7 days after rash appears
Mononucleosis	Saliva and blood/4-6 weeks	Yes	Varies by individual; health provider assessment needed
Mumps	Direct contact with saliva and respiratory secretions, droplet contact/12-25 days	Yes	From 12-26 days after exposure or until 9 days after onset of parotitis
Pertussis	Direct contact with saliva and respiratory secretions, droplet contact/1-2 weeks	Yes	Until 7 days of effective therapy given
Rubella	Direct, droplet, airborne/ 16-18 days	Yes	At least 4 days after rash onset

Staphylococcus aureus (skin lesions)	Direct contact	Yes	Until lesions are resolved
Streptococcal throat (group A, beta-hemolytic)	Direct contact, rarely indirect/1-3 days	Yes	After 24-48 hours of antibiotics use
Tuberculosis (active)	Droplet contact and airborne/4-12 weeks	Yes	When three consecutive sputum smears are negative along with clinical response to treatment†

†Henderson DK: HIV-1 In the health care setting. In Mandell GL, Douglas RG Jr, Bennett JE, editors: Principles and practice of infectious diseases, ed 4, New York, 1995, Churchill Livingstone.

Managing Significant Health Care Worker Exposures

Although the numbers of occupational exposures can be significantly reduced through the use of universal precautions, work practice controls, and engineering controls, the possibility of HCW exposure to bloodborne pathogens cannot be completely eliminated as long as bleeding patients are treated and needles and sharp instruments are used in the delivery of care. Infection with bloodborne pathogens has been documented as a result of both percutaneous (needle stick/cut) and mucocutaneous (splash/aerosol) exposures.

First Aid

Immediately after exposure, the site should be vigorously scrubbed with a disinfectant solution such as 10% povidone iodine. Contaminated mucous membranes should be irrigated for 10 minutes with normal saline or running tap water. Although these first aid measures have not been documented to decrease risk of infection, they may help to remove HIV cells from the site.[16] Immediately after receiving first aid, the exposed HCW should report the exposure to the appropriate supervisor or to an occupational medicine service. Reporting should not wait until the next shift or next day; if antiretroviral chemoprophylaxis (zidovudine) is indicated for HIV exposure, it should be initiated within 1 to 2 hours.[17]

Postexposure Follow Up

According to the OSHA (1991) regulations, employers must arrange postexposure medical evaluation and follow up at no charge to employees. The medical evaluation must contain the following elements: documentation of the exposure route and circumstances surrounding the exposure, testing and documentation of the source individual in accordance with state laws, disclosure to the HCW of the source individual's testing results following applicable confidentiality laws, and follow up of the exposed HCW according to current recommendations of the U.S. Public Health Service (USPHS).[8] Figure 8-1 shows a diagram for percutaneous exposure follow up that may also be used for mucocutaneous exposures.[18] Although the USPHS does not currently recommend follow up for exposed HCWs beyond 6

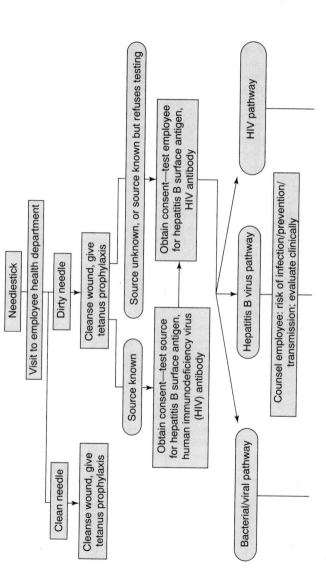

Continued

Figure 8-1.
Percutaneous exposure follow up. Adapted from Critikon, 1991.

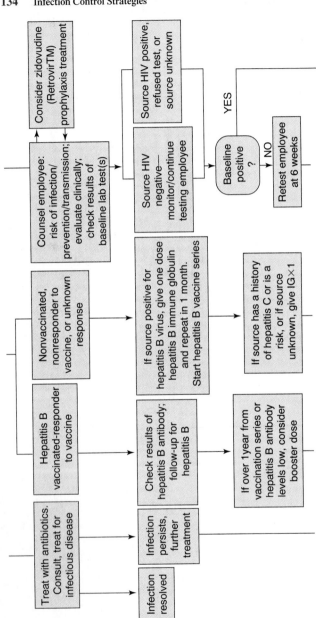

Counsel employee: risk of infection/prevention/transmission; evaluate clinically; check results of baseline lab test(s)

Consider zidovudine (Retrovir™) prophylaxis treatment

Source HIV positive, refused test, or source unknown

Source HIV negative—monitor/continue testing employee

Baseline positive ?

YES

NO → Retest employee at 6 weeks

Nonvaccinated, nonresponder to vaccine, or unknown response

If source positive for hepatitis B virus, give one dose hepatitis B immune globulin and repeat in 1 month. Start hepatitis B vaccine series

If source has a history of hepatitis C or is a risk, or if source unknown, give IG×1

Hepatitis B vaccinated-responder to vaccine

Check results of hepatitis B antibody, follow-up for hepatitis B

If over 1 year from vaccination series or hepatitis B antibody levels low, consider booster dose

Treat with antibiotics. Consult, treat for infectious disease

Infection persists, further treatment

Infection resolved

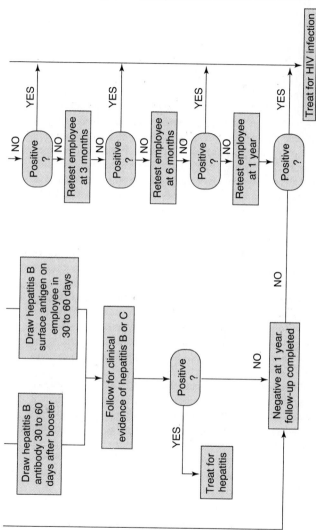

Figure 8-1, cont'd.
Percutaneous exposure follow up. Adapted from Critikon, 1991.

months, 1-year follow up serologies may be considered because of the possibility of delayed seroconversions in a high-risk exposure situation.[16]

HCW follow up should include baseline serological testing for HIV and HBV if the HCW consents. The HCW may choose to have the baseline test blood held for up to 90 days to make an informed decision about HIV testing.[8] Serological testing for hepatitis C may also be included in baseline evaluation. The health care provider who conducts the HCW evaluation must submit a written opinion to the employer documenting only that the HCW has been informed of the medical evaluation results and if HBV vaccine was indicated and was given.[8] The employer may not be informed of serological testing results or of any other findings related to the HCW evaluation.[8]

Counseling

Although prospective studies demonstrate a low rate (0.2%) of HIV infection per percutaneous exposure, the possibility of contracting this fatal infection as a consequence of an exposure can be a great stressor to an HCW.[19] Ongoing confidential contact with a counselor and an opportunity to ask questions and discuss concerns during the follow-up period is important. Exposed HCWs should be encouraged not to discuss their exposure with coworkers; in the event of infection the HCWs may not want their seropositive status known.

HIV/HBV counseling should include the sensitive issue of sexual practices, including the possible use of barrier precautions during sexual relations in the follow up period to protect partners against infection should HIV seroconversion or HBV infection occur. Exposed HCWs should also be counseled to recognize and report symptoms that may represent acute HBV or HIV infection such as fever, upper respiratory infection, malaise, lymphadenopathy, gastrointestinal symptoms, and rash.[16]

Zidovudine Treatment

Postexposure antiretroviral chemoprophylaxis with zidovudine may be offered to HCWs who experience percutaneous or mucocutaneous occupational exposure to documented HIV-positive sources. If the source individual is suspected of having HIV, zidovudine may be offered until serological results are available.

Because data from animal and human studies are inadequate to establish the efficacy or safety of this drug for postexposure prophylaxis, providers cannot make recommendations for or against the use of the zidovudine. HCWs considering the drug must be counseled regarding the rationale for prophylaxis, the risk of HIV from the exposure, the limits of knowledge related to efficacy of the drug for postexposure use, the known toxicity of the drug, and the need for serological follow up regardless of whether the drug is taken.[17]

Although there is little documentation of the efficacy of one dosage schedule over another, the common routine is 200 mg of zidovudine every 4 hours for 4 to 6 weeks.[17] Some institutions omit the 4 A.M. dose.[17] The most common side effects of zidovudine are gastrointestinal, such as nausea, vomiting, and diarrhea. HCWs electing zidovudine treatment should have hematologic parameters (including white cell differentials) and blood chemistry studies evaluated at baseline, at 2-week intervals during treatment, and at 2 weeks following treatment.[16]

Summary

The prevention of infection in HCWs requires careful adherence to OSHA requirements for work practice controls, engineering controls, tuberculosis testing, and HBV vaccine and attention to CDC recommendations for other routine immunizations and isolation techniques. HCWs who demonstrate symptoms of communicable illness must adhere to work restriction guidelines as communicated by their facilities. Finally, HCWs must report exposures to blood or bloody body fluids to initiate OSHA-mandated follow up and treatment.

References

1. American Nurses Association: Needlesticks put RNs at risk, *Am Nurse* December: 2, 1990.
2. Krasinski K, LaCouture R, Holzman RS: Effect of changing needle disposal systems on needle puncture injuries, *Infect Control* 8(2):59, 1987.
3. Makofsky D: Installing needle disposal boxes close to the bedside reduced needle-recapping rates in hospital units, *Infect Control Hosp Epidemiol* 14(3):140, 1993.

4. Martin LS: A model for biosafety level 2: HBV/HIV. Paper presented at Third National Symposium on Biosafety, Atlanta, March, 1994.
5. Younger B et al: Impact of a shielded safety syringe on needlestick injuries among health-care workers. *Infect Control Hosp Epidemiol* 13(6):349, 1992.
6. Gartner K: Impact of a needleless intravenous system in a university hospital, *Am J Infect Control* 20(2):75, 1992.
7. Rutowski J, Peterson SL: A needleless intravenous system: an effective risk management strategy, *Infect Control Hosp Epidemiol* 14(4):226, 1993.
8. Department of Labor/OSHA. Occupational exposure to bloodborne pathogens: final rule, *Federal Register* 56(235):64004, 1991.
9. U.S. Food and Drug Administration: FDA safety alert: needlestick and other risks from hypodermic needles on secondary IV administration sets—piggyback and intermittent IVs, April, 1992.
10. Centers for Disease Control: *Immunization recommendations for health-care workers*, Atlanta, 1987, U.S. Department of Health and Human Services, Public Health Service.
11. Centers for Disease Control: General recommendations on immunization: recommendations of the Immunization Practices Advisory Committee (ACIP), *MMWR* 38:205, 1989.
12. Fedson DE: Immunizations for health-care workers and patients in hospitals. In Wenzel RP, editor: *Prevention and control of nosocomial infections*, ed 2, Baltimore, 1993, Williams & Wilkins.
13. Sherertz RJ, Marosok RD, Streed SA: Infection control aspects of hospital employee health. In Wenzel RP, editor: *Prevention and control of nosocomial infections,* ed 2, Baltimore, 1993, Williams & Wilkins.
14. Centers for Disease Control: Guidelines for preventing the transmission of tuberculosis in health-care facilities, 1994, *Federal Register* 59(208):54242, 1994.
15. Tierney LM, McPhee SJ, Papadakis, MA: *Current medical diagnosis and treatment*, East Norwalk, Conn, 1994, Appleton & Lange.
16. Fahey BJ et al: Managing occupational exposures to HIV-1 in the healthcare workplace, *Infect Control Hosp Epidemiol* 14(7):405, 1993.
17. Centers for Disease Control: Public health service statement on management of occupational exposure to human immunodeficiency virus, including considerations regarding zidovudine use, *MMWR* 39(RR-1):1, 1990.
18. Critikon, Inc.: *Clinical implication and financial impact of needlesticks*, Conn, 1991, Critikon.
19. Henderson DK: HIV-1 in the health care setting. In Mandell GL, Douglas RG Jr, Bennett JE, editors: *Principles and practice of infectious diseases*, ed 4, New York, 1995, Churchill Livingstone.

Cleaning, Disinfecting, and Sterilizing

9

Medical and surgical devices may serve as vehicles for the transmission of infectious agents to susceptible hosts. Nearly 150 years ago, Louis Pasteur proved the germ theory of disease transmission. Joseph Lister put this theory to practical use with his use of carbolic acid (phenol) as a means of preventing surgical wound infection. Lister's early attempts at antisepsis marked the beginning of efforts to control microorganisms in the health care environment. Now, our knowledge and experience involving microbial inactivation using disinfection or sterilization processes is sophisticated. These major advances in patient safety are in large measure a result of the ever-increasing understanding of the microbial environment.[1]

Hospital, ambulatory care, and home health agencies establish policies identifying the appropriate methods for cleaning and disposal of patient care equipment. Cleaning, disinfection, and sterilization procedures are based on the intended use of the items. Appropriate care and disposal of instruments and equipment is vital to prevent the transmission of nosocomial infection to patients and to health care providers.

Definitions

It is important to have a clear understanding of the terms and classifications used in this process to choose the most appropriate procedure for the item or surface in question.

Cleaning removes all visible foreign material (dust, soil) on objects, environmental surfaces, and skin using soap, water, and friction. *Decontamination* (similar to cleaning) removes most pathogenic, or disease-producing microorganisms and foreign matter from an object, rendering it safe for handling. There are five purposes for decontamination procedures:[1,2]

1. To prevent the spread of infection via patient equipment or environmental surfaces
2. To remove visible soil
3. To remove invisible soil (microorganisms and film)
4. To prepare all surfaces for direct contact with sterilants or disinfectants
5. To protect personnel and patients

All instruments or patient care objects must be decontaminated using soap, water, and friction before they are subjected to disinfection or sterilization methods.

Disinfection destroys or kills most of the pathogenic organisms on an object or instrument, except bacterial spores, by using liquid chemical compounds or wet pasteurization. The outcome of the disinfection process is affected by several factors:

1. Organic load (bioburden) present on the object
2. Type and level of microbial contamination
3. Prior cleaning/decontamination of the object
4. Disinfectant concentration and exposure time
5. Physical structure of the object
6. Temperature and pH of the disinfection process[1,3]

There are three levels of disinfection: high, intermediate, and low. *High-level disinfection* kills all microorganisms with the exception of bacterial spores. *Intermediate-level disinfection* kills bacteria, most viruses, and most fungi but not bacterial spores. *Low-level disinfection* kills most bacteria, some viruses, and some fungi but cannot be relied on to kill resistant microorganisms such as tubercle bacilli or bacterial spores.[3-5]

Germicides are chemical compounds that kill microorganisms on both living tissue and inanimate objects. *Antiseptics* kill organisms on skin and living tissue. *Disinfectants* are used on inanimate objects only, not on living tissue. Not all disinfectants function alike, so they are classified according to their level of kill: low, intermediate, or high. The choice of disinfectant depends on the category of instrument use (noncritical, semicritical, critical), length of the exposure or procedure, type of object, and the method needed to achieve the correct level of disinfection or sterilization. Table 9-1 uses the instrument categories and levels of disinfection to recommend the appropriate method of disinfection or sterilization.[3] Many types of disinfectants are available for use in health care settings: alcohol; chlorine and chlorine compounds; formaldehyde and glutaraldehyde; hydrogen peroxide; iodophors; peracetic acid; phenolics; quaternary ammonia; and combinations of these types. Table 9-2 depicts the characteristics of each disinfectant solution. Information from both tables may be used to choose the most appropriate disinfectant for the work needed and the setting. Users of chemical disinfectants must be aware of the correct way to use the chemical to protect themselves from injury. Personal protective equipment (PPE) is required for preventing both exposure to disease (from the cleaning procedure) and for exposure to chemical injury. Proper ventilation may be required for the disinfectant as well.[1,3]

Sterilization completely eradicates all microorganisms, including bacterial spores, on an object that has been properly decontaminated. This is an absolute state and is accomplished by physical or chemical means: pressurized steam, dry heat, ethylene oxide gas, or chemicals. Chemical disinfectants are classified as chemical sterilants if they can kill bacterial spores. This normally requires a prolonged exposure time from 6 to 10 hours. Sterilization may occur in outpatient clinics, mobile clinics, surgical areas, or respiratory therapy areas. It is vital that sterilization procedures outside of a central processing department promote the same level of safety and efficiency. Requirements include routine biological, mechanical, and chemical monitoring to ensure that all parameters of sterilization are met before using the instrument on or in a patient. The type of item to be sterilized affects the method used. For example, pressurized steam sterilizes surgical instruments, and ethylene oxide gas (ETO) sterilizes rubber and plastic items.[1,4,5]

Medical devices, equipment, and surgical materials may be classified into three categories based on the potential risk of infection involved in their use: noncritical, semicritical, or critical.

1. *Noncritical* items come in contact with intact skin but not with mucous membranes. They rarely, if ever, transmit disease and can be cleaned with a detergent and a low level disinfectant solution. Refer to Table 9-2 for the levels of disinfectants. The following are examples of noncritical objects.

   a. Bedpans, commodes, urinals
   b. Blood pressure cuffs, percussion hammers, bandage scissors

Text continued on p. 148.

Table 9-1   Methods of sterilization and disinfection[a]

Object	Sterilization Critical Items (Will Enter Tissue or Vascular System, or Blood Will Flow Through Them) Procedure	Exposure Time (hr)	Disinfection High Level: Semicritical Items (Will Come in Contact with Mucous Membrane or Nonintact Skin) Procedure (Exposure Time ≥ 20 min)[b,c]	Intermediate Level: Some Semicritical Items[a] and Noncritical Items Procedure (Exposure Time ≤ 10 min)	Low Level: Noncritical Items (Will Come in Contact with Intact Skin) Procedure (Exposure Time ≤ 10 min)
Smooth, hard surface[d]	A[e]	MR	C	I	I
	B	MR	D	K	J
	C	MR	E	L	K
	D	6	F		L
	E	6	G[f]		M
	F	MR	H		
Rubber tubing and catheters[c]	A	MR	C		
	B	MR	D		
	C	MR	E		
	D	6	F		
	E	6	G[d]		
	F	MR			

From Rutala W: Disinfection, sterilization and waste disposal. In Wenzel R, editor: *Prevention and control of nosocomial infections*, Baltimore, 1993, Williams & Wilkins.

[a]Modified from Simmons BP: CDC guidelines for the prevention and control of nosocomial infections: guidelines for hospital environmental control, *Am J Infect Control*, June 11(3):97-120, 1983.

[b]The longer the exposure to a disinfectant, the more likely it is that all microorganisms will be eliminated. A 10-minute exposure is not adequate to disinfect many objects, especially those that are difficult to clean because they have narrow channels or other areas that can harbor organic material and bacteria. A 20-minute exposure is the minimal time needed to reliably kill *M. tuberculosis* and nontuberculous mycobacteria with glutaraldehyde.

[c]Tubing must be completely filled for disinfection; care must be taken to avoid entrapment of air bubbles during immersion.

[d]Mayhall CG: Surgical infections including burns. In Wenzel RP, editor: *Prevention and control of nosocomial infections*, Baltimore, 1993, Williams & Wilkins.

[e]   A. Heat sterilization, including steam or hot air (see manufacturer's recommendations).

    B. Ethylene oxide gas (see manufacturer's recommendations).

    C. Glutaraldehyde-based formulations (2%). (Caution should be exercised with all glutaraldehyde formulations when further in-use dilution is anticipated.)

    D. Demand-release chlorine dioxide (will corrode aluminum, copper, brass, series 400 stainless steel and chrome with prolonged exposure).

    E. Stabilized hydrogen peroxide 6% (will corrode copper, zinc, and brass).

    F. Peracetic acid, concentration variable, but ≤1% is sporicidal.

    G. Wet pasteurization at 75°C for 30 minutes after detergent cleaning.

    H. Sodium hypochlorite (1000 ppm available chlorine; will corrode metal instruments).

    I. Ethyl or isopropyl alcohol (70%-90%).

    J. Sodium hypochlorite (100 ppm available chlorine).

    K. Phenolic germicidal detergent solution (follow product label for use-dilution)

    L. Iodophor germicidal detergent solution (follow product label for use-dilution).

    M. Quaternary ammonium germicidal detergent solution (follow product label for use-dilution).

    MR. Manufacturer's recommendations.

[f]Pasteurization (washer disinfector) of respiratory therapy and anesthesia equipment is a recognized alternative to high level disinfection. Some data challenge the efficacy of some pasteurization units.

Continued.

Table 9-1 Methods of sterilization and disinfection—cont'd

	Sterilization		Disinfection		
	Critical Items (Will Enter Tissue or Vascular System, or Blood Will Flow Through Them)		High Level: Semicritical Items (Will Come in Contact with Mucous Membrane or Nonintact Skin)	Intermediate Level: Some Semicritical Items[a] and Noncritical Items	Low Level: Noncritical Items (Will Come in Contact with Intact Skin)
Object	Procedure	Exposure Time (hr)	Procedure (Exposure Time ≥ 20 min)[b,c]	Procedure (Exposure Time ≤ 10 min)	Procedure (Exposure Time ≤ 10 min)
Polyethylene tubing and catheters[c,g]	A	MR	C		
	B	MR	D		
	C	MR	E		
	D	6	F		
	E	6	G[f]		
	F	MR			

Lensed instruments	B	MR	C
	C	MR	D
	D	6	E
	E	6	F
	F	MR	
Thermometers (oral and rectal)[h]			I[h]
Hinged instruments	A	MR	C
	B	MR	D
	C	MR	E
	D	6	F
	E	6	
	F	MR	

[g]Thermostability should be investigated when appropriate.
[h]Do not mix rectal and oral thermometers at any stage of handling or processing.

Table 9-2 Some common disinfectants with their use dilutions, properties, and cost

Germicide	Use Dilution	Level of Disinfection*	Inactivates†,‡						Important Characteristics									Approximate Cost (in dollars)	
			Bacteria	Lipophilic Viruses	Hydrophilic Viruses	M. tuberculosis	Mycotic Agents	Bacterial Spores	Shelf Life < 1 Week	Corrosive/Deleterious Effects	Residue	Inactivated by Organic Matter	Skin Irritant	Eye Irritant	Respiratory Irritant	Toxic	Easily Obtainable	Purchase ($)/gal	Cost ($)/gal at Use Dilution
Isopropyl alcohol	60%–95%	Int	+	+	–	+	+	–	+	±	–	+	±	+	–	+	+	3.70 (70%)	3.70 (70%)
Hydrogen peroxide	3%–25%	CS/High	+	+	+	+	+	±	+	–	–	±	+	+	–	+	+	24.50 (6%)	24.50 (6%)
Formaldehyde	3%–8%	High/Int	+	+	+	+	+	±	+	–	+	–	+	+	+	+	+	38.42 (37% wt)	3.84 (3.7% wt)

Quaternary ammonium compounds	0.4%-1.6% aqueous	Low	+	+	−	−	−	±	−	+	−	−	+	+	+	−	+	+	10.77	0.04 (0.4%)
Phenolic	0.4%-5% aqueous	Int/Low	+	+	±	+	±	−	+	−	+	±	+	+	−	+	+	9.70-15.70	0.6(0.4%)-0.08(0.8%)
Chlorine	100-1000 ppm free chlorine	High/Low	+	+	+	+	+	±	+	+	+	+	+	+	+	+	+	1.00 (5.25%)	0.10 (0.5%)
Iodophors	30-50 ppm free iodine	Int	+	+	+	±	±	−	+	±	+	+	+	±	+	+	+	10.10 (10%)	0.05 (0.05%)
Glutaraldehyde	2%	CS/High	+	+	+	+	+	+	+	−	+	+	+	+	+	+	+	6.50-14.00	6.50-14.00

From Rutala W: Disinfection, sterilization and waste disposal. In Wenzel R, editor: *Prevention and control of nosocomial infections*, Baltimore, 1993, Williams & Wilkins. Modified originally from Laboratory Biosafety Manual. World Health Organization, 1983.

*Int, intermediate; CS, chemosterilizer.

†+, yes; −, no; ±, variable results.

‡Inactivates all indicated microorganisms with a contact time of 30 minutes or less except bacterial spores, which require 6 to 10 hours of contact time.

   c. Linens
   d. Work surfaces
   e. Carpets[2,4,6]
2. *Semicritical* items come in contact with mucous membranes
   and require decontamination and either intermediate- or
   high-level disinfection or sterilization (Tables 9-1 and 9-2).
   Examples of semicritical objects follow:
   a. Thermometers
   b. Diaphragm fitting rings
   c. Specula: aural, vaginal, anal, nasal
   d. Tonometers
   e. Endoscopes[2,4,6]
3. *Critical* items enter directly into the bloodstream or into
   other normally sterile areas of the body. Needles, intravenous
   equipment, and urinary catheters are normally disposable
   items sterilized by the manufacturer. Reusable items must be
   decontaminated, then sterilized. Examples of these are as
   follows:
   a. Surgical instruments
   b. Cautery tips, needle electrodes
   c. Biopsy forceps (used with endoscopes)[2,4,6]

Placing instruments and equipment in one of these categories
assists in choosing the proper level of disinfection or sterilization
needed to protect the patient and the provider. It is important to
understand that all reusable items must be cleaned or decontaminated before disinfection or sterilization for the disinfectant or the
sterilant to work properly.

Equipment Decontamination and Disinfection Procedures

Thorough equipment cleaning or decontamination is required to
reduce the bioburden of the object to be disinfected or sterilized.
The sterilant (steam or gas) or the chemical disinfectant must be
able to contact all surfaces. Cleaning the object involves the use of
detergents and water and the mechanical removal of soil and
organic material (friction). Decontaminating a reusable contaminated object is the most important first step of the whole
disinfection and sterilization process. Disinfection normally includes soaking the items in a dilute or full-strength chemical

solution for varied periods of time, depending on the object and on the chemical solution.

Specific Infection Risks and Prevention Strategies

A contaminated object is a risk to anyone who comes in contact with it. A nosocomial infection may occur if another patient comes in contact with an ineffectively decontaminated, disinfected, or sterilized object. Health care providers are placed at risk by exposure to organisms on a contaminated object during and after use and during decontamination. They are also at risk for chemical exposure when using disinfectant solutions. Utility gloves and PPE such as protective face wear and gowns are required for decontaminating objects contaminated with blood or body fluids. Utility gloves are recommended because latex or vinyl gloves rip easily and can get caught in instrument or equipment hinges. Clean or sterile latex or vinyl gloves should be used to remove disinfected items from the chemical.[7] See Chapter 7 for specific protection guidelines.

Preparation

Gather the following equipment:
1. For decontaminating:
   a. PPE: utility gloves, eye/face protection, waterproof apron or gown (as needed)
   b. Detergent and water; low-sudsing detergents allow for maximum visualization of items
   c. Basin (or sink)
   d. Soft bristle scrub brush or tooth brush; abrasive scrub pads may damage instruments
2. For disinfecting
   a. PPE
   b. Soaking container with lid
   c. Tap water or sterile or distilled water, depending on the item; follow manufacturer's directions
   d. Chemical disinfectant; carefully follow manufacturer's directions for dilution—more is not better, and too much can be dangerous.[2,6]

Decontamination Procedure

1. Put on utility gloves and other PPE.
2. Rinse the contaminated object with tepid running water to

remove organic matter. (Hot water makes protein in organic material coagulate and adhere to the object.)

3. Wash the object with warm water and soap to reduce the surface tension of the water and to emulsify the organic material.
4. Use the brush to remove the organic material from all surfaces including all seams and grooves. Scrub below the level of the water to decrease splashing or spraying onto the face or clothing.
5. Rinse thoroughly in warm water.
6. Air dry articles.
7. Change detergent solution at least daily.
8. Clean the brush and the sink.
9. Remove PPE before going on to disinfection or sterilization processing.
10. Wash hands.[2,6]

Disinfection Procedure

1. Completely submerge decontaminated articles in correctly diluted disinfectant solution. Refer to Table 9-1 for contact time; solutions can corrode metal instruments if left soaking for more than 30 minutes. Always read the label and follow the manufacturer's recommendations.
2. Put lid on soaking container.
3. Wear clean or sterile gloves when removing articles to protect hands from chemical irritation and to decrease solution contamination.
4. Rinse item copiously in tap water or sterile water after soaking.
5. Air dry.[2]

Waste Disposal

Health care workers have a professional responsibility to dispose of all medical waste in a manner that poses minimal hazard to patients, other health care workers, and the public. Waste disposal from patient care activities is part of a comprehensive waste management program that conforms to federal, state, and local regulations.

The Centers for Disease Control and Prevention (CDC) designates several types of medical waste as potentially infectious: microbiologic, pathologic, blood, and sharps.[7]

Specific Infection Risks and Prevention Strategies

The CDC guidelines recommend the following:

1. Place all sharp items such as needles in a puncture-resistant container located as close as possible to the point of use.
2. Bag grossly contaminated articles to prevent human or environmental exposure to blood and body fluids. Bags must be impervious, sturdy, and large enough to hold the materials without contaminating the outside or breaking the bag.
3. Wash hands after handling medical waste.

Procedure Preparation

Gather color-coded (usually red or orange) impervious bags and PPE such as latex or utility gloves, depending on the task.

Procedure

1. Place soiled, disposable equipment and garbage in plastic waste bags that line the waste container. Dry items may be separated for incineration according to agency policy.
2. Place contaminated, nondisposable equipment in a labeled bag before removing it from the patient's room. Use two bags if the first bag is not impervious or if it is soiled on the outside. Send the bags to central processing for decontamination and further processing.
3. Disassemble special procedure trays, and discard disposable components (especially sharps). Return bagged nondisposable items to central processing for further decontamination and sterilization.
4. Handle soiled linen as little as possible to prevent contamination of the environment or personnel. Place soiled linen in covered laundry bags.
5. Place laboratory specimens in leak-proof containers. No special precautions are needed if the container is not contaminated on the outside.
6. Disinfect or destroy any item that is visibly or grossly contaminated, such as books or toys.
7. Wash hands after handling medical waste products.[7-9]

Environmental Control

All environments harbor pathogens. Items within the health care environment including air and water filters, baths, sinks, and

Text continued on p. 160.

Table 9-3   Reservoirs of infectious agents in the environment

Reservoir	Associated Pathogens	Transmission	Significance*	Prevention/Control
Air filters	Aspergillus	Airborne	Moderate	Replace soiled filters periodically
Chutes	Pseudomonas, Staphylococci	Airborne	Low	Proper design and placement
False ceilings	Rhizopus	Airborne	Low	Barrier protection during reconstruction Add fungicide to moist material
Fireproof materials	Aspergillus	Airborne	Low	
Humidifiers/ nebulizers	Acinetobacter, Legionella, Pseudomonas	Airborne, large droplet	High	Avoid when possible; use sterile water; disinfect between use
Outside construction plus inadequate ventilation	Rhizopus, Aspergillus	Airborne	High	Use at least 95% efficiency filters in hospital; filter all hospital air
Pigeon droppings	Aspergillus	Airborne	Low	Maintain filter efficiency; filter all hospital air

Inhaled medications	*Pseudomonas, Klebsiella, Serratia*	Inhalation	Moderate	Sterile preparation by pharmacy
Showers	*Legionella*	Inhalation	Low	Prohibit in immunocompromised patients
Ventilators	*Pseudomonas*	Inhalation	Moderate	Follow current CDC guidelines
Bronchoscopes	*Serratia, Pseudomonas, Mycobacteria*	Contact	Moderate	Pseudoepidemics common; follow disinfection guidelines
Contaminated germicides	*Pseudomonas*	Contact	High	Avoid extrinsic contamination and seek verification of manufacturer's microbiocidal efficacy claims
Dialysis water	GNR	Contact	Moderate	Follow guidelines: dialysate ≤ 2000 organisms/ml; water ≤ 200 organisms/ml

From Weber D, Rutala W: Environmental issues and nosocomial infections. In Wenzel R, editor: *Prevention and control of nosocomial infections*, Baltimore, 1993, Williams & Wilkins.

CDC, Centers for Disease Control and Prevention; *GNR*, gram-negative rods; *ECG*, electrocardiogram; *IV*, intravenous; *ICU*, intensive care unit.

*High, multiple well-described outbreaks due to this reservoir; *moderate*, occasional well-described outbreaks; *low*, rare, well-described outbreaks; *none*, actual infection not demonstrated.

Continued.

Table 9-3   Reservoirs of infectious agents in the environment—cont'd

Reservoir	Associated Pathogens	Transmission	Significance	Prevention/Control
ECG electrodes	S. aureus, GNR	Contact	None	Disinfect after use or use disposable leads
Elasticized bandages	Zygomycetes	Contact	Moderate	Avoid in immunocompromised patients or over nonintact skin
Electronic thermometers	C. difficile	Contact	Low	Probe cover, disinfect each day
Endoscopes	Salmonella, Pseudomonas	Contact	High	Follow proper disinfection procedures
Faucet aerators	Pseudomonas	Contact, large droplet	Low	No precautions necessary
Ice baths	Staphylococcus, Ewingella	Contact	Moderate	Avoid direct contact with ice to cool IV solution and syringes; use closed system for thermodilution
Intraaortic balloon pump	Pseudomonas	Contact	Low	Add germicide to water reservoir

Mattresses	*Pseudomonas, Acinetobacter*	Contact	Moderate	Use intact plastic cover, disinfect between patients
Plaster	*Pseudomonas, Bacillus, Cunninghamella, Clostridia*	Contact	Moderate	Use judiciously in immunocompromised patients or over non-intact skin
Potable water	*Pseudomonas, Mycobacteria, Flavobacteria, Serratia, Acinetobacter, Legionella*	Contact	Moderate	Follow public health guidelines
Pressure transducers	*Pseudomonas, Enterobacter, Serratia*	Contact	Moderate	Disinfect transducer between patients and replace disposable dome; use good aseptic technique

Continued.

Table 9-3   Reservoirs of infectious agents in the environment—cont'd

Reservoir	Associated Pathogens	Transmission	Significance	Prevention/Control
Sinks	*Pseudomonas*	Contact, large droplet	Low	Use separate sinks for hand washing and disposal of contaminated fluids
Suction apparatus	*Klebsiella, Salmonella, Pseudomonas, Proteus*	Contact, large droplet	Low	Avoid backflow; avoid aerosolization; disinfect between patient use
Thermometers (glass)	*Salmonella*	Contact	Moderate (rectal only)	Disinfect between use
Tub immersion	*Pseudomonas*	Contact	Moderate	Add germicide to water; drain and disinfect after each use
Urine-measuring devices	*Serratia*	Contact	Moderate	Disinfect between patients; use good hand washing technique

Water baths	Pseudomonas, Acinetobacter	Contact	Moderate	Add germicide to water bath or use plastic overwrap
Electric breast pumps	Pseudomonas, Klebsiella, Serratia	Ingestion	Moderate	Follow guidelines
Enteral feeds	GNR	Ingestion	Low	Use sterile commercial feeds or aseptically prepared feeds; refrigerate; minimize manipulation; use closed administration set
Food	Salmonella, S. aureus, Clostridia, Vibrios, hepatitis A, Norwalk virus	Ingestion	High	Follow local health guidelines
Ice/ice machines	Legionella, Enterobacter, Pseudomonas, Salmonella	Ingestion, Contact	Moderate	Periodic cleaning

Continued.

Table 9-3   Reservoirs of infectious agents in the environment—cont'd

Reservoir	Associated Pathogens	Transmission	Significance	Prevention/Control
Air-fluidized beds	—	—	None	Follow manufacturer's recommendations
Carpets	—	—	None	Prudent to avoid in areas of heavy soiling
Flowers	GNR	—	None	Prudent to avoid in the ICU and immunocompromised patients' rooms
Fresh vegetables	Aerobic gram-negative rods, *Listeria*	—	None	Prudent to avoid in immunocompromised patients

Pets	Salmonella	—	None	Prudent to avoid in hospital setting (except seeing eye dogs)
Stethoscopes	Staphylococci	—	None	Prudent to clean periodically with alcohol
Toilets	—	—	None	Use good hand washing technique
Medical waste	—	—	None	Follow state and federal regulations

potable water may serve as reservoirs for infectious agents. Table 9-3 depicts the possible hospital reservoirs, their associated pathogens, modes of transmission, significance, and methods of control and prevention.[10] Specific guidelines to reduce reservoirs of infection for care activities are listed here.

1. Bathing: Use soap and water to remove drainage, secretions, perspiration, or sediments.
2. Dressing materials: Change dressings that are wet and soiled.
3. Contaminated articles: Place items in impervious bags.
4. Contaminated needles: Place syringes and uncapped needles in puncture-resistant containers.
5. Bedside unit: Keep table surfaces clean and dry.
6. Bottled solutions: Date bottles when opened; keep tightly closed; do not leave open longer than necessary.
7. Surgical wounds: Keep drainage tubes and collection bags patent.
8. Drainage bags and containers: Routinely empty containers; maintain the drainage system below the level of the site being drained unless it is clamped.

Summary

Cleaning and decontaminating a reusable contaminated object is the most important first step of the whole disinfection or sterilization process. Choosing the right level of disinfection or sterilization is directly related to the use of the item, and choosing the correct chemical disinfectant is related to the level of disinfection needed: low, intermediate, or high. Not all items require high-level disinfection. Using the correct level protects people using the chemical disinfectant and provides adequate preparation of the item to prevent nosocomial transmission. Handling contaminated medical waste appropriately further protects patients, health care provider, and the public.

References

1. Reichert M, Young J: *Sterilization technology for the health care facility*, Gaithersburg, Md, 1993, Aspen.
2. Heroux D et al: *Ambulatory care infection control manual*, Seattle, 1993, Group Health Cooperative Businesses.
3. Rutala W: Disinfection, sterilization and waste disposal. In Wenzel R, editor: *Prevention and control of nosocomial infections*, Baltimore, 1993, Williams & Wilkins.
4. Rutala W: APIC guideline for selection and use of disinfectants, *Am J Infect Control* 18 (2):99, 1990.
5. Soule B, editor: *The APIC curriculum for infection control practice*, vol 1, Dubuque, Iowa, 1983, Kendall/Hunt.
6. Potter P, Perry A: *Fundamentals of nursing: concepts, process & practice*, ed 3, St Louis, 1993, Mosby.
7. Centers for Disease Control: Guidelines for prevention of transmission of human immunodeficiency virus and hepatitis B virus to health care and public safety workers, *MMWR* 39:1, 1989.
8. Kozier B et al: *Techniques in clinical nursing*, Redwood City, Calif, 1993, Addison-Wesley.
9. Weinstein S et al: Bacterial surface contamination of patient's linen: isolation precautions versus standard care, *Am J Infect Control* 17 (5):264, 1989.
10. Weber D, Rutala W: Environmental issues and nosocomial infections. In Wenzel R, editor: *Prevention and control of nosocomial infections*, Baltimore, 1993, Williams & Wilkins.

Surgical Asepsis 10

Surgical asepsis is the preparation and maintenance of a sterile environment to prevent infection during an operation or procedure. Components of surgical asepsis include preparation of the equipment, supplies, environment, and personnel who are involved in the specific procedure as well as preparation and monitoring of the patient who is undergoing the procedure.

Surgical aseptic techniques are designed to create a safe environment by controlling four main sources of infectious organisms: the patient, personnel, equipment, and environment. These sources of infection may be endogenous (acquired from organisms within the body) or exogenous (acquired from organisms in the environment). The patient is the major source of endogenous infection; personnel, equipment, and the environment are the primary sources of exogenous infection.

Specific techniques to follow in establishing and maintaining surgical asepsis are discussed further in this chapter and include the following:

1. Staff considerations: surgical hand scrub, gowning, gloving, and the removal of soiled gowns and gloves.
2. Patient considerations: skin cleansing/scrub, skin shaving/depilatory, and wound covering.
3. Environmental considerations: room preparation and sterilization of equipment and supplies.
4. Establishing and maintaining a sterile field.
5. Standards for practice.

Staff Considerations

Practices aimed at controlling exogenous infection include completing a surgical hand scrub, donning a sterile gown, and wearing sterile gloves. The surgical hand scrub reduces the transfer of microbes from personnel to the patient. The sterile gown and gloves provide a barrier to pathogens.

Surgical Hand Scrub

Although sterile gloves are worn for invasive procedures, the skin of the hands and forearms should be scrubbed to lessen the number of microorganisms. Specifically, there are three purposes of the surgical hand scrub:

1. To remove debris and transient microorganisms from the nails, hands, and forearms
2. To reduce the resident microbial count to a minimum
3. To inhibit rapid rebound growth of microorganisms[1]

Preparation

The attire that is worn should promote a high level of cleanliness and hygiene and should protect the patient and the health care worker. Attire may include scrub clothes, hair covering, masks, protective eyewear, and other barriers to contamination. Rings, watches, and bracelets should be removed so that contaminants are not harbored on the hands and arms. Fingernails should be short and clean. Although the Association of Operating Room Nurses recommends that nail polish not be worn in the operating room,[1] it does not appear that the use of nail polish is associated with increased microbial counts, especially when the nails are kept short and clean.[2] The hands and forearms should be free of open lesions and breaks in the skin.

Equipment

A packaged scrub brush containing an antimicrobial cleaning agent approved by the facility's infection control committee should be used. Povidone-iodine (e.g., Betadine) or chlorhexidine (e.g., Hibiclens) are common agents. A nail cleaner is also contained in most packaged scrub brush kits. Some brushes contain no chemical cleaner, allowing the nurse to use an antimicrobial agent of choice from a dispenser.

A water faucet with an automatic start-stop mechanism allows the nurse to perform the hand scrub without contaminating the hand to turn off the water. If this is not available, the water must be turned off by another person.

Procedure

1. Turn on the water and adjust the temperature.
2. In preparation for the formal scrub, moisten the hands and

forearms, wash, and rinse to remove gross contamination and loosen superficial debris.

3. Open the top of the package containing the scrub brush (or sponge) to expose the nail cleaner and brush. Remove the nail cleaner, and clean the subungual areas under running water (Fig. 10-1).

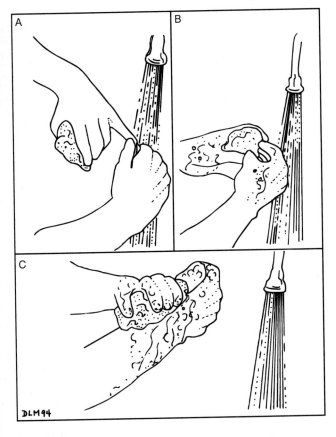

Figure 10-1.
Surgical scrub technique. **A**, Cleaning nails with plastic nail cleaner. **B**, Holding brush perpendicular to nails facilitates thorough scrubbing of undersides of nails. **C**, Holding brush lengthwise along arm covers maximum area with each stroke.

4. After the nails are cleaned, remove the brush from its package. Clean one hand and arm in a circular fashion using friction. Clean the other hand and arm in a similar manner. The entire process should take 5 to 10 minutes.
5. During washing, hold the hands higher than the elbows so that water and cleansing debris drip away from the hands into the sink.
6. Upon completion of the scrub, discard the brush appropriately; allow excess moisture to drip toward the elbows and into the sink. Do not touch any part of the sink, faucet, or clothing.
7. Dry the hands and don the sterile gown and gloves.

Gowning
Preparation

Gown once a hand scrub has been performed and the appropriate equipment has been gathered. Gowning is recommended when splashes, spray, or splatter of blood or other body fluids are likely to occur. The gown is considered personal protective equipment according to the Occupational Safety and Health Administration 1991 Standard and is a component of standard precautions. (See Chapter 2.)

Equipment

A sterile gown and gloves (discussed in the next section) are required. Open the outer wrapper of the sterile gown on a flat surface to expose the enclosed gown and drying towel.

Gowning Procedure

Upon completion of the surgical hand scrub, approach the sterile gown and towel that have been opened aseptically and placed on a table or counter. Use the following procedure:
1. Without touching or dripping water onto the sterile gown or gloves, lift the towel off the gown. The towel should not touch your clothing.
2. Dry one hand and arm with half the towel, moving from fingers to elbow (Figure 10-2). Use the other half of the towel to dry the other hand and arm, and discard the towel into the appropriate container.
3. Pick up the gown (which comes folded inside-out) by the inside of the garment near the shoulder areas. Allow the gown to open, and slip your hands into the armholes (Figure 10-3). Hold the hands at chest level and away from the body.

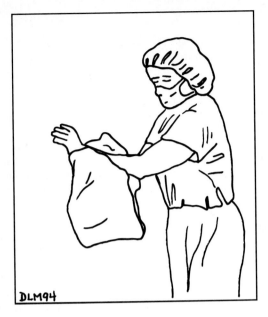

Figure 10-2.
Drying hands and forearms. Fingers and hands should be
dried thoroughly before forearm is dried. Extending arms reduces possibility of contaminating towel or hands.

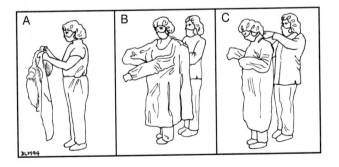

Figure 10-3.
Gowning procedure. **A**, Sterile nurse keeps hands on inside
of gown while unfolding it at arm's length. **B**, Unsterile
nurse reaches under flap of gown to pull sleeves on scrub
nurse. **C**, Unsterile nurse closes neckline of gown, touching
only snap area of neckline.

4. Advance the hands and arms into the sleeves. If the closed gloving technique (described in the next section) is to be performed, the arms should not extend beyond the cuff of the sterile gown.
5. An "unsterile" nurse stands behind the "sterile" nurse and pulls the gown over the shoulders and ties or clasps the neckline. The unsterile nurse then grasps the inner waist ties, taking care not to touch the outer portion of the gown, and ties the inside of the gown.

Gloving: Closed Technique

Preparation

Gloves are donned once cleansing of the hands and arms has taken place and the gown is in place. The gloves should have been opened aseptically and placed on a table or counter.

Equipment

A pair of sterile gloves is necessary. The gloves should fit properly without bagging or looseness. Selection of specific types of gloves depends on sensitivity to latex, rubber, or vinyl. Latex sensitivity is considered to be a true allergic condition and may be more common than previously thought.[3-6] Alternatives to latex gloves are available; for example, Tactylon, a nonlatex, nonvinyl, thermoplastic elastomer, is available in sterile and nonsterile examination gloves.[7]

Procedure

1. Keep hands inside the cuff of the gown (Figure 10-4, *A*).
2. Place the first glove palm side down on top of the other, cuff-covered hand. The glove fingers should be pointing toward the elbow (Figure 10-4, *B*).
3. Securely hold the glove cuff by the hand (Figure 10-4, *C*) on which it has been placed, and with the other hand pull it over the opening of the sleeve and the cuff.
4. As the glove cuff is pulled back, place the fingers into the finger cots (Figure 10-4, *D*).
5. Position the remaining glove on the opposite forearm with the gloved hand, and apply it in the same manner as in steps 3 and 4 (Figure 10-4, *E*).
6. Adjust the gloves, and wipe them clean with a sterile moist pad;

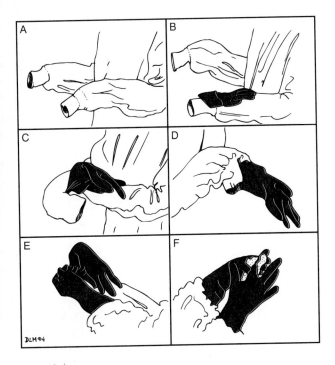

Figure 10-4.
Closed gloving technique. **A**, Keep hands inside sleeve cuffs.
B, Lift first glove by grasping it through fabric of sleeve.
Cuff on glove facilitates easier handling of glove. Place glove
palm down along forearm of matching hand, with thumb
and fingers of glove pointing toward elbow. Glove cuff lies
over gown wristlet. **C**, Hold glove cuff securely with the
hand on which it is placed, and, with other hand, stretch
the cuff over opening of sleeve to cover gown wristlet
entirely. **D**, Draw cuff back onto wrist, directing fingers into
their spaces in the glove. **E**, Use gloved hand to position
remaining glove on opposite sleeve in same fashion. Place
glove cuff around gown cuff. Draw second glove onto hand,
and pull cuff into place. **F**, Adjust fingers of gloves, and
wipe gloves with wet pad to remove glove powder.

the nonsterile nurse can open a sterile dressing sponge and wet it with sterile saline to remove glove powder (Figure 10-4, *F*).

Removing Soiled Gown and Gloves

To protect the hands, forearms, and nurse's clothing from microorganisms that may be present on the gown and gloves, apparel is removed before leaving the work area to confine contaminants. The gown is removed before the gloves so that the nurse's bare hands do not come into contact with contaminants on the gown. Gross blood and other debris is wiped off the gloves with a clean, moist pad.

Procedure

1. The unsterile nurse unfastens the back closures of the gown.
2. The gowned nurse grasps the shoulder seams of the gown and pulls the gown and sleeves forward and over the gloved hands, turning the gown inside out and everting the cuffs of the gloves (Figure 10-5, *A* and *B*).
3. Fold the gown inside out and into a ball, and discard it in the appropriate container.
4. Remove the gloves, placing a gloved hand on the outer portion of the glove covering the second hand. Pull the glove off the hand so that the glove is everted and the skin is not touched by the soiled glove (Figure 10-5, *C*).
5. Remove the second glove by placing the bare fingers on the everted edge (i.e., the inner, "clean" area) of the remaining glove, pulling the glove off the hand and everting it (Figure 10-5, *D*).
6. Discard the gloves into an appropriate container.

Patient Considerations

The patient, and in particular the patient's skin, is a major source of endogenous microbial contamination. When the integrity of the skin is broken by the insertion of percutaneous devices such as intravenous lines or by a surgical incision, the patient is exposed to microorganisms that can invade the body and cause infection. Cleansing of the skin, skin scrubs, and removal of excess hair are common methods employed to lower the number of bacteria on the skin's surface. Sterilization of the skin is unfeasible because bactericidal chemicals may also destroy living tissues.[8] Draping the

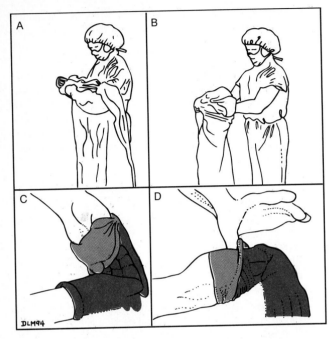

Figure 10-5.
Removal of soiled gown and gloves. **A**, To protect clothing and arms from microorganisms on gown, grasp the gown without touching clothes. **B**, Turn outer side of soiled gown away from body, avoiding touching body with gown. **C**, To prevent outer side of soiled gloves from touching hands, place gloved fingers of one hand under everted cuff of other glove, and pull it off hand and fingers. **D**, To prevent contact of ungloved hand with remaining soiled glove, hook bare thumb on inner side of glove and pull glove off.

patient and covering the wound complete the patient considerations.

Skin Cleansing/Scrub

Preparation

Surgical aseptic preparation of the patient's skin begins by skin cleansing done before admission for the operation or procedure.

The patient needs instruction in the use of specific antimicrobial soap solutions and the use of friction to reduce the number of microorganisms. This superficial cleansing may be followed by one or more skin scrubs to reduce bacteria on skin surfaces. These microorganisms can be removed or reduced with antiseptic agents. The purpose is to remove external dirt, debris, and skin microorganisms, thereby decreasing the risk of postoperative wound infections.[9] The antimicrobial agent used for cleansing may also leave a film or layer of protection that inhibits the growth of microorganisms for a period of time. Cleansing should never be vigorous enough to cause abrasions or skin breakdown.

Equipment

Antimicrobial soap, a washcloth, and a towel are gathered. Access to a shower or other source of running water is provided.

Procedure

1. Turn on the water and adjust the temperature.
2. Moisten the body parts.
3. Lather the antimicrobial soap on the washcloth.
4. Wash the body parts thoroughly using ample soap and friction.
5. Rinse the body parts with running water.
6. After washing and rinsing, pat dry with the towel.

Skin Shaving/Depilatory
Preparation

Although surgical preparation of the skin used to include shaving a wide area surrounding the operative site, this practice has recently been reconsidered.[10] Shaving may cause small nicks and breaks in skin integrity and may be the source of infection. A wet or dry shave may be done. A wet shave is done with antimicrobial soap and water; a dry shave may remove fewer epithelial cells. If hair must be removed, a depilatory cream may be used. Also, hair may be clipped very short. If shaving is necessary, it should be done in the operating room or immediately before the procedure to reduce the risk of infection. Specific orders or institutional guidelines are followed for the type of shave and area of skin to be prepared.

Equipment

A razor with a sharp blade, antimicrobial soap, warm water, a small basin, and a towel are gathered. Alternately, to use a depilatory cream, a washcloth and towel are gathered. Depilatory creams contain chemicals; the patient should be screened for sensitivities. Label directions are followed for use of the depilatory.

Procedure for wet shave

1. Assemble equipment at the patient's bedside.
2. Wash your hands and dry them thoroughly.
3. Expose the area to be shaved, protecting the patient's privacy with drapes and covers.
4. Wet and lather the area to be shaved.
5. Using firm, quick strokes, shave across the area in overlapping strokes.
6. Rinse the razor frequently to avoid hair buildup. Change the blade as necessary to avoid dullness.
7. Rinse the area well.
8. Towel dry the area.
9. Clean the equipment, discarding the razor blade in a contaminated sharps container.

Wound Covering

Preparation

After the operation or procedure is completed, a dressing is applied to the incision. The wound covering may be a gauze, a semiocclusive, or an occlusive dressing. Most surgical dressings have three layers—a contact (primary) layer, an absorbent layer, and an outer protective layer.[11]

Equipment

Sterile 4 × 4s, abdominal pads, nonadhesive dressings, and tape are assembled as needed for the specific site.

Procedure

1. Cover the incision with a sterile dressing before removing the sterile drapes.
2. Remove the drape, taking care not to dislodge the dressing.
3. Reinforce the dressing with additional pads.
4. Cover the dressing with tape.
5. Cover the exit sites of drains or tubes with dressings, taking care not to dislodge the drains or tubes.

Environmental Considerations

The environment in which an operation or procedure takes place makes a crucial difference in preventing or minimizing the risk of infection. Two major concerns are the operating room itself and the maintenance of sterility in the field.

Operating Room Considerations

Surgical suites are designed to minimize contamination with the use of foot pedals or automatic electric controls at sinks, through control of traffic patterns to reduce the number of personnel who enter and exit patient areas, and with the use of controlled airflow patterns.

The door to the operating room should be closed at all times to avoid mixing corridor air with the operating room air, which would increase the number of microorganisms. The temperature of the room should be maintained at between 20°C and 27°C (68°F-80°F). The humidity should be maintained at about 50% for comfort and to inhibit microbial growth.[12] Excess personnel should be restricted from entering the room, and the total number of persons allowed in the room should be limited. Additional personnel who wish to view the operation can be accommodated in surgical viewing suites, when available.

Establishing and Maintaining a Sterile Field

To restrict the transfer of microorganisms to the wound and to protect the sterility of instruments, equipment, supplies, and gloved hands of personnel, a sterile field must be established. This is accomplished by placing sterile drapes around the wound or site of intervention.

Preparation

The size dimensions of the sterile field are determined by the scope and complexity of the intervention. In addition to the sterile field created on the patient, other sterile fields may be established on tables or counters to maintain the sterility of equipment and supplies. Practices employed to protect and maintain the sterility of the field are listed in the box on p. 174.

Equipment

Draping materials must create an effective barrier against the passage of microorganisms from the nonsterile to the sterile areas.

Considerations for Maintaining a Sterile Field

- Only sterile items should be used within a sterile field.
- Sterile items introduced onto a sterile field should be opened, dispensed, and transferred in a manner that maintains their sterility.
- Items located below the level of the draped patient are considered unsterile.
- Unsterile persons do not reach across a sterile field or touch items within the sterile field.
- Sterile persons do not lean over an unsterile field or touch unsterile items.
- Sterile gown should be considered sterile in front from the chest to the level of sterile field, and the sleeves are sterile from 2 inches above the elbow to the cuffs.
- Areas of the surgical gown considered unsterile include the neckline, shoulders, underarms, back, and sleeve cuffs.
- The edges of a package containing a sterile item are considered unsterile.
- Unsterile persons should face sterile areas on approach to avoid inadvertent contamination of sterile areas during movement.
- Unsterile persons should not walk between two sterile fields.

They may be made from natural or synthetic material, and they come in a variety of sizes and configurations. Waterproof drapes prevent the wicking action that can transport microorganisms from moistened, nonsterile materials to the sterile area. Drapes should also be as lintfree as possible and meet fire safety standards.

Procedure

1. To create a sterile field on a flat surface (e.g., a table or counter), an unsterile nurse opens the package containing a sterile sheet. This nurse grasps the edges of the sheet, without touching the inner sterile portion, and pulls open the sheet to cover the surface.
2. Once this sterile surface is created, the unsterile nurse opens containers of required sterile items and transfers the contents onto the sterile field.

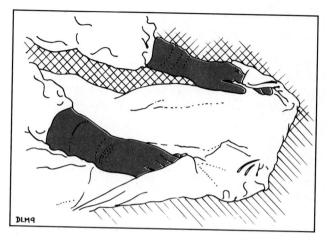

Figure 10-6.
Sterile drape. When placing sterile drape on unsterile surface, sterile nurse rolls corners of drape over hands to avoid contamination.

3. The sterile nurse (gowned and gloved) approaches the sterile field and arranges the sterile items to be used.
4. Sterile drapes are applied to the patient, taking care not to contaminate the nurse's or physician's gown and gloves. One method to reduce the possibility of contamination is to make a cuff with the drape (Figure 10-6). Additional sterile fields may be created with drapes from the original sterile field.

Monitoring and Evaluating Surgical Asepsis
Patient Monitoring

Patients are monitored preoperatively and postoperatively for wound infections. Recently, the prophylactic use of antibiotics has been recommended for specific surgical cases.[13] Statistics are maintained by institutions on the incidence of surgical infections. If the infection rate is considered too high, an investigation into the possible causes is conducted.

Staff Monitoring

Personnel who work in health care settings are routinely screened for infectious diseases. (See Chapter 8.) All health care workers are encouraged to receive hepatitis B vaccination and must attend annual reviews on meeting standards for occupational safety. Persons who are ill, have open wounds, or have been exposed to communicable diseases should not be in contact with patients.

Standards for Practice

Standards are authoritative statements describing the responsibilities for which nurses are accountable. Professional standards direct and evaluate nursing practice and reflect the values and priorities of the profession. Standards developed by the American Nurses' Association and the Association of the Operating Room Nurses describe a competent level of nursing practice and professional performance designed to achieve desired patient outcomes.[1]

The Association of Operating Room Nurses' recommended practices guide nurses in the optimum performance of their practice.[14] Compliance is voluntary, and implementation of the practices should be integrated into existing institutional policies and procedures.

Standards for the operating room and for maintenance of a sterile environment are also established by regulatory agencies such as the Joint Commission on Accreditation of Healthcare Organizations. Local, state, and federal agencies, such as the Occupational Safety and Health Administration, enforce regulations designed to protect consumers and health care professionals. Other agencies, such as the Centers for Disease Control and Prevention, provide guidelines to maintain the health of the community and investigate diseases threatening the public well-being (Chapter 2).

By following the principles of surgical asepsis, nurses protect both the patient and themselves from infection. Strict adherence to the standards and procedures set forth in this chapter will help ensure a safe and secure environment for nursing practice.

References

1. Association of Operating Room Nurses, Inc: *Standards and recommended practices*, Denver, 1993, AORN.

2. Baumgardner CA et al: Effects of nail polish on microbial growth of fingernails: Dispelling sacred cows, *AORN J* 58(1):84, 1993.

3. Wolf BL: Anaphylactic reaction to latex gloves (letter), *N Engl J Med* 329(4):279, 1993.

4. Gonzalez E: Latex hypersensitivity: a new and unexpected problem, *Hosp Pract* 27(2):137, 1992.

5. Arellano R, Bradley J, Sussman G: Prevalence of latex sensitization among hospital physicians occupationally exposed to latex gloves, *Anesthesiology* 77(5):905, 1992.

6. Lagier F et al: Prevalence of latex allergy in operating room nurses, *J Allergy Clin Immunol* 90(3:1):319, 1992.

7. Hamann C: Alternatives for health care workers with latex glove allergies (letter), *JAMA*, 269(18):2368, 1993.

8. Kleinbeck SV: Principles and practices of surgical asepsis. In Meeker MH, Rothrock JC, editors: *Alexander's care of the patient in surgery,* ed 9, St Louis, 1991, Mosby.

9. Macheca MK: Surgical client. In Potter PA, Perry AG, editors: *Fundamentals of nursing: concepts, process and practice*, ed 3, St Louis, 1993, Mosby.

10. Ellis JR, Nowlis EA, Bentz PM: *Modules for basic nursing skills*, vol II, ed 5, Philadelphia, 1992, JB Lippincott.

11. Cole S: Clients with wounds. In Potter PA, Perry AG, editors: *Fundamentals of nursing: concepts, process and practice*, ed 3, St Louis, 1993, Mosby.

12. Boehnlein MJ: Intraoperative interventions. In Long BC, Phipps WJ, Cassmyer VL, editors: *Medical-surgical nursing: a nursing process approach*, ed 3, St Louis, 1993, Mosby.

13. Page CP et al: Antimicrobial prophylaxis for surgical wounds: Guidelines for clinical care, *Arch Surg* 128:79, 1993.

14. Association of Operating Room Nurses, Inc: Recommended practices: universal precautions in the perioperative practice setting, *AORN J* 57:554, 1993.

INFECTION PREVENTION AND NURSING PROCEDURES III

Collecting Blood and Body Fluid Specimens

11

The collection of blood and body fluid specimens plays a major role in the diagnosis and treatment of many patients. How specimens are collected determines their usefulness in directing the course of treatment. If specimens are collected incorrectly, health care providers may make inaccurate diagnoses, and patients may suffer delayed or inappropriate treatment.

At the same time, obtaining, handling, transporting, and processing specimens place health care workers (HCWs) at risk for infection or disease. HCWs must know and practice standard precautions, as outlined in Chapter 7. Hand washing before and after the collection of each specimen and using gloves are the primary protective strategies for this group of procedures.

Key Steps to Consider During Collection of Specimens

Once the order for a procedure is documented and the patient is properly identified, the procedure should be explained to the patient. Signed consent forms should be obtained, if required. The most beneficial information for patients is a description of the sensations they may experience during the procedure.[1,2] The patient should be encouraged to ask any and all questions about a procedure, even those that seem trivial.[1] Descriptions of nonpainful as well as painful sensations that might be experienced during the procedure such as tightness from a tourniquet application should be provided.[2] Because of cultural taboos, some patients may be embarrassed about the collection of body excreta, such as feces or urine. Sensitivity during explanations, the careful selection of terminology, and protection of the patient's privacy mitigate social awkwardness encountered in specimen collection.

In collecting any blood or body fluid specimen, HCWs must anticipate what parts of their own bodies and clothing may be exposed to the patient's blood or body fluid during the collection process. The more assistance the patient requires during the collection of specimens, the more vigilant HCWs must be about self-protection. Standard precautions to prevent the transmission of pathogens should apply to the collection of all specimens (see Chapter 7). Hand washing, personal protective equipment (e.g., gloves), and prevention of self-injury with contaminated sharps or equipment are the primary methods of protection.

To collect any specimen for laboratory analysis, the HCW must know the purpose of the analysis and understand the correct amount and proper way to obtain, transfer, and store the specimen. By knowing the purpose of specimen collection, the HCW can avoid hazards and interpret the meaning of the results.

Specimen containers must be carefully labeled, properly closed, and free of possible contaminants on the outside surfaces. Specimens should be enclosed in sealed plastic bags to ensure safe transfer and handling.

In addition, the HCW must know how to prepare and care for the patient before, during, and after specimen collection. Does the patient require assistance with positioning, comfort, breathing, or muscle control during specimen collection?

The HCW should document the time and date of the specimen collection procedure, describe the specimen obtained, describe the patient's response to specimen collection, and note any unusual requirements or occurrences on the patient's health record.

Blood Specimens

Definition

Samples of blood may be obtained from capillaries, arteries, and veins, depending on the diagnostic test and the age of the patient. Capillary samples obtained from finger sticks in children and adults and from heel sticks in infants yield small amounts of blood commonly used for glucose testing. Arterial samples, usually obtained by arterial puncture by respiratory or laboratory

Table 11-1 Step-by-step guide for collection of blood specimens

Specimen	Infection Risk		Preparation for Collection	Procedure
	Patient	Health Care Workers		

Blood specimen	Microbial contamination from own skin or HCW's skin
	
	Bacteremia from indwelling arterial or vascular catheters
	
	Types of organisms that threaten bloodstream: *Escherichia coli, Klebsiella, Staphylococcus aureus, S. epidermis, Corynebacterium,* and *Candida albicans*
		All blood from all patients poses risk for bloodborne pathogens: HIV, HBV, HCV.	1. Identify special requirements for specific patients.
			2. Assemble all properly labeled collection tubes, cleansing swabs, tourniquet, sterile cotton balls, pads, and tape.
			3. Select appropriate gauge needle.
			4. Label tubes with name, date, and HCW's initials.
				1. Wash hands.
				2. Put on gloves.
				3. Position the arm with support.
				4. Apply tourniquet to puncture site, asking patient to make a fist.
				5. Palpate and locate puncture site (antecubital area, etc.).
				6. Cleanse site:
				  ■ Apply 2% povidone iodine or alcohol (30%-70%)
				  ■ Cleanse in circular motion.

Continued.

HCW, health care worker; *HIV,* human immunodeficiency virus; *HBV,* hepatitis B virus; *HCV,* hepatitis C virus.

Table 11-1   Step-by-step guide for collection of blood specimens—cont'd

Specimen	Infection Risk	Preparation for Collection	Procedure
Patient	Health Care Workers		7. Allow to dry.
			8. Do not palpate once the skin is clean.
			9. Enter the skin at 45-degree angle, bevel of needle upward.
			10. Relocate vein and insert needle into vein.
			11. Release tourniquet and relax fist.
			12. Collect blood in appropriate specimen tubes.
			13. Remove gloves.
			14. Wash hands.

technicians or drawn from indwelling arterial lines, are used for measuring blood gases. Venous samples are obtained from needle puncture of an accessible vein or from intravenous catheters. Table 11-1 provides a step-by-step guide for collection of blood specimens.

Specific Considerations
Children

After obtaining a medical order, a local anesthetic cream with a plastic film should be applied for 60 minutes for patients with lightly pigmented skin and 120 minutes for patients with heavily pigmented skin (the dense and compact character of the stratum corneum of dark skin may slow the absorption of any topical agent).[3] This intervention avoids the pain of venipuncture for children[3] and adults.

If blood is drawn from small veins, specific techniques may be helpful. Pressing the vein beyond the point of the needle or placing the bevel of the needle lightly against the wall of the vein minimizes the risk of vein collapse. Small-gauge "butterfly" infusion needles may also prevent collapse.[4]

Infants

It has been shown that the recommended puncturing depth of 2.4 mm for newborn heels is excessive. For an experienced phlebotomist, a lancet of 1.8 mm is sufficient to obtain an adequate blood sample and will avoid bone injury.[5] In addition, warming the puncture site increases blood flow and facilitates a successful procedure. To avoid burns, a small cloth soaked in tap water warmed to no more than 42°C (check with a thermometer) can be used.[5] Disposable heel warmers are available commercially. Retractable lancets are now available to protect the HCW.

Intravascular catheters

Although drawing blood from indwelling intravascular catheters avoids the discomfort of venipuncture and may reflect total body composition more accurately, patients with intravascular catheters in place lose more blood volume to frequent diagnostic sampling than do those who do not have catheter lines in place.[7] Patients in intensive care units are particularly susceptible to nosocomial anemia.[8] The nurse can minimize blood loss by coordinating diagnostic testing and by withdrawing the minimum acceptable amount for laboratory purposes.[7,8] Samples of blood are considered to be reliable after the catheter dwell volume plus one additional milliliter of blood is discarded.[7] The destruction of red cells with resulting erroneous readings is minimized by drawing blood at a steady, even rate of 1 ml per 5 to 10 seconds.[7]

If the cap on a central venous catheter is removed to attach a syringe to withdraw blood samples, a clamp must be attached to the catheter above the cap to prevent air from entering the catheter. A sterile drape under the cap and the use of povidone-iodine or alcohol wipe to cleanse the hub minimize contamination. Gloves must be worn to protect both the patient and the HCW.

Arterial samples

Arterial samples for blood gas measurement should immediately be immersed in ice water for transport to minimize cellular glycolysis.[5] A one-handed scoop method or a recapping device should be used to guard against injury.

Blood for culture

Blood cultures are taken by venipuncture or from indwelling intravascular lines. Intravascular catheter specimens are frequently contaminated with normal skin flora or pathogens.[8] Changing the venipuncture needle before inoculation of culture media has no effect on sample contamination and is therefore unnecessary.[9] Special vacuum tubes with prepared culture media are now available for use.[4]

Finger puncture

The distal phalanx of the second, third, or fourth fingers should be cleansed with an Isopropanol/water absorbent pad. Dry the site with a sterile absorbent pad. The thumb is placed below and well away from the puncture site to guard against injury. Retractable lancets are now available to protect the HCW. The puncture is made in one smooth, quick motion at a 90-degree angle. The initial drop of blood contains interstitial and intercellular fluid as well as surface debris and should be wiped away with a dry sterile pad.[5]

Home care

The effect of distance between the patient's home and the laboratory must be considered in the transport of blood specimens.

Table 11-2 Step-by-step guide for collection of sterile urine specimens

Specimen	Infection Risk		Preparation for Collection	Procedure
	Patient	Health Care Workers		
Urine	Organisms responsible for most urinary tract infections: *E. coli, Klebsiella, Proteus, Enterococcus, Enterobacter*	Risk is if blood is visible in urine. If the patient needs assistance, gloves should be worn to avoid contamination	Instruct patient to cleanse his/her periurethral area to collect a midstream specimen. Specify amount of urine required. Instruct patient to wash hands before and after the procedure.	**Male Patients** Clean the glans from meatus up in a circular motion with antiseptic soaked gauze pad. After beginning urinary stream, pass the specimen container into the stream to collect 1-2 ounces of urine. **Female Patients** Spread the labia minora with the thumb and forefinger of nondominant hand. Cleanse by wiping from the urethral orifice to the anus in one downward stroke, once each side and then

Continued.

Table 11-2 Step-by-step guide for collection of sterile urine specimens—cont'd

Specimen	Infection Risk	Preparation for Collection	Procedure
Patient	Health Care Workers		**Female Patients** down the middle (changing cleansing pads for each wipe). After urinary stream has begun, pass the specimen container into the stream to collect 1-2 ounces of urine. Cleanse any urine from the external surface of the collection container and place in plastic box or bag. Label with name of patient, date, and time. Transport specimen to the laboratory within 15 minutes or refrigerate.

Therefore the type of specimen collector tube (with or without preservative), the mixing technique, and the optimum transport temperature with regard to the purpose of the specimen must be determined before the home visit for specimen collection. Safe sharps disposal and safe specimen transport is also a consideration to guard against HCW injury.

Urine Specimen
Definition

Samples of urine may be collected by a natural procedure, a clean-voided (midstream) procedure, or a sterile procedure. A natural or random urine specimen may be tested for specific gravity, pH, or glucose level.[10] A clean-voided or midstream urine specimen is used to measure bacteriuria and to perform a culture and sensitivity.[10,11] Recent research indicates that perineal cleansing for midstream specimens with nonsterile wipes is as effective as sterile wipes.[12] A sterile specimen is collected from an indwelling catheter. Table 11-2 provides a step-by-step guide for collection of sterile urine specimens.

Special Considerations
Children and infants

Young children may be reluctant to urinate in unfamiliar containers and strange bathrooms. Special collection devices for young children and infants who cannot control urination are available. Plastic collecting devices with adhesive edges can be placed over a child's cleansed urethra.[10]

Indwelling catheters

Because bacteria grow rapidly in urinary drainage bags, a sterile needle and syringe should be used to collect a fresh specimen from the end of rubber, self-sealing catheter sample ports. Clean the catheter port with an antimicrobial swab before inserting the needle into the catheter.[10] Silastic, plastic, or silicone catheters cannot be punctured by needles. These catheters usually have a special port to remove urine specimens.[10]

Cultures

The growth of bacterial colonies from urine specimens is not measurable for the first 24 hours. Identification of specific organisms takes 48 hours. Initial readings of white blood cells in the urine cannot be relied upon in women, because a large percentage of women have small numbers of white blood cells present in the urine most of the time.

Stool Specimens
Definition

Bowel contents can be readily collected and tested for blood, abnormal metabolic products, bacteria, viruses, ova, and parasites. Only a small amount of feces is required for most analyses—approximately 1 inch, or the size of a walnut. One ounce of a dilute, liquid stool should be collected for a specimen.[10] Table 11-3 provides a step-by-step guide for the collection of stool specimens.

Specific Considerations
Children and infants

Fecal specimens can be collected with a wooden spatula directly from the diaper of infants.

Ileostomy and colostomy

Fecal samples can be readily collected with temporary plastic ostomy bags.

Cultures

Once a specimen is collected as described in Table 11-3, a sterile swab can be inserted into the sample and then into the culture tube to obtain a fecal sample for culture.

Sputum Specimens
Definition

Sputum is comprised of secretions of the respiratory tract and can be confused with saliva and mucus from the oral cavity. It is important that the nurse hear the deep, productive cough behind the expectoration of sputum to be certain of obtaining the correct specimen. One to two teaspoons of sputum is sufficient for analysis. The common tests of sputum are culture and sensitivity, acid-fast bacillus, and cytology.[10] Table 11-4 provides a step-by-step guide for obtaining a sputum specimen.

Text continued on p. 195.

Table 11-3 Step-by-step guide for collection of stool specimens

Specimen	Infection Risk		Preparation for Collection	Procedure
	Patient	Health Care Workers		
Stool (bowel contents)	Gastroenteritis from self-contamination, e.g., transference of *E. coli* from the lower GI tract to the upper GI tract	Hand washing and gloves should be used for specimen procurement and handling to avoid hepatitis A, salmonella, shigella, and other bowel pathogens. HIV and hepatitis B and C risk is present if stool is bloody.	1. Verify any diet or medicinal restrictions before test. 2. Instruct patient to wash hands and to avoid cross-contamination from urine or menstrual flow. 3. Instruct patient to defecate in a specific collecting receptacle (bedpan, or device attached to toilet seat). 4. Wash hands after specimen collection.	1. Put on gloves. 2. Obtain specimen from patient. 3. Wearing gloves, use a wooden spatula and transfer 1 ounce or 1 inch of fecal material to the labeled specimen container. Wrap spatula in a paper towel before discarding. Be sure outside of specimen container does not become contaminated. 4. Remove gloves and wash hands.

Continued.

GI, gastrointestinal; *HIV,* human immunodeficiency virus.

Table 11-3   Step-by-step guide for collection of stool specimens—cont'd

Specimen	Infection Risk	Preparation for Collection	Procedure
Patient	Health Care Workers		5. Place specimen container in a plastic bag and send to laboratory. Refrigerate if "holding" or unable to send to laboratory. 6. Follow up includes charting any unusual symptoms encountered during defecation; use air freshener if needed.

Table 11-4 Step-by-step guide for collection of sputum specimens

Specimen	Infection Risk	Preparation for Collection	Procedure
Sputum	**Patient**	1. Collect in early morning when respiratory secretions have accumulated during sleep.	1. Ask patient to cough productively and to expectorate directly into the container.
	Potential risk if suctioning required	2. Instruct patients not to brush their teeth because it can alter the bacteria present.	2. Cover container immediately to prevent release of airborne or droplet pathogens.
	Health Care Workers	3. Instruct patient to do deep breathing.	3. Wash outside of container with soap and water and dry with paper towel before placing in plastic bag.
	Use airborne precautions (see Chapter 7). Wear an approved respirator, protective eye wear, and gloves.	4. Positioning, postural drainage, and percussion may be needed to assist the patient to produce the sputum.	4. Send specimen immediately to laboratory or refrigerate.
	Airborne organisms such as mycobacterium can spread during sputum induction caused by coughing.		5. Provide mouth care to patient.
	All cough-producing procedures by patients who may have TB		*Continued.*

TB, tuberculosis.

Table 11-4 Step-by-step guide for collection of sputum specimens—cont'd

Specimen	Infection Risk	Preparation for Collection	Procedure
Patient	Health Care Workers	5. Instruct patient to avoid touching the inside of the sputum container.	
	should be performed using local exhaust ventilation devices (e.g., booths or special enclosures) or if that is not feasible, in a room that meets ventilation requirements for TB isolation.*		

*From Centers for Disease Control: Guidelines for preventing the transmission of tuberculosis in health-care facilities, 1994, *Federal Register* 59(208):54242, 1994.

Specific Considerations

Children

The nurse will need to position and percuss children who are unable to produce sputum with a cough.

Infants

Infants who lack mature cough reflexes will likely require suctioning to obtain a sputum specimen.

Tracheostomy

Patients with fresh tracheostomies will require suctioning to obtain sputum specimens.

Cultures

Sputum samples for culture are derived directly from the container in the laboratory. Once the specimen is obtained, it should be transferred to the laboratory immediately.

Elderly patients

Many elderly persons cannot produce an effective cough in a standing or semi-Fowler's position and cannot tolerate normal head-down postural drainage positions. These patients must be supported carefully by over-bed tables and pillows in modified positions to accomplish a productive cough without undue fatigue. This may become a very slow process to be successful.

Surgical patients

Patients with incisions anywhere on the trunk require support of the incision while attempting to cough. The strongest support is provided by the nurse, who places a gloved hand firmly on each side of the incision while the patient coughs.

Neutropenic patients

If the patient is neutropenic, the condition must be indicated on the laboratory request so that laboratory personnel do not discard the specimen as inadequate (this may occur if there are no white blood cells in a sputum specimen).

Table 11-5 Step-by-step guide for collection of cerebral spinal fluid (CSF) Specimens

Specimen	Infection Risk		Preparation for Collection	Procedure
	Patient	Health Care Workers		
Cerebral spinal fluid	Contamination from needle inserted into the subarachnoid space with skin flora from their own skin or from organisms transferred by health care worker's skin, break in technique, or contaminated equipment	Standard precautions apply (gowns, gloves, masks, protective eye wear). (See Chapter 7.)	1. Obtain patient consent form. 2. Perform neurological assessment. 3. Have patient urinate before procedure. 4. Position patient in fetal position (knees and head brought forward). 5. Prepare sterile field.	1. Physician dons gloves, cleanses skin, and punctures site with sterile lumbar-puncture needle. 2. Once specimens are obtained, label and send to lab. 3. Cover puncture site with sterile dry dressing. 4. Keep patient flat for 8-24 hours to avoid headache. 5. Monitor neurological status for 24 hours.

Cerebral Spinal Fluid Specimens
Definition

Cerebrospinal fluid specimens are obtained during a lumbar puncture that is performed by a physician. Table 11-5 provides a step-by-step guide for collection of cerebral spinal fluid.

Specific Considerations

Children, infants, and neurologically impaired adult patients may require special restraint equipment, sedatives, and staff assistance. Protective face wear is necessary whenever there is potential risk of splash contamination, as might occur from a spinal tap of a patient with increased intracranial pressure.

Wound Specimens
Definition

Wound specimens should contain viable infective organisms, not the cellular exudate, slough, or debris from the healing process. Optimal samples of organisms should be obtained after a vigorous saline rinsing of the wound.[13,14] Table 11-6 provides a step-by-step guide for collection of wound specimens. In chronic wounds, loose necrotic slough should be debrided before a culture specimen is obtained. Viable infective organisms are likely located in highly vascular tissue rather than in wound debris.[15]

Specific Considerations

Because wounds are contaminated by multiple normal skin flora, it is often difficult to interpret the results of wound cultures with a clinical assessment of the wound. The standard of 10^5 colony forming units per gram of tissue for a specific organism is based on the premise that wound healing is severely compromised when the number of organisms exceeds this level. However, β-*hemolytic streptococcus* impairs healing below this level.[14] Laboratory personnel need to know the type and site of specimen collected and any topical or systemic skin treatment.[15]

Aspiration cultures are commonly used with closed wounds or abscesses. Tissue biopsies with specific laboratory processing and quantitative analyses of organisms are more likely performed during surgical procedures.[15] Swab cultures are obtained with a

Table 11-6 Step-by-step guide for collection of wound specimens

Specimen	Infection Risk		Preparation for Collection	Procedure
	Patient	Health Care Workers		
Wounds	Contamination of a swab inserted into the wound with skin flora from their own skin or from organisms transferred by health care worker's skin, break in technique, or contaminated equipment	Standard precautions are recommended (gloves are always indicated; masks and eyewear are needed if irrigation is performed). (See Chapter 7.)	1. Wash hands. 2. Put on protective equipment. 3. Cleanse wounds of superficial debris with normal saline.	1. See Figure 11-1 for appropriate swab technique. 2. Swab with sterile applicator in rotary and clockwise fashion. 3. Scrape ulcer base or deep section of wound with sterile curette after debriding any superficial exudate. 4. If anaerobic culture is needed, insert immediately into sterile collecting tubes. Do not refrigerate anaerobic cultures.

5. Collect a minimum of 0.25 cc specimen.
6. Place culture tubes in plastic bag.
7. Remove protective equipment.
8. Wash hands.
9. Transfer specimen to laboratory within 12 hours.

Culturing Technique

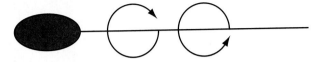

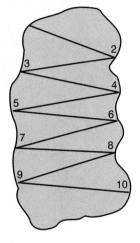

- Thoroughly rinse wound with sterile saline before culturing

- Do not use pus to culture

- Do not swab over hard eschar

- Use sterile Ca Alginate swab or rayon (not cotton) swab

- Rotate swab

- Swab wound edges and 10-pt coverage

Figure 11-1.
Culturing technique.
(From Alvarez O, Rozint J, Meehan M: Principles of moist wound healing: indications for chronic wounds. In Krasner D, editor: *Chronic wound care: a clinical source book for healthcare professionals,* King of Prussia, Pa, 1990, Health Management Publications.)

calcium alginate swab and transport medium. Swab cultures should not be obtained on dry skin surfaces because this yields only skin contaminants.[15] Figure 11-1 shows the culturing technique.

Summary

By following these strategies for the collection of blood and body fluids, nurses protect both themselves and their patients from infection risk. Nurses also ensure that quality specimens are collected for the diagnosis and treatment of patients.

References

1. Thrasher SB: What I didn't know really hurt me, *RN* 52:49, 1989.
2. Bardewick AM, Johnson JE: Preference for information and involvement, information seeking and emotional response of women undergoing colposcopy, *Res Nurs Health* 13(1):1,1990.
3. Hellgren U et al: Local anaesthetic cream for the alleviation of pain during venepuncture in Tanzanian schoolchildren, *Br J Clin Pharmacol* 28:205, 1989.
4. Weinstein SM: *Plumer's principles and practices of intravenous therapy,* ed 5, Philadelphia, 1993, JB Lippincott.
5. Meites S: Skin-puncture and blood-collecting technique for infants: update and problems, *Clin Chem* 34(9):1890, 1988.
6. Carlson KK et al: Obtaining reliable plasma sodium and glucose determinations from pulmonary artery catheters, *Heart Lung* 19(6): 613, 1990.
7. Tiffin J, Jacobs P: The Dracula factor—red cell loss due to repeated blood sampling, *S Am Med J* 79:627, 1991.
8. Douard MC et al: Quantitative blood cultures for diagnosis and management of catheter-related sepsis in pediatric hematology and oncology patients, *Intensive Care Med* 17:17, 1991.
9. Isaacman DJ, Karasic RB: Lack of effect of changing needles on contamination of blood cultures, *Pediatr Infect Dis J* 9(4):274, 1990.
10. Potter PA, Perry AG, editors: *Fundamentals of nursing: concepts, process and practice,* ed 3, St Louis, 1993, Mosby.
11. Brown J, Meikle J, Webb C: Collecting midstream specimens of urine—the research base, *Nurs Times* 87(13):49, 1991.
12. Jones E: In search of a fine specimen, *Nurs Times* 88(6):62, 1992.
13. Alvarez O, Rozint J, Meehan M: Principles of moist wound healing: indications for chronic wounds. In Krasner D, editor: *Chronic wound care: a clinical source book for healthcare professionals,* King of Prussia, Pa, 1990, Health Management Publications.
14. Doughty DB: Principles of wound healing and wound management. In Bryant RA, editor: *Acute and chronic wounds: nursing management,* St Louis, 1992, Mosby.
15. Cuzzell JZ: The right way to culture a wound, *Am J Nurs* 93(5):48, 1993.

The Immuno-compromised Patient

12

The purpose of this chapter is to provide nurses with succinct guidelines for management of the immunocompromised patient at risk for infection. A brief discussion of conditions that interfere with immune function, identification of individuals at highest risk for the development of sequelae resulting from immune dysfunction, description of standards of care for the immunocompromised patient, and integration of relevant research findings are described. The Oncology Nursing Society's Outcome Standards for Cancer Nursing Practice provide a general framework for organizing approaches to the care of immunocompromised patients.[1] Discussion of the immune system is beyond the scope of this chapter; see Chapter 5.

A competent human immune system protects the body from a variety of microorganisms and malignant growths.[2] A wide range of opportunistic infections and tumors may occur when the immune system is compromised. Nurses need to understand the underlying causes of immune dysfunction and disease states that cause or contribute to illness in the affected individual. Nurses also must be cognizant of patient and environmental variables that contribute to an increased risk of infection. These variables may include treatments, procedures, or factors related to the patient's medical condition. The degree of immunosuppression is directly related to the type and aggressiveness of treatment.[3] For example, a patient receiving adjuvant chemotherapy is less likely to be as severely immunosuppressed as an individual receiving high dose ablative chemotherapy for bone marrow transplantation. Therefore nurses must be equipped to readily and thoroughly assess each individual and to plan appropriate intervention strategies designed to minimize the potential risk of infection to an immunocompromised patient.

Terminology

The terms *immunosuppression* and *immunocompromise* are frequently used interchangeably to refer to an individual whose immune system function is decreased. However, the two terms are not synonymous. The box below presents definitions of terms used in this chapter. The box on pp. 204-205 presents categories of immune deficiency disorders so that care providers may identify the many sources of immunosuppression in patients and understand when to institute measures that protect immunocompromised patients.

Definition of Terms

Immunosuppression is an artificial reduction of immune response that involves the suppression of the production of antibodies or sensitization of lymphocytes, for example, giving drugs to prevent transplant rejection.

Immunocompromise refers to a state in which the individual is at an increased risk for infection as a result of an ineffective host state. The individual who is immunosuppressed often is also immunocompromised.

Immunocompetence refers to the ability to mount an immune response.

Opportunistic infections are infections caused by microbes that cannot be defeated by a weakened immune system. Examples include tuberculosis, candidiasis, *P. carinii* pneumonia, and cytomegalovirus.

Opportunistic tumors are tumors that may develop when the immune system is suppressed. Examples include Kaposi's sarcoma, non-Hodgkin's lymphoma, and lymphoma.

From Hotter AN: Wound healing and immunocompromise, *Nurs Clin North Am* 25(1):193, 1990; Schindler LW: Understanding the immune system, National Cancer Institute & National Institute of Allergy and Infectious Diseases, NIH Publication No 88-529, U.S. Department of Health and Human Services/PHS/NIH, 1988; Bartlett JG, Finkbeiner AK: *The guide to living with HIV infection*, Baltimore, 1991, Johns Hopkins University Press.

Immune Deficiency Disorders

Primary Immunodeficiency Disorders

Immunodeficiency disorders associated with B cells or antibody

- X-linked infantile agammaglobulinemia
- Transient hypogammaglobulinemia
- Common variable hypogammaglobulinemia (e.g., autoimmune diseases such as hemolytic anemia and systemic lupus erythematosus)
- Selective immunoglobulin disorders (e.g., IgA deficiency)

Immunodeficiency disorders associated with T cells and cell-mediated immunity

- Congenital thymic aplasia (e.g., DiGeorge Syndrome)

Secondary Immunodeficiency Diseases

Diseases in which the immune dysfunction is secondary to other diseases

- Loss of T or B lymphocytes from leukemia or other malignant disorders
- Tumor invasion of bone marrow
- Sequelae from surgery, trauma, anesthesia, burns; result of chronic diseases such as diabetes, renal failure, cirrhosis

Treatment of cancer

- Chemotherapeutic agents
- Radiation therapy
- Bone marrow transplant

Organ transplantation or graft vs. host disease
Other factors

Acquired Immunodeficiency Syndrome (AIDS)

Human immunodeficiency virus–related diseases

- Reduction of CD4$^+$ helper lymphocyte cells and functional impairment

Severe combined immunodeficiency disease (SCID)

- Heterogeneous group of immune disorders in which stem cells fail to differentiate into T or B cells (high susceptibility to any type of microbial infection)

Phagocytic dysfunctions

- Deficiency of antibodies, complement components or lymphokines or defects in phagocytic cell metabolic pathways (e.g., Chediak-Higashi syndrome and chronic granulomatous diseases)

Diseases caused by abnormalities in complement system

- May result in recurrent bacterial infections and increased susceptibility to autoimmune diseases

- Age
- Stress
- Malnutrition
- Radiation exposure

Modified from Benjamini E, Leskowitz S: *Immunology: a short course,* ed 2, New York, 1991, Wiley-Liss; Lewis SM, Collier IC: *Medical-surgical nursing: assessment and management of clinical problems,* St Louis, 1992, Mosby.

Specific Infection Risks

Individuals who are immunocompromised from any of the listed immune deficiency disorders are at an increased risk of developing infection because their impaired immune system does not provide adequate protection against invading microorganisms (bacteria, viruses, fungi). Normal mechanical defense mechanisms may be affected (respiratory, gastrointestinal systems). Body flora that are normally harmless (such as *Candida*) may become pathogenic and may become a source of infection for immunocomprised patients.

Additional risk factors for patients who already are immuno-compromised include physiological and psychological health status, age, existence of comorbid conditions, invasive procedures (e.g., venous access), and treatments (e.g., chemotherapy, radiation therapy, bone marrow transplantation, and complementary therapy). The weakened immune system can cause the individual to be susceptible to common everyday infections, such as influenza and *Staphylococcus aureus,* as well as the more exotic organisms, such as histoplasmosis and toxoplasmosis.

Standards of Nursing Care for Immunocompromised Patients

Infection and sepsis are the primary causes of morbidity and mortality among immunocompromised persons.[4] Accurate and rapid assessment of the client is essential to ensure correct diagnosis and appropriate intervention. The Oncology Nursing Society's Outcome Standards enable nurses to assess both potential and real problems of client management and include concepts relevant to health promotion and disease prevention. The standards for prevention and early detection, protection, nutrition, and potential for physiological alterations are of prime consideration for the immunocompromised patient. Factors such as client age, underlying disease and comorbid conditions, psychosocial and demographic variables, need for spirituality, and ability to carry out daily living activities may influence nurses' assessments and decisions concerning intervention strategies designed to contribute to client well-being. The importance of recognizing the influence of these factors to total client well-being is assumed to be incorporated into any nursing assessment. Therefore specific intervention strategies are discussed only for those standards as they relate to the client's

Text continued on p. 213.

Table 12-1 Standards of nursing care for immunocompromised individuals

Standards of Care	Clinical Manifestations	Risk Factors and Infection Potential	Intervention Strategies	Expected Outcomes
Prevention and Early Detection				
Identification of risk groups and factors for disseminated infection and sepsis	**Risk Groups** ■ HIV-related illness ■ Bone marrow transplant ■ Hematologic malignancy ■ Older age ■ Cancer ■ Drug-induced suppression ■ Radiation therapy	Knowledge deficit related to lack of information concerning health maintenance and prevention of infection Potential for multisystem infectious complications	See box on home care infection prevention Monitor vital signs as appropriate to condition Observe for minor temperature elevations	Patient is free of infectious complications. Patient, family, and HCW have sufficient information to be knowledgeable of risk factors for infection. Client, family, and HCW implement appropriate preventive strategies (see box on p. 216).

Compiled from the following sources: Buschel PC: Managing infections in the neutropenic oncology patient, *Proceedings of the Sixth National Conference on Cancer Nursing,* American Cancer Society publication 4503.02-PE, 1992; Workman ML, Ellerhorst-Ryan J, Hargrave-Koertge V: *Nursing care of the immunocompromised patient,* Philadelphia, 1993, WB Saunders; Ezzone S, Camp-Sorrell D: *Manual for bone marrow transplant nursing: recommendations for practice and education,* Pittsburgh, 1994, Oncology Nursing Press.

HIV, human immunodeficiency virus; *HCW,* health care worker; *IV,* intravenous.

Continued.

Table 12-1 Standards of nursing care for immunocompromised individuals—cont'd

Standards of Care	Clinical Manifestations	Risk Factors and Infection Potential	Intervention Strategies	Expected Outcomes
	Clinical Manifestations Opportunistic infections (tuberculosis, candidiasis, pneumocystis pneumonia, cytomegalovirus) Opportunistic tumors (Kaposi's sarcoma, lymphoma)			Patient seeks early intervention Patient adopts and maintains a healthy lifestyle (see Table 12-3).
Protection from Infection Immune system	Neutrophil count below 1000/mm^3; fever, subtle signs and symptoms not easily identified with pathologic condition (e.g., a general malaise; diaphoresis; night sweats, fatigue)	Potential for multibody system infection (e.g., respiratory [pneumonia], blood [septicemial], genitourinary, gastrointestinal, skin,	Careful inspection of any access site Blood cultures of venous access sites when indicated Institution of appropriate empiric therapy as soon as	Patient remains free of systemic infection. Patient and family describe early signs and symptoms of neutropenic infection.

soft tissue, and mucous membrane) Potential for endogenous infection (normal flora becomes pathogenic)	cultures drawn Avoid contact with persons with communicable diseases such as influenza Institute neutropenia precautions for neutrophil counts below 500 mm^3 (screen visitors for communicable diseases, assess oral mucosa daily, provide meticulous skin and mouth care, avoid unnecessary invasive procedures) Monitor vital signs and other basic needs (e.g., nutrition, elimination)	Patient maintains normal physiologic needs for nutrition, elimination, and other bodily functions. Maintain comfort, mobility, and safety as appropriate to condition.

Continued.

Table 12-1   Standards of nursing care for immunocompromised individuals—cont'd

Standards of Care	Clinical Manifestations	Risk Factors and Infection Potential	Intervention Strategies	Expected Outcomes
Integumentary system	Pain, urticaria, rashes, fever, redness, swelling	Potential for skin infection from disease process or venous or urinary access devices Normal flora becomes pathogenic	Monitor skin and oral mucosa Encourage fluids Catheter care (see Chapter 14) Nasogastric tube care (see Chapter 18) IV site care (see Chapter 17)	Patient remains free of skin infection. Patient describes clinical manifestations of alteration of skin integrity.
Nutrition	Weight loss Poor hydration and diet intake Loss of skin turgor and muscle tone Myalgia	Potential for malnutrition Increased risk for infection from contaminated food Decreased mobility Dehydration Decreased skin integrity	Monitor weight Nutrition consultation Encourage adequate food and fluid intake Cook all foods thoroughly Wash or peel all fresh fruits and vegetables	Patient will maintain sufficient food and fluid intake. Patient eats balanced diet. Patient maintains adequate weight.

Elimination	Alteration in elimination (e.g., nausea, diarrhea, constipation, urinary disturbances)	Decreased gastrointestinal motility Decreased mucous membrane integrity Skin breakdown Dehydration Urinary catheterization	Measure intake and output Monitor signs and symptoms of dehydration (e.g., decreased urinary output and specific gravity, increased serum sodium, increased heart rate, decreased skin turgor, dry mucous membranes) Educate patient and family concerning community resources	Patient maintains normal patterns of elimination.

Continued.

Table 12-1   Standards of nursing care for immunocompromised individuals—cont'd

Standards of Care	Clinical Manifestations	Risk Factors and Infection Potential	Intervention Strategies	Expected Outcomes
			Encourage fluids, fiber, and exercise Administer antidiarrheal medications or stool softeners as indicated Provide skin and oral care	
Physiological functioning	Signs and symptoms related to affected circulatory system	Potential alteration in pulmonary or cardiovascular systems	Monitor vital signs Assess lungs and cyanosis Monitor laboratory data	Patient maintains optimal physiologic patterns. Patient and family are knowledgeable about potential risk factors.

potential risk for infection. Table 12-1 presents selected standards of care, lists clinical manifestations and risk factors, identifies potential patient care issues or problems, suggests intervention strategies, and lists expected outcomes.

Infection Prevention

Hospitalized patients are at increased risk for the development of nosocomial infections. Risk of these infections can be markedly reduced through practice of simple intervention strategies. Table 12-2 suggests methods designed to reduce the risk of nosocomial infection for the immunocompromised patient.

Home Care Considerations

With changes in the health care system, it is increasingly likely that patients who are immunocompromised will be cared for in the home setting. It is important that the patient and family members learn strategies to prevent infection in the patient and prevent transmission of infection to family members. For the patient, maintaining nutrition, skin care, and oral hygiene and avoiding persons with respiratory infections are important strategies. For the family, learning methods for household disinfection and safe disposal of wastes, including disposal of needles and other sharp objects, is critical (see box on p. 216).

Standard Precautions in the Home

Standard precautions must be used at all times (see Chapter 7). In some home situations, running water may be unavailable. An alcohol hand rinse or commercial solution for hand cleaning should be used. A referral for adequate housing for clients should be made if the home is grossly inadequate or unsafe. The use of disposable, single-use examination gloves is required when working with body fluids. Gowns, masks, and protective eye wear are not needed unless there is copious drainage or excessive secretions when suctioning.

Text continued on p. 223.

Table 12-2 Methods to reduce the risk of nosocomial infection

Procedure	Precautionary Measure
Direct Patient Contact	
General patient contact	Do a 10-second hand wash before and after patient contact. OSHA-approved particulate respirator required if client has active tuberculosis.
Handling blood or body fluids	Wear gloves and remove immediately after tasks involving contact with blood or body fluids. Wash hands after glove removal.
Likelihood of soiling clothes or arms	Wear a fluid-resistant gown or apron; discard or launder after use.
Likelihood of splash to the face	Wear a mask and protective eyewear.
Phlebotomy, insertion of intravenous catheter	Wear gloves; do not recap, bend, or cut needle; discard needles and sharps in a puncture-resistant container located at point of use.
Arterial puncture or cannulation	Wear gloves, mask, and protective eyewear.

Handling of Soiled Linen and Disposable Equipment	Blood or body fluid contaminated linen and disposable equipment should be marked as such and handled or disposed of in accordance with OSHA guidelines.
Handling of Reusable Equipment and Devices	
Device that enters the bloodstream or normally sterile body cavity	Wash thoroughly and sterilize (see Chapter 9).
Device that touches intact mucosa but does not penetrate sterile body cavities	Wash thoroughly and use an intermediate level or high level disinfectant, depending on equipment (see Chapter 9).
Device that touches only intact skin	Clean with soap and water. Use a low level disinfectant (see Chapter 9).

Modified from Libman H, Witzburg RA: *HIV infection: a clinical manual,* Boston, 1993, Little, Brown.

OSHA, The Occupational Safety and Health Administration.

Infection Prevention in Home Care Settings

Avoidance of Needlestick or Sharp Object Injury

- Place needles/sharps in a labeled, puncture proof, non-breakable container with a closed lid (e.g., bleach bottle, plastic soda bottle, or coffee can).
- Keep away from children.
- When containers are full, fill with 1:10 dilution of household bleach.
  - Seal lid with tape.
  - Place in paper bag.
  - Place directly in garbage on day of pickup.*

Avoidance of Potentially Infectious Materials

- Place dressings, bandages, and contaminated tissues in a plastic, leakproof bag.*
- Dispose of feces, urine, sputum, and vomitus into the toilet and flush. Do not discard in sink or garbage. Be aware of potential for splashing.
- Ordinary soiled laundry does not have to be washed separately. Add 1 cup of bleach with detergent to washing machine if linen is soiled with blood or body fluids. Use a cold-water rinse followed by a hot-water wash with bleach.
- Wear household rubber gloves for cleaning surfaces contaminated with body fluids. Intact household gloves can be reused if they are washed with soap and water, rinsed in a 1:10 dilution of household bleach, and hung to dry.
- Wash contaminated surfaces with soap and water and a 1:10 dilution of household bleach. Take special care to rinse toys well to remove disinfectant.

* In disposing contaminated sharps or needles and waste material, check with the local Health Department for specific regulations.

Table 12-3 Health maintenance suggestions for patients

Health Factors	Self-Care Actions	Rationale
Physical and dental examinations	Seek early medical and dental treatment.	Prompt care may maintain health.
	Inform the HC team of your immune status.	Treatment may need to be adjusted accordingly.
	Do not accept vaccinations without the advice of your HC team.	Live virus may promote illness.
	Report any change in health status as soon as possible.	Early intervention may decrease sequelae.
Skin care	Shower daily. Avoid tub baths.	Decrease secondary infections from one part of the body to another.
	Use mild soap or emollient cream.	Harsh skin products may cause dryness.
	Observe cuts and abrasions for healing.	Health maintenance.
Hair care	Wash hair gently.	Gentle hair care may inhibit hair loss.
	Use mild soap and conditioner.	
	Avoid drying sprays and gels.	
	Cover head while in bed.	
	Comb hair, do not brush.	

From Flaskerud JH, Ungvarski PJ: *HIV/AIDS: a guide to nursing care*, Philadelphia, 1992, WB Saunders; Durham JD, Cohen FL: *The person with AIDS: nursing perspectives*, New York, 1991, Springer.

HC, health care; *HIV*, human immunodeficiency virus; *HBV*, hepatitis B virus.

Continued.

Table 12-3 Health maintenance suggestions for patients—cont'd

Health Factors	Self-Care Actions	Rationale
Mouth care	Use nonabrasive toothpaste. Brush tooth surface only (avoid gums). Use soft toothettes for gum care. Perform mouth care at least three times a day.	Limit secondary infection. Avoid gingival bleeding.
Environmental cleaning and safety	Clean body fluid contaminated surfaces with daily prepared bleach solution (5.25% sodium hypochlorite) diluted 1:10 with water. Use full-strength bleach in laundry for body fluid soiled linen. Throw used needles and sharps in proper container; use plastic bags to contain wetness when discarding items soiled with body fluids.	Kills bacteria and viruses (e.g., HIV, HBV). Guarantees safe disposal of contaminated waste.
Pet care	Assign pet care to nonimmunocompromised person. Wash hands after handling pet.	Microorganisms from pet excreta may be harmful (e.g., litter boxes, cages, aquariums).
Sexual practices	A healthy sexual relationship is beneficial. Learn and incorporate safe sexual practice.	Safe sexual expression promotes emotional well being and inhibits disease transfer.

Procreation	Thorough consideration of the risks versus the benefits of pregnancy should be explored with the HC team.	Medications and treatment may be harmful to the fetus; the risk of perinatal transfer of HIV is approximately 25%.
Intravenous drug use	Attempt drug treatment. Use sterile works whenever possible; to clean needles, use full strength bleach then rinse with water before using; if using in a group, you go first.	Decrease the incidence of secondary infection and transmission. Use of harm reduction techniques may have a positive effect on health.
Hand washing	Frequently wash hands with warm water and soap. Use soap pump dispenser. Rinse well. Apply emollient cream. Wear household rubber gloves when cleaning.	Proper hand washing may decrease incidence of infection and cross contamination.

Continued.

Table 12-3 Health maintenance suggestions for patients—cont'd

Health Factors	Self-Care Actions	Rationale
Nutrition	Keep kitchen clean. Wash hands before and after handling food. Scrupulously wash or peel fresh fruit and vegetables. Prepare fresh fruits and vegetables before handling raw meat, fish, and poultry. Always wash utensils and cutting boards used with raw meat, fish, and poultry with soap and water before using on uncooked foods. Eat high-protein and high-calorie diet (6 small meals a day).	Clean surfaces decrease microbe growth.

Prepare well-cooked meats, fish, poultry.

Do not thaw frozen foods to room temperature.

Use only pasteurized foods.

Do not use raw milk or raw cider.

Serve hot foods hot and cold foods cold.

Check expiration dates; when in doubt, throw it out.

Well-cooked, nutritious foods may increase strength and maintain health.

Complete cooking destroys bacteria and parasites.

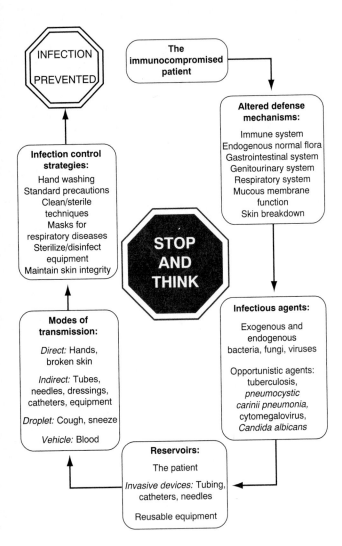

Figure 12-1.
Factors affecting the immunocompromised patient, leading
to the selection of the correct infection control strategies
to prevent infectious complications

Health Maintenance Strategies

Although the primary focus of this chapter is nursing care for the patient who requires direct care, it is also important to consider strategies to prevent infection in the immunocompromised individual whose self-care abilities are intact. Overall health maintenance strategies that may be taught to patients and families are listed in Table 12-3.

Summary

Although infection control strategies such as handwashing, standard precautions, and disinfection are important for all patients, they are especially critical for individuals whose immune systems are altered by primary immunodeficiency disorders, secondary immunodeficiency disorders, and human immunodeficiency virus infection. This chapter has presented strategies to prevent infection for immunocompromised individuals in hospital and home care settings as well as for those who are able to provide their own care. It is important for the nurse and other care providers to stop and think about altered defense mechanisms, infectious agents, reservoirs, modes of transmission, and infection control strategies to prevent infection in the immunocompromised individual (Figure 12-1).

References

1. Task Force to Develop Standards for Oncology Nursing Practice: *Standards of oncology nursing practice,* Kansas City, 1987, American Nurses Association.

2. Lewis SM, Collier IC: *Medical-surgical nursing: assessment and management of clinical problems,* St Louis, 1992, Mosby.

3. Buchsel PC: Managing infections in the neutropenic oncology patient, *Proceedings of the Sixth National Conference on Cancer Nursing,* American Cancer Society publication 4503.02-PE, (1992).

4. Workman ML, Ellerhorst-Ryan J, Hargrave-Koertge V: *Nursing care of the immunocompromised patient,* Philadelphia, 1993, WB Saunders.

Surgical Procedures

13

A major cause of morbidity and mortality among hospitalized surgical patients is nosocomial infection.[1] Medical and surgical patients may require devices such as chest tubes and tracheostomy tubes, which increase the patient's risk for acquiring an infection. Other procedures commonly performed on patients include thoracentesis, paracentesis, bone marrow biopsy, and endoscopy. Guidelines for infection control for all these procedures is described in this chapter.

Chest Tubes
Description

The insertion of a chest tube into a patient's chest removes air, fluid, or blood from the intrapleural space.[2] A chest tube is indicated in the case of a pneumothorax or hemothorax. Chest trauma, thoracic surgery, mechanical ventilation with barotrauma, or an iatrogenic pneumothorax caused by central line placement may create a need for a chest tube. Heart surgery often necessitates a mediastinal chest tube for draining blood.

Placement of the chest tube depends on the location of the patient's intrapleural problem; for example, the second intercostal space is appropriate for a pneumothorax, and typically the sixth to eighth intercostal space is used for a hemothorax. The chest tube is connected to a water seal drainage system.[3] The insertion procedure requires an aseptic technique. Surgical asepsis deters pathogens from coming into contact with a surgical wound. Chapter 10 discusses surgical aseptic techniques at length.

Two methods of chest tube insertion are the blunt-dissection method and trocar insertion.[2] Both require local anesthesia and a small skin incision. In the blunt-dissection method, the pleural space is penetrated by a forceps through a skin incision. An alternate method inserts a chest tube through a hollow trocar that penetrates the pleural space.[2]

Specific Infection Risks

To prevent the introduction of microorganisms into the patient's pleural cavity and the open wound, the procedure is done under aseptic technique. (See Chapter 10 for specific procedures.) Invasion of the skin, tissue, and lungs with tubes and trocars provides a pathway for microorganisms to enter and infect the patient. Chest tube sites and dressings provide areas for microbial growth as well.

For health care workers, there is a risk of contact with blood and secretions from the patient; therefore standard precautions must be followed. (See Chapter 7 for specific procedures.) Risks from sharps and trocars are minimized by careful handling and placement in appropriate puncture-resistant containers.

Preparation

Assemble a sterile chest tube tray containing the following equipment:

1. Two pairs of sterile gloves, gowns, and masks
2. Sterile drapes
3. Antiseptic skin prep and swabs (povidone-iodine)
4. Local anesthetic (1% lidocaine)
5. 1.25-inch, 18- to 20-gauge needle to draw up anesthetic
6. 5/8-inch 18- to 20-gauge needle to administer the anesthetic
7. 10-ml syringe
8. Scalpel with #11 blade
9. Alcohol wipes
10. Hemostat
11. Trocar
12. Forceps
13. Chest tube(s): sizes 16-24 or 28-36, depending on need
14. Thoracic drainage system with sterile connector and 6-foot drainage tubing
15. Suture material with cutting needle
16. Dressing materials — 4 × 4 gauze pads, petrolatum gauze, tape
17. Kelly clamps
18. Suction source

Procedure for Infection Prevention

Table 13-1 details the specific steps, rationale, and infection prevention strategies important in chest tube placement.[2]

Text continued on p. 231.

Table 13-1 Procedure for chest tube insertion

Steps	Rationale	Special Considerations
1. Wash hands.	Reduces transmission of microorganisms	
2. Open the chest tube tray using sterile technique.	Reduces transmission of microorganisms	
3. Assist the physician with preparation of the insertion site.	Inhibits the growth of bacteria at the insertion site	
a. Pour antiseptic solution into the basin using aseptic technique.	Used to saturate gauze pads for cleansing	
b. Wipe the top of the vial of local anesthetic with an alcohol swab.	Disinfects the surface of the vial	
c. Invert the vial so that the physician can withdraw the anesthetic solution into the syringe.	Maintains sterility	
4. Assist the physician with insertion of the chest tube.		Sterile procedure is performed by the physician; the nurse monitors and reassures the patient.
a. The physician infiltrates the insertion site with the anesthetic agent.	Results in loss of sensation and reduction of pain during insertion of the chest tube	

b. The physician makes a small incision at the insertion site, using a "tunnel" approach to dissect the subcutaneous tissue and intercostal muscle.

Admits the diameter of the chest tube

c. The physician perforates the pleura using a trocar.

Ensures that the opening is large enough for the chest tube and decreases the incidence of extrapleural positioning; relieves air and fluid

d. The physician advances the chest tube through the incision and into the pleural space.

Places the chest tube in the correct position

A trocar or hemostat may be used to facilitate insertion of the chest tube; listen for the return of a rush of air as it escapes, and observe an initial fogging of the chest tube on normal exhalation, which indicates proper placement.

Continued.

Modified from Boggs RL, Wooldridge-King M: *AACN procedure manual for critical care,* ed 3, Philadelphia, 1993, WB Saunders.

Table 13-1 Procedure for chest tube insertion—cont'd

Steps	Rationale	Special Considerations
5. Remove the adapter from the end of the 6-ft length of latex connecting tube, keeping the exposed end of the tube sterile and connected to the chest tube.	Maintains sterility and creates a closed system	Length of connecting tube must be sufficient to allow patient movement and to decrease the chance that a deep breath by the patient will draw chest drainage back into the pleural space. The chest drainage system should be placed below the level of the patient's chest to promote gravity drainage and to prevent backflow; if two chest tubes are placed, a Y connector may be used to join them to a single drainage system.
6. Tape all connection points in the chest drainage system.	Keeps the tubes together; prevents air leaks into the pleural space	Parham bands may be used to secure connections instead of tape.
a. One-inch tape is placed horizontally extending over connections (a portion of the connector	Secures connections but allows visualization of drainage	

may be left unobstructed by the tape).	
b. Reinforce the horizontal tape with tape placed vertically so that it encircles both ends of the connector.	Secures connections
7. Instruct the patient to take a deep breath and exhale slowly.	Facilitates drainage and reexpansion of the lung
8. Assist the physician with suturing the chest tube to the skin.	Prevents displacement of the chest tube; the skin next to the tube is sutured and the ends of the suture are wrapped around the tube, anchoring the tube to the chest wall
9. Apply occlusive dressing.	Provides for an airtight seal around the insertion site
a. Apply split drain sponges around the chest tube, one over the top and one from underneath the tube.	Creates an airtight system A petrolatum gauze may be wrapped around the tube close to the insertion site if the air leak is large; however, this may cause maceration of the skin.

Continued.

Table 13-1   Procedure for chest tube insertion—cont'd

Steps	Rationale	Special Considerations
b. Apply 2 to 3 gauze pads (4×4) on top of the split drain sponges.	Creates an airtight system	
c. Tape the dressing to the skin.	Secures the dressing	Determine that the patient is not allergic to the tape.
10. Tape the chest tube to the skin.	Prevents side-to-side movement and accidental dislodgment of the chest tube	
11. If prescribed turn on suction source. (Physician will determine the amount of suction necessary.)	Assists in pulling drainage from the pleural cavity	
12. Coil latex connecting tube and secure to sheet.	Drainage accumulating in dependent loops obstructs chest drainage into the collecting system	Allow enough length for patient movement.
13. Order a stat portable chest x-ray per physician instruction/protocol.	Verifies correct placement and position of the chest tube	
14. Dispose of equipment in appropriate receptacle.	Standard precautions	
15. Wash hands.	Reduces transmission of microorganisms	

Follow Up Assessment

Respiratory status should be assessed, and chest tube placement should immediately be checked by x-ray. Kinking of the chest tube should be prevented by carefully coiling the tubing on top of the bed and securing it to the bed linen, leaving room for the patient to turn. The patient should be evaluated frequently for signs of pneumothorax or subcutaneous emphysema. Integrity of the thoracic drainage system should be maintained.

Tracheostomy Care
Description

A tracheostomy is typically performed to allow a patent airway, long-term intubation, and mechanical ventilation or to effectively remove tracheobronchial secretions. The procedure is best done in the operating room under sterile conditions. At times the procedure is performed at the critically ill patient's bedside or in the emergency room, but even then, skilled operating room personnel including the physician, nurse, and anesthesiologist are recommended to be in attendance.[2] Surgical gowns, masks, and gloves are needed for this sterile procedure. Tracheostomy care maintains patency of the tube, cleans the stoma site, and prevents infection.

Specific Infection Risks and Prevention Strategies

There is a risk of introducing microorganisms into the patient's trachea and lung when suctioning the tube, handling the inner cannula, and caring for the insertion site. In critically ill patients, invasive devices such as tracheostomy tubes increase the patient's vulnerability to nosocomial infection.[4-6] The tube bypasses the upper airway, decreasing the body's mechanical cleaning functions (i.e., cilia, mucous membranes, and cough, sneeze, gag reflexes). The tube also provides an open pathway into the lungs. Smoking, advanced age, and underlying disease are all considered potential risk factors for a patient undergoing a tracheostomy tube placement.

Contact with patient secretions occurs with a tracheostomy, so nurses should follow standard precautions. There is direct contact and potential splash secondary to expelled secretions with suctioning; therefore gown, mask, protective face wear, and gloves are needed.

Preparation

Collect a tracheostomy care kit or the following supplies:

1. Suction supplies
2. Mask and goggles
3. Two pairs of sterile gloves
4. Sterile normal saline solution
5. 3% hydrogen peroxide
6. Twill tape or tracheostomy ties
7. Prepackaged sterile tracheostomy dressing
8. Sterile cotton swabs
9. Sterile brush
10. Scissors
11. Sterile basin and towel

Procedure

1. Explain procedure to patient.
2. Wash hands. Aseptic technique for respiratory tract manipulations is imperative to prevent nosocomial infection.[6]
3. Remove old tracheostomy dressing. Wash hands.
4. Hyperoxygenate the lungs.
5. Put on gloves, and suction trachea using sterile technique.
6. Remove gloves. Wash hands.
7. Fill sterile solution container with 100 ml of 1:1 normal saline and 3% hydrogen peroxide.
8. Fill a second solution container with normal saline for rinsing.
9. Put on sterile gloves, and remove the inner cannula, placing it in the solution of hydrogen peroxide and normal saline.
10. Use the sterile brush to gently clean the inner cannula. (Disposable inner cannulae do not require this step.)
11. Rinse the inner cannula in normal saline and reinsert it into the tracheostomy tube.
12. Reconnect the oxygen source.
13. Gently clean around the stoma site with 4 × 4 gauze and swabs with 3% hydrogen peroxide. Wipe only once with each gauze or swab to prevent contamination.
14. Rinse with normal saline and dry.
15. Change tracheostomy ties by getting assistance from another staff member to avoid dislodging the tube.
16. Cut tracheostomy ties with scissors and replace ties using a square knot.
17. Apply dry (prepackaged) tracheostomy dressing under face

plate of tracheostomy. Do not cut a 4×4 gauze pad for use as a tracheostomy dressing because the edges fray and may provide a source for infection.[2]

18. Discard equipment in the appropriate receptacle to prevent transmission of microorganisms.

19. Wash hands.

Follow Up Assessment

The patient's respiratory and comfort status is assessed. Any signs of infection around the tracheal stoma are documented and reported.

Home Care Considerations

Patients who are discharged home with a tracheostomy or family members may be taught to use a nonsterile or clean technique in suctioning and caring for the tracheostomy. Supplies for tracheostomy care at home include a mirror, a clean bowl or basin, 3% hydrogen peroxide, warm tap water, 4×4 gauze sponges, cotton-tip swabs, and pipe cleaners. Wash hands before beginning the procedure. Pour 1/2 hydrogen peroxide and 1/2 warm tap water into a bowl. Unlock the inner cannula, and place it in the bowl. Remove the tracheostomy dressing. Moisten a swab with hydrogen peroxide, and clean the stoma and outer plate of the tracheostomy tube. Moisten a swab with warm water, and rinse the area. Apply a clean tracheostomy dressing. Scrub the inner cannula using a pipe cleaner folded in half, and rinse thoroughly with tap water. Dry the inner cannula with gauze, and reinsert and lock it in place.

Paracentesis
Description

Paracentesis removes fluid from the peritoneal cavity to relieve respiratory distress or discomfort from an elevated diaphragm. Fluid may also be removed for diagnostic purposes.

Specific Infection Risks and Infection Prevention Strategies

Microorganisms may enter the patient's peritoneal cavity if the procedure is not performed with sterile technique and sterile equipment. Potential contact with body fluids warrants the use of standard precautions for personnel.

Procedure Preparation

Gather the following equipment:

1. Sterile gloves
2. Povidone-iodine solution
3. Sterile towels or sterile drape
4. Local anesthetic
5. Sterile paracentesis tray containing a needle, trocar, cannula, and three-way stopcock
6. Sterile tubes for specimens
7. Syringes: two 10-cc syringes and two 50-cc syringes
8. Sterile 1-L collection bottle with connecting tubing
9. Suture material
10. Hemostat
11. Four to six sterile 4×4 gauze pads
12. Personal protective equipment as needed or anticipated[2,3]

Procedure

1. Position the patient upright so that fluid accumulates in the lower abdomen.
2. Explain the procedure, and ensure that the bladder is decompressed.
3. Wash hands.
4. Open the sterile paracentesis tray using aseptic technique.
5. After injecting the patient with a local anesthetic, the physician uses a scalpel to make a small incision before inserting the trocar or needle.
6. Attach a syringe or stopcock and tubing to withdraw peritoneal fluid.
7. Record the amount and characteristics of fluid, and send for analysis as appropriate.
8. Apply a sterile dressing to the wound site after closure.
9. Wash hands after disposing of all materials in appropriate containers.[2,3]

Follow Up Assessment

The patient should be observed for any signs of perforation of bowel or bladder or peritoneal fluid leak. Blood pressure and pulse, skin color, weight, and abdominal girth should be observed. The puncture site is checked for signs of infection.

Thoracentesis

Description

Thoracentesis withdraws fluid or air from the pleural space. Fluid may be removed for diagnostic or therapeutic purposes. Chemotherapeutic agents or other medications may be administered via a thoracentesis.[3]

Specific Infection Risks and Infection Prevention

Sterile technique and sterile equipment are required to prevent introducing microorganisms into the pleural space.

Contact with patient fluids necessitates the use of standard precautions.

Preparation

A thoracentesis tray that includes sterile gloves, sterile drapes, povidone-iodine solution, local anesthetic, 5-ml syringe with 21-gauge and 25-gauge needles for anesthetic injection, 17- gauge thoracentesis needle for aspiration, 50-ml syringe, three-way stopcock and tubing, sterile specimen containers, sterile hemostat, sterile 4 × 4 gauze pads, and drainage bottles is assembled.[3]

Procedure

The procedure is explained to the patient, and the person is placed in a sitting position, often with arms and head resting on an overbed table. The physician dons sterile gloves, cleans the site with an antiseptic solution, and administers the local anesthetic.[7] A syringe or stopcock is attached to the aspirating needle and is inserted into the pleural cavity through the intercostal space. A 50-ml syringe may be attached to the needle, and a hemostat may be used to hold the needle in place and prevent pleural tear or lung puncture; or, a teflon catheter may be introduced into the needle, the needle removed, and the fluid drained into a syringe or drainage tubing to prevent the risk of lung puncture.[3] After the fluid and needle are withdrawn, pressure is applied to the puncture site using a 4 × 4 gauze pad. A new sterile gauze pad is applied and taped in place.

Follow Up Assessment

The patient's blood pressure, pulse, respiration rate, and skin color are monitored. The site is checked for fluid leak.

Bone Marrow Biopsy

Description

A bone marrow biopsy is the removal of a specimen of bone marrow to allow diagnosis of abnormal blood cell development.[7]

Specific Infection Risks

Bone marrow biopsy carries a risk of infection to the bone. Sterile technique and equipment are required.

The risk of contact with the patient's blood and body fluids is decreased with the use of standard precautions.

Preparation

Assemble a bone marrow biopsy tray containing the following:

1. Sterile drapes
2. Antiseptic to clean skin
3. Local anesthetic
4. Ten 4×4 gauze pads and 2×2 gauze pads
5. Two 12 ml syringes
6. 22-gauge 1-inch or 2-inch needle
7. A scalpel
8. A sedative
9. Specimen containers
10. Bone marrow needle
11. 70% isopropyl alcohol
12. 1% lidocaine
13. Adhesive tape
14. Sterile gloves
15. Glass slides for the specimen[3,7]

Procedure for Infection Prevention

1. Explain the procedure to the patient, and administer the sedative as ordered.
2. Position the patient for appropriate site: sternum or posterior superior or anterior iliac crest.
3. Using sterile technique, cleanse and drape the site.
4. The site is anesthetized down to the periosteum in a circular motion, withdrawing the needle each time.
5. After the anesthetic takes effect, a scalpel may be used to make a small stab incision to accommodate the bone marrow needle.

This helps reduce infection risk by avoiding pushing skin into the bone marrow.

6. The biopsy needle is directed into the bone marrow cavity, and a plug of tissue is removed.

7. The nurse puts on gloves, cleanses the area around the site with alcohol to remove the povidone-iodine solution, and exerts firm pressure with a sterile 2×2 gauze pad to control bleeding. The nurse then applies a dry sterile dressing.[3]

Follow Up Assessment

The site is assessed for bleeding and infection. Analgesics are provided if needed to control site pain.

Endoscopy
Description

Endoscopy is a category of diagnostic procedures that permits direct visualization of hollow organs. Fiberoptic endoscopes are flexible, easily maneuvered, and used to investigate certain body interiors such as the gastrointestinal (GI), genitourinary (GU), or respiratory tracts.[7] Bronchoscopy procedures are used to examine the lungs. Esophagogastroduodenoscopy procedures are used to examine the esophagus, stomach, and duodenum, respectively, and are considered clean procedures. The latter procedure permits diagnosis, biopsies, and coagulation of bleeding. Colonoscopy and sigmoidoscopy of the lower GI tract are increasingly common procedures, especially in ambulatory care settings.

Specific Infection Risks and Infection Prevention

When there is a risk of contamination of sterile body cavities with microorganisms, as in a bronchoscopy and cystoscopy, sterile technique is required. This risk is not the same for the GI and upper respiratory tract, and clean technique is recommended. However, data suggest that manually disinfected endoscopes and automated disinfection methods do not consistently eliminate all bacteria, missing specifically nontuberculous mycobacteria or coliform bacteria.[8] There have been sporadic outbreaks of infections related to inadequately disinfected endoscopes. Recent guidelines on infection prevention for flexible endoscopy provide specific information from experts to limit infection risks to patients.[9]

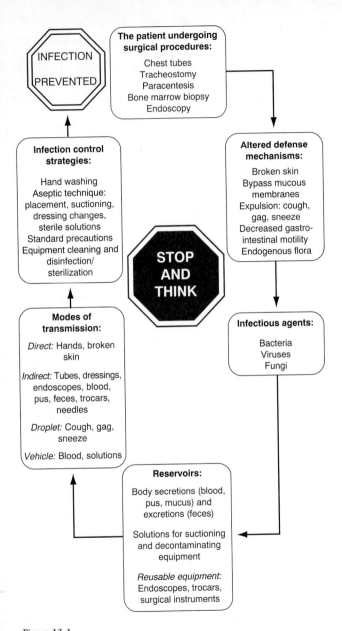

Figure 13-1.
Factors affecting the patient undergoing surgical procedures,
leading to the selection of the correct infection control
strategies to prevent complications.

Standard precautions should be followed because of direct contact with blood or body fluids. (See Chapter 7 for specific guidelines.)

Preparation

Preparation for an endoscopy depends on the specific site being visualized. For example, a sterile bronchoscopy tray is necessary to view the lung. Each endoscopy procedure follows specific guidelines for equipment and care. Several GI endoscopic procedures require nothing by mouth status for the patient or a bowel cleansing regimen. These procedures include esophagogastroduodenoscopy and colonoscopy, among others.

Procedure

After explaining the procedure and preparation to the patient, the nurse may give the patient a sedative, depending on the specific procedure. Guidelines for precise procedures to be followed depend on the endoscopic examination.

Follow Up Assessment

Blood pressure, pulse, and respiratory rate are monitored after the procedure. The site is checked for bleeding. If a sedative was given, the level of consciousness is monitored and the nurse ensures that the airway is patent.

Summary

All of these procedures directly invade the body and provide direct access to normally sterile body cavities. Normal body defense mechanisms and cleansing functions may be totally bypassed, such as in a tracheostomy. Invasive devices play an important role in providing access for microorganisms. Figure 13-1 summarizes the risk factors and prevention strategies for surgical procedures.

References

1. Horan T et al: The National Nosocomial Infections Surveillance (NNIS) system: nosocomial infections in surgical patients in the United States, January 1986-June 1992, *Infect Control Hosp Epidemiol* 14:73, 1993.
2. Boggs RL, Wooldridge-King M: *AACN procedure manual for critical care*, ed 3, Philadelphia, 1993, WB Saunders.
3. *Nursing procedures, student version*, Springhouse, Pa, 1993, Springhouse Corporation.

4. Maki DG: Risk factors for nosocomial infection in intensive care, *Arch Intern Med* 149:30, 1989.

5. Martin MA: Nosocomial infections in intensive care units: an overview of their epidemiology, outcome, and prevention, *New Horizons* 1:162, 1993.

6. George DL: Epidemiology of nosocomial ventilator-associated pneumonia, *Infect Control Hosp Epidemiol* 14:163, 1993.

7. Kozier B, Erb G, Olivieri R: *Fundamentals of nursing: concepts, process and practice*, ed 4, Redwood City, Calif, 1991, Addison-Wesley.

8. Fraser VJ et al: A prospective randomized trial comparing manual and automated endoscope disinfection methods, *Infect Control Hosp Epidemiol* 14:383, 1993.

9. Martin MA, Reichelderfer M: APIC guideline for infection prevention and control in flexible endoscopy, *Am J Infect Control* 22:19, 1994.

Catheterization 14

Infection of the urinary tract is caused by microbial invasion of any portion of the urinary system: kidneys (pyelonephritis), bladder (cystitis), prostate (prostatitis), urethra (urethritis), or urine (bacteriuria). Once bacteria invade any portion, all other areas are at risk. Urinary tract instrumentation by a catheter increases the risk of infection.[1]

Catheterization of the urinary bladder carries a high risk of urinary tract infection (UTI) and is considered one of the leading causes of nosocomial infections. UTIs account for about 40% of all nosocomial infections reported by acute care hospitals per year. Approximately 10% of hospitalized patients are catheterized, providing a large population at risk for catheter-associated UTI.[2,3] Studies demonstrate that most nosocomial UTIs (66%-86%) follow urinary tract instrumentation, primarily urinary catheterization.[2] Some clinical indications for urinary catheterization are to completely empty the bladder; decompress it during surgery; prevent distention; relieve retention, distention, or pressure; measure residual urine; drain and irrigate; or instill medication.[3]

This chapter discusses indwelling, straight (intermittent), and condom catheterization procedures, their risk for infecting patients, and infection prevention strategies.

Specific Infection Risks

The ability to empty the bladder completely is one of the best defense mechanisms the body has to prevent UTIs. If the bladder empties completely during the voiding process, bacteria do not have an opportunity to invade tissue or to grow and multiply. The bladder itself has an intrinsic antibacterial capability. Some researchers believe that mucoprotein present on the mucosal surface of the bladder contributes to this defense mechanism.[1] Host factors that increase the risk of urinary infection include advanced age, general debilitation, female gender, the postpartum state, and meatal colonization by urinary pathogens.[2]

Except for the distal urethra, the urinary system is normally sterile. A urinary catheter bypasses the urinary clearing mechanism, introduces organisms from the urinary meatus or urethra, provides a route of entry for microorganisms, and may serve as a focus for infection.[2] Gram-negative organisms are commonly associated with UTIs. Found in the colon, they include *Escherichia coli, Klebsiella* organisms, *Enterobacter* organisms, group D *streptococci, Pseudomonas* species, and *Candida albicans.*[4] Risk of septicemia is increased when bacteria are present in urine at the time of instrumentation.[2]

There is a direct relationship between the method and duration of catheter use and the risks of infection. Long-term, indwelling catheterization is generally associated with a higher infection rate than is short-term, intermittent or condom catheterization.[1-3]

Procedure Risks

1. Trauma during instrumentation
2. Improper or inadequate meatal site care
3. Trauma to the meatus or urethra or contamination of the drainage system by inexperienced or unknowledgeable personnel
4. Faulty aseptic technique allowing pathogenic organisms into the bladder during catheter insertion
5. Forceful catheter introduction or incorrect catheter size causing trauma to the urethral mucosa (also for male subjects, trauma from catheter introduction at an incorrect angle or forceful introduction through a stricture)
6. Transfer of organisms on the hands of personnel[2,3]

Indwelling Catheter Risks

1. Movement of the catheter in and out of the urethra causing friction, irritation, and tissue trauma at the meatal orifice (from bacteria on the catheter's exterior surface that gain access into the bladder or from secretions from the trauma site that provide a growth medium for organisms that have colonized the site)
2. Contamination of a bag's drainage port with hands, urinometers, or urine measuring containers
3. Disconnection of the catheter from drainage tubing for sampling or irrigation

4. If the catheter is taped to the leg of a male, development of a fistula at the penoscrotal junction
5. Backflow of contaminated urine from the drainage bag if the bag is raised above the level of the bladder
6. Kinked or obstructed tubing interfering with urine flow and causing stasis
7. Accumulation of exudate, feces, or encrustation around an indwelling catheter causing irritation or enhancing bacterial growth[1,2]

Straight and Intermittent Catheter Risks

There is less risk with straight and intermittent catheterization than with indwelling catheterization. As with any invasive procedure, improper technique causes risk. Failure to catheterize as necessary can cause distention, which, if greater than 500 ml may lead to tissue trauma and bacterial invasion.[2]

Condom Catheter Risks

Condom catheters also can cause UTIs. Risk is reduced because the patient is not instrumented. However, tissue excoriation can occur when the nurse removes the tape, if the catheter is not changed every 24 hours and if the penis is not dried thoroughly before applying the catheter. If an inelastic or rigid fastening system is used, erections may lead to necrosis and ischemia.[2]

Indwelling and Straight Catheterization
Procedure Description

Catheterization of the bladder is accomplished by insertion of a red rubber or plastic tube through the urethra and into the bladder. The catheter allows urine to drain from the bladder for those patients unable to void voluntarily when accurate urine output is essential. Catheterization should be done only when medically warranted because it increases the patient's risk of infection.

Procedure

Table 14-1 details specific equipment, steps, rationale, and infection prevention strategies important when placing a straight or indwelling urinary catheter.

Text continued on p. 261.

Table 14-1   Inserting a straight or indwelling catheter

Steps	Rationale
1. Assess status of patient.	
a. Time that patient last voided	May indicate likelihood of bladder fullness
b. Level of awareness or developmental stage	Reveals patient's ability to cooperate during procedure
c. Mobility and physical limitations (to see if additional nursing personnel needed to assist with procedure)	Affects way that the patient will be positioned.
d. Patient's age	Determines catheter size to use (No. 8-10 Fr is generally used for children and 14-16 for women. No. 12 may be considered for young women. No. 16-18 is used for men unless larger size is ordered by physician.)
e. Distended bladder	Can indicate need to insert catheter if patient is unable to void independently (Patients at risk for distension include women after childbirth, patients after surgery, and men with prostatic hypertrophy.)
f. Pathological condition that may impair passage of catheter (e.g., enlarged prostate gland)	May prevent passage of catheter through urethra into bladder
g. Allergies	Determines allergy to antiseptic, tape, or rubber
h. Review of the physician's order for catheterization	Physician's order required (Physician may order catheterization after surgery or childbirth if the client has not voided for 8 hours.)

Continued.

2. Prepare necessary equipment and supplies.

a. Sterile gloves*	Procedure considered sterile
b. Sterile drapes, one fenestrated	
c. Lubricant*	Minimizes urethral trauma during insertion
d. Antiseptic cleaning solution*	
e. Cotton balls or gauze squares*	
f. Forceps*	
g. Prefilled syringe with sterile water*	Used to inflate balloon of indwelling catheter
h. Catheters of correct size and type for procedure* (intermittent or indwelling)	
i. Flashlight or gooseneck lamp	Helps in seeing woman's urinary meatus
j. Bath blanket	Promotes privacy
k. Waterproof absorbent pad	
l. Trash receptacle	
m. Perineal hygiene supplies: disposable gloves, basin with warm water, soap, face cloth, and towel	Helps reduce risk of UTI; provides opportunity to examine woman's urethral meatus or to retract foreskin of uncircumcised man
n. Sterile drainage tubing and collection bag (may be preattached to catheter), tape, safety pin, elastic band	Helps secure position of indwelling catheter, thus preventing trauma to external urethral sphincter

Modified from Potter P, Perry A: *Fundamentals of nursing: concepts, process and practice,* St Louis, 1993, Mosby.

*These items may be contained on catheterization tray or may need to be added after sterile field is established. This depends on whether disposable or nondisposable trays are used by the institution. Check outer label on prepackaged container for contents.

Table 14-1   Inserting a straight or indwelling catheter—cont'd

Steps	Rationale
o. Receptacle or basin (usually bottom of tray)	Provides area for urine to drain when straight or indwelling catheter is used
p. Sterile specimen container	For obtaining a sterile urine specimen to determine presence of bacteria
3. Explain procedure to patient. Also describe pressure sensation that will be felt during catheter insertion.	Reduces anxiety and promotes cooperation
4. Arrange for extra nursing personnel to assist, if appropriate.	May be necessary to assist with positioning dependent client; promotes use of correct body mechanics and safety
5. Wash hands.	Reduces transmission of infection
6. Raise bed to appropriate working height.	Promotes use of proper body mechanics
7. Facing patient, stand on left side of bed if right-handed (on right side if left-handed). Clear bedside table and arrange equipment.	Allows successful catheter insertion from a comfortable position with easy access to all equipment
8. Raise side rail on opposite side of bed.	Promotes patient safety
9. Close cubicle or room curtains.	Reduces patient's embarrassment and aids in relaxation
10. Place waterproof pad under patient.	Prevents soiling of bed linen

11. Position patient.

    a. *Female:* Assist to dorsal recumbent position (supine with knees flexed). Ask patient to relax thighs so as to externally rotate them (legs may be supported with pillows), or position patient in side-lying (Sims') position with upper leg flexed at knee and hip if unable to be supine (optional).

        Provides good view of perineal structures. Use an alternate position if patient cannot adduct leg at hip joint (e.g., because of arthritic joints). Also, this position may be more comfortable for patient. Support patient with pillows, if necessary, to maintain position.

    b. *Male:* Assist to assume supine position with thighs slightly abducted.

        Supine position prevents tensing of abdominal and pelvic muscles.

12. Drape client.

    a. *Female:* Drape with bath blanket. Place blanket diamond fashion over client; one corner at neck, side corners over each arm and side, and last corner over perineum. Raise gown above hips.

        Avoids unnecessary exposure of body parts and maintains comfort.

    b. *Male:* Drape upper trunk with bath blanket and cover lower extremities with bed sheets, exposing only genitalia.

13. Wash hands and apply disposable gloves. Wash perineal area with soap and water as needed; dry.

        Reduces presence of microorganisms near urethral meatus

Continued.

Table 14-1 Inserting a straight or indwelling catheter—cont'd

Steps	Rationale
14. Position lamp to illuminate perineal area. (When using flashlight, have assistant hold it.)	Permits accurate identification and good view of urethral meatus
15. Remove and dispose of gloves. Wash hands.	Prevents transmission of microorganisms
16. Open catheterization kit and catheter (if packaged separately) according to directions, keeping bottom of container sterile.	Prevents transmission of microorganisms from table or work area to sterile supplies
17. Apply sterile gloves.	Allows handling of sterile supplies without contamination
18. Organize supplies on sterile field. Open inner sterile package containing catheter. Pour sterile package of antiseptic solution in correct amount containing sterile cotton balls. Open packet containing lubricant. Remove specimen container (cap should be loosely placed on top) and prefilled syringe from collection compartment of tray, and set them aside on sterile field.	Maintains surgical asepsis and organizes work area (All activities requiring use of both hands must be completed before cleansing urethral meatus.)
19. Before inserting indwelling catheter, test balloon by injecting fluid from prefilled syringe into balloon valve. Balloon should inflate fully without leaking. Withdraw fluid and leave syringe on port of catheter. (See illustration.)	Checks integrity of balloon (Replace catheter if balloon leaks or inflates improperly.)

Continued.

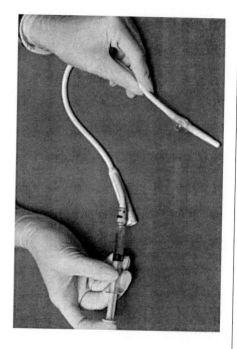

Table 14-1 Inserting a straight or indwelling catheter—cont'd

Steps	Rationale

20. Apply sterile drape.
  a. *Female:* Allow top edge of drape to form cuff over both hands. Place drape down on bed between patient's thighs. Slip cuffed edge just under buttocks, taking care not to touch contaminated surface with gloves. Pick up fenestrated sterile drape, and allow it to unfold without touching unsterile object. Apply drape over perineum, exposing labia and being sure not to touch contaminated surface.
  b. *Male:* Apply drape over thighs just below penis. Pick up fenestrated sterile drape. Allow it to unfold, and drape it over penis with fenestrated slit resting over penis.
	Maintains sterility of work surface (Outer surface of drape covering your hands remains sterile until touched by buttocks. Sterile drape against sterile gloves is sterile.)

21. Place sterile kit and its contents on sterile drape between patient's thighs, and open urine specimen container, keeping top sterile.	Provides easy access to supplies during catheter insertion; prepares container for transfer of urine

22. Apply lubricant along sides of catheter tip.
  a. *Female:* 2.5-5 cm (1-2 in)
  b. *Male:* 7.5-12.5 cm (3-5 in)
	Allows easy insertion of catheter tip through urethral meatus

23. Cleanse urethral meatus.

a. *Female:*

(1) With nondominant hand, carefully retract labia to fully expose urethral meatus. Maintain position of nondominant hand throughout procedure.

Provides full visualization of meatus (Full retraction prevents contamination of meatus during cleansing. Closure of labia during cleansing requires that procedure be repeated because area has become contaminated.)

(2) With dominant hand, pick up cotton ball with forceps and clean perineal area, wiping front to back from clitoris toward anus. Use new clean cotton ball for each wipe: along near labial fold, along far labial fold, directly over meatus.

Reduces number of microorganisms at urethral meatus (Use of single cotton ball for each wipe prevents transfer of microorganisms. Preparation moves from area of least contamination to that of most contamination. Dominant hand remains sterile.)

b. *Male:*

(1) If client is not circumcised, retract foreskin with nondominant hand. Grasp penis at shaft just below glans. Retract urethral meatus between thumb and forefinger. Maintain nondominant hand in this position throughout catheter insertion.

Minimizes chance of erection (If erection develops, discontinue procedure. Accidental release of foreskin or dropping of penis during cleansing requires process to be repeated because area has become contaminated.)

Continued.

Table 14-1　Inserting a straight or indwelling catheter—cont'd

Steps	Rationale
(2) With dominant hand pick up cotton ball with forceps and clean penis. Begin at meatus. Using circular motion, advance down toward base (shaft). Repeat this process three times, changing cotton ball each time.	Reduces number of microorganisms at meatus and moves from area of least to most contamination (Dominant hand remains sterile.)
24. Pick up catheter with gloved dominant hand approximately 5 cm (2 in) from catheter tip. Hold end of catheter loosely coiled in palm of dominant hand. Place distal end of catheter in urine tray receptacle unless already attached to drainage bag.	Prevents soiling of bed linen and allows accurate measurement of urinary output
25. Insert catheter.	
a. *Female* (see illustration): Grasp catheter in dominant hand with nondominant hand continuing to retract labia.	

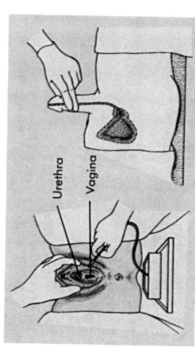

(1) Ask patient to take deep breath and slowly insert catheter through meatus. (If no urine appears, catheter may be in the vagina. If catheter is in the vagina, leave it in place; obtain and insert another catheter, then remove first catheter.) Repeat cleansing steps if it is necessary to remove nondominant hand to obtain new catheter.

Aids in insertion of catheter through relaxation of external sphincter (Catheter in the vagina is no longer sterile. Leaving first catheter in place helps prevent inserting second catheter in vagina.)

Continued.

Table 14-1 Inserting a straight or indwelling catheter—cont'd

Steps	Rationale
(2) Advance catheter approximately 5-7.5 cm (2-3 in) in adult, 2.5 cm (1 in) in child, or until urine flows out catheter's end. If inserting retention catheter, advance another 5 cm (2 in) after urine appears. Do not force catheter against resistance.	Prevents trauma to urethra (Female urethra is short. Appearance of urine indicates that catheter tip is in bladder or lower urethra. Further advancement of catheter ensures bladder placement. Balloon of retention catheter must be advaned into bladder. Forceful insertion may traumatize urethra.)
(3) Release labia, and hold catheter securely with nondominant hand.	Helps prevent expulsion (Bladder or sphincter contraction may cause accidental expulsion of catheter.)
b. *Male* (see illustration): Lift penis to position perpendicular to client's body and apply light traction upward:	Straightens urethral canal to ease catheter insertion
(1) Ask patient to bear down as if voiding and slowly insert catheter through meatus.	Aids in insertion of catheter through relaxation of external sphincter
(2) Advance catheter 17.5-22.5 cm (7-9 in) in adult, 5-7.5 cm (2-3 in) in young child, or until urine flows out catheter's end. If resistance is felt, withdraw catheter; do not force it through urethra.	Ensures proper placement (Adult male urethra is long. Appearance of urine indicates that catheter tip is in bladder or urethra. Resistance to catheter passage may be caused by strictures or enlarged prostate.)
If inserting retention catheter, advance another 5 cm (2 in) after urine appears.	Ensures that balloon is advanced into bladder.

(3) Release penis and hold catheter securely with dominant hand.	Helps prevent expulsion (Bladder or sphincter contraction may cause accidental expulsion of catheter.)
26. Collect urine specimen as needed: Fill specimen cup or jar to desired level (20-30 ml) by holding end of catheter in dominant hand over cup (or collect specimen from sterile drainage bag). With dominant hand, pinch catheter to stop urine flow temporarily, and then release catheter to allow remaining urine in bladder to drain into collection tray. Cover specimen cup and set it aside for labeling.	Allows sterile specimen to be obtained for culture analysis
27. Allow bladder to empty fully, about 750-1000 ml (unless institution policy restricts maximal volume of urine to drain with each catheterization).	Minimizes infection opportunity (Retained urine may serve as reservoir for growth of microorganisms. Rapid emptying of large volume of urine may cause engorgement of pelvic blood vessels and hypovolemic shock.)
28. Remove straight single-use catheter. Withdraw catheter slowly but smoothly until removed.	Minimizes patient discomfort

Continued.

Table 14-1   Inserting a straight or indwelling catheter—cont'd

Steps	Rationale
29. Inflate balloon of indwelling catheter.	
a. While holding catheter at urinary meatus with dominant hand, take end of catheter; place it between first two fingers of nondominant hand.	Allows catheter to be anchored while syringe is manipulated
b. Take dominant hand and attach syringe to injection port at end of catheter. (In some sets, syringe is already connected.)	Port connects to lumen, leading to inflatable balloon
c. Slowly inject total amount of solution. If client complains of sudden pain, aspirate solution and advance catheter further. Inject no more fluid than balloon size indicates.	Inflates balloon within bladder (If balloon is malpositioned in urethra, pain occurs during inflation.)
d. After inflating balloon fully, release catheter with nondominant hand and pull gently to feel resistance (see illustration). Then move catheter slightly back into bladder. Disconnect syringe.	Anchors catheter tip in place above bladder outlet to prevent removal of catheter (Gentle pulling ensures proper placement and anchoring. Advancing catheter upward minimizes pressure on bladder neck.)

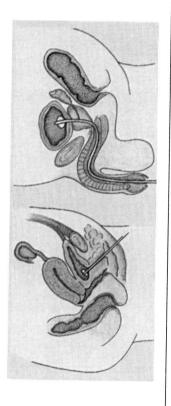

Continued.

Table 14-1 Inserting a straight or indwelling catheter—cont'd

Steps	Rationale
30. Attach end of catheter to collecting tube of drainage system, unless already connected to bag. Place drainage bag in dependent position (see illustration). Do not place bag on side rails of bed.	Establishes closed system for urine drainage (Dependent position of drainage bag promotes flow of urine away from bladder. Bags attached to side rails may be raised above level of bladder if rail is raised.)

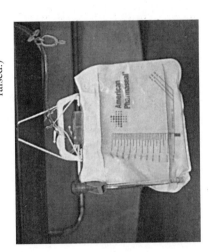

31. Tape catheter.	
a. *Female:* Tape catheter to inside of thigh with strip of nonallergenic tape. Allow for slack so that movement of thigh does not create tension on catheter.	Minimizes trauma to urethra and meatus during movement (Catheter positioned over thigh prevents kinking. Nonallergenic tape prevents skin breakdown.)
b. *Male:* Tape catheter to top of thigh or lower abdomen (with penis directed toward abdomen). Allow some slack in catheter so that movement does not create tension on catheter.	Should prevent necrosis (Anchoring catheter to lower abdomen is thought to reduce pressure on urethra at junction of penis and scrotum, thus reducing possibility of tissue necrosis.)
32. Be sure there are no obstructions or kinks in tubing. Place excess coil of tubing on bed, and fasten it to bottom sheet with clip from drainage set or with rubber band and safety pin.	Allows free drainage of urine by gravity and prevents backflow of urine into bladder
33. Remove gloves and dispose of equipment, drapes, and urine in proper receptacles. Wash hands.	Prevents transmission of infection
34. Assist patient to comfortable position. While wearing clean gloves, wash and dry perineal area as needed.	Maintains patient's comfort and security

Continued.

Table 14-1 Inserting a straight or indwelling catheter—cont'd

Steps	Rationale
35. Instruct patient on ways to lie in bed with catheter: side-lying facing drainage system with catheter and tubing draped over lower thigh or side-lying facing away from system, catheter and tubing extending between legs.	Prevents obstruction (Urine should drain freely without obstruction. Placing catheter under extremities can result in obstruction from compression of tubing from client's weight. When client is on one side facing away from system, catheter should not be placed over upper thigh; this forces urine to drain uphill.)
36. Caution patient against pulling on catheter.	Reduces trauma to urethral meatus
37. Wash hands.	Reduces spread of infection
38. Palpate bladder and ask if patient is uncomfortable.	Determines whether distention is relieved
39. Observe character and amount of urine in drainage system.	Determines whether urine is flowing adequately
40. Report and record type and size of catheter inserted, amount of fluid used to inflate balloon, and characteristics and amount of urine.	Communicates pertinent information to all members of health care team

Follow Up Assessment

The comfort level of the patient should be assessed frequently. The amount and character of the urinary drainage is observed and recorded. Kinking of the tubing is prevented by attaching excess coils to the bottom sheet of the bed. The patient should be reassessed frequently to prevent obstructed urine flow. The patient should be assessed for signs of UTI including dysuria, fever, chills, nausea, vomiting, and malaise.[5]

Indwelling Catheter Care
Procedure Description

Catheter care prevents infection and maintains adequate urinary flow. The accumulation of perineal secretions at the urethra places the patient at risk for infection. Cleaning the perineal tissues with soap and water and applying antiseptic ointment is recommended three times daily and following defecation or incontinence.[5]

Procedure

Table 14-2 details the specific equipment, steps, rationale, and specific infection prevention strategies in care of the indwelling catheter.

Follow Up Assessment

The patient is assessed for signs of UTI including dysuria, fever, chills, nausea, vomiting, and malaise. Routine catheter care is provided as long as the patient is catheterized.[5]

Condom Catheterization
Procedure Description

A condom catheter may be used as an alternative to urethral catheterization for incontinent or comatose men who completely and spontaneously empty their bladders. The condom is a rubber sheath with an outflow tube that is placed over the penis. A strip of elastic tape fits around the top of the condom catheter to hold it in place. Standard adhesive tape does not expand and should not be used to secure the condom. The end of the outflow tube attaches to a plastic drainage bag that is then attached to the bed or the patient's

Text continued on p. 269.

Table 14-2 Indwelling catheter care

Steps	Rationale
1. Assess for episode of bowel incontinence or patient's report of discomfort at catheter insertion site.	Considers accumulation of secretions or feces causing irritation to perineal tissues and acting as site for bacterial growth
2. Prepare necessary equipment and supplies.	Ensures orderly procedure
a. Catheter care kit:	
(1) Gloves	
(2) Cotton balls or application swabs	
(3) Clean washcloth or towel	
(4) Warm water and soap	
(5) Antibiotic ointment (e.g., neomycin)	
b. Bath blanket	Drapes patient
c. Waterproof absorbent pad	Prevents soiling of bed linen
3. Explain procedure to patient. Offer opportunity to perform self-care if patient is able.	Reduces anxiety and promotes cooperation (Embarrassment may motivate patient to perform own hygiene.)
	Maintains patient's self-esteem
4. Provide privacy by closing door or bedside curtain.	
5. Wash hands.	Reduces transmission of infection
6. Position patient.	
a. *Female:* dorsal recumbent position	Ensures easy access to perineal tissues
b. *Male:* supine position	

7. Place waterproof pad under client.	Protects bed linen from soiling
8. Drape bath blanket on bed clothes so that only perineal area is exposed.	Prevents unnecessary exposure of body parts
9. Apply gloves.	
10. Remove anchor tapes to free catheter tubing.	
11. Use nondominant hand.	
a. *Female:* Gently retract labia to fully expose urethral meatus and catheter insertion site, maintaining position of hand throughout procedure.	Provides full visualization of urethral meatus (Full retraction prevents contamination of meatus during cleansing. Accidental closure of labia or dropping of penis during cleansing requires process to be repeated.)
b. *Male:* Retract foreskin if client is not circumcised and hold penis at shaft just below glans, maintaining position of hand throughout procedure.	
12. Assess urethral meatus and surrounding tissues for inflammation, swelling, and discharge. Note amount, color, odor, and consistency of discharge. Ask patient if burning or discomfort is felt.	Determines presence of local infection and status of hygiene
13. Cleanse perineal tissue.	
a. *Female:* Use clean cloth and soap and water; clean toward anus. Repeat process to cleanse labia minora, and then cleanse around urethral meatus, moving down catheter. Be sure to	Reduces number of microorganisms at urethral meatus (Use of clean cloth prevents transfer of microorganisms. Cleansing moves from area of least to most contamination.)

Continued.

Modified from Potter P, Perry A: *Fundamentals of nursing: concepts, process and practice*, St Louis, 1993, Mosby.

Table 14-2   Indwelling catheter care—cont'd

Steps	Rationale
cleanse each side. Dry area well.	Determines whether cleansing is complete
b. *Male:* While spreading urethral meatus, cleanse around catheter first, and then wipe in circular motion around meatus and glans.	Reduces presence of secretions or drainage on outside catheter surface
14. Reassess urethral meatus for discharge.	
15. With towel, soap, and water, wipe in circular motion along length of catheter for 10 cm (4 in).	Further reduces growth of microorganisms at insertion site
16. Apply antiseptic ointment at urethral meatus and along 2.5 cm (1 in) of catheter if ordered by physician.	
17. Place client in safe, comfortable position.	Promotes comfort
18. Remove gloves. Dispose of contaminated supplies, and wash hands.	Prevents spread of infection
19. Record and report condition of perineal tissues, time procedure was performed, patient's response, and abnormalities noted.	Provides data to document procedure and informs staff of patient's condition

Table 14-3 Applying a condom catheter

Steps	Rationale
1. Assess status of patient to determine need for condom catheter.	Assesses need (Patient continuously incontinent of urine is at risk for skin breakdown.)
2. Prepare necessary equipment and supplies.	
a. Rubber condom sheath (proper size)	
b. Strip of elastic tape and skin preparation (e.g., tincture of benzoin)	
c. Urinary collection bag with drainage tubing or leg bag and straps	Allows patient to remain mobile with urinary leg bag
d. Basin with warm water and soap	
e. Towels and wash cloths	
f. Disposable gloves	Protects hands; reduces patient's risk of infection
g. Bath blanket	
h. Razor (optional)	
3. Explain procedure to patient.	Reduces anxiety and promotes cooperation
4. Wash hands.	Reduces transmission of infection
5. Provide privacy by closing door or bedside curtain.	Maintains patient's self-esteem
6. Assist client into supine position. Place bath blanket over upper torso. Fold sheets so that lower	Promotes patient comfort and prevents unnecessary exposure of body parts

Continued.

Modified from Potter P, Perry A: *Fundamentals of nursing: concepts, process and practice*, St Louis, 1993, Mosby.

Table 14-3 Applying a condom catheter—cont'd

Steps	Rationale
extremities are covered; only genitalia should be exposed.	
7. Assess condition of penis.	Provides baseline to compare changes in condition of skin after condom application
8. Apply disposable gloves. Provide perineal care and dry thoroughly. Clip hair at base of penis.	Removes irritating secretions (Rubber sheath rolls onto dry skin more easily. Hair adheres to condom and pulls during condom removal.)
9. Prepare urinary drainage collection bag and tubing or prepare leg bag for connection to condom, if necessary. Clamp off drainage exit ports. Secure collection bag to bed frame or client's leg; bring drainage tubing up through side rails onto bed.	Provides easy access to drainage equipment after condom is in place
10. Apply skin preparation to penis and allow to dry (approximately 30-60 sec).	
11. With nondominant hand, grasp penis along shaft. With dominant hand, hold condom sheath at tip of penis and smoothly roll sheath onto penis.	Prepares penis for easy condom placement

12. Allow 2.5-5 cm (1-2 in) of space between tip of glans penis and end of condom catheter.
13. Encircle penile shaft with strip of elastic adhesive. Strip should touch only condom sheath. Apply snugly but not tightly.
14. Connect drainage tubing to end of condom catheter. Be sure that condom is not twisted (see illustration).

Allows free passage of urine into collecting tubing when patient passes urine
Ensures position (Condom must be secured so that it is snug and will stay on but not too tight to cause constriction of blood flow.)
Allows urine to be collected and measured; keeps client dry (Twisted condom obstructs urine flow.)

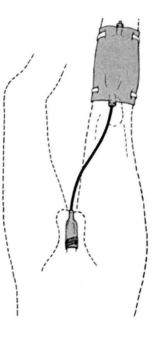

Continued.

Table 14-3 Applying a condom catheter—cont'd

Steps	Rationale
15. Place excess coiling of tubing on bed and secure to bottom sheet.	Prevents looping of tubing and promotes free drainage of urine
16. Place patient in safe, comfortable position (lying down or sitting but not obstructing urine drainage).	Promotes patient's comfort
17. Remove gloves. Dispose of contaminated supplies and wash hands.	Prevents spread of infection
18. Return in 30-60 min to observe for urinary drainage.	Determines whether normal voiding is occurring
19. Regularly inspect skin on penile shaft for signs of breakdown or irritation.	Indicates whether condom or urine is causing irritation or whether adhesive is too restrictive
20. Record and report time of catheter application, condition of skin, and voiding pattern.	Provides data to determine change in elimination status

leg. Although this is a noninvasive procedure, infections can occur. Infection risks are associated with the accumulation of secretions around the urethra, trauma to the urethra, or increased pressure in the outflow tube. Catheter care includes checking for skin irritation and cleaning the urethral meatus and penis.[6]

Procedure

Table 14-3 describes the specific equipment, steps, rationale, and specific infection prevention strategies important when applying the condom catheter.

Follow Up Assessment

Regular assessment of the quantity and character of the urinary output is necessary. The penis is inspected for signs of skin breakdown. The catheter is changed daily and the skin is inspected. Twisting of the catheter and obstruction of urinary drainage should be prevented.

Home Care Considerations

Procedures for the placement and care of indwelling or condom catheters do not differ in the home setting. If a family caregiver is performing the care, adequate instruction must include procedures to prevent infection for both the patient and the caregiver. When a patient is discharged home with a catheter in place, include the following instructions.

1. Avoid tension on the catheter.
2. Check for patency.
3. Avoid clamping or kinking the tubing.
4. Avoid reflux (backflow) from the drainage bag.
5. Use the following techniques to take care of collection bags, leg bags, and tubing.
   a. Wash bags and tubing daily with soap and water.
   b. Soak bags and tubing in mild vinegar solution for 15 minutes.
   c. Rinse bags and tubing with lukewarm water.
   d. Keep the ends of the catheter clean with a piece of clean gauze.
6. Attach the collection bag securely to the bed or chair, below the level of the bladder. If the patient is ambulatory, remember to unfasten the bag before the patient moves.

Tips for Preventing Infection in Catheterized Patients

- Follow good hand washing techniques.
- Do not allow the spigot on the drainage bag to touch a contaminated surface.
- If the drainage tubing becomes disconnected, do not touch the ends of the catheter or tubing. Wipe the ends of the tube with antimicrobial solution before reconnecting.
- Ensure that each patient has a separate receptacle for measuring urine to prevent cross-contamination.
- Prevent pooling of urine and reflux of urine into the bladder.
- Avoid raising the drainage bag above the level of the patient's bladder.
- If it becomes necessary to raise the bag during transfer of the patient to a bed or stretcher, clamp the tubing.
- Avoid allowing large loops of tubing to dangle from bedside.
- Before the patient exercises or ambulates, drain all urine from tubing into bag.
- Avoid prolonged clamping or kinking of the tubing (except during bladder conditioning).
- Empty the drainage bag at least every 8 hours. However, if large outputs are noted, empty it more frequently.
- Remove the catheter as soon as possible after conferring with the physician.
- Perform routine perineal hygiene per agency policy and after defecation or bowl incontinence.

From Potter P, Perry A: *Fundamentals of nursing: concepts, processes and practice,* St Louis, 1993, Mosby.

7. Report anuria, leaks around the catheter, accidental catheter removal, back pain, cloudy urine, and elevated temperatures.[7]

Infection Prevention Strategies

Procedures shown to be most effective in reducing UTI include hand washing, aseptic techniques for insertion and care of devices, closed urinary catheter systems, and decreased duration of indwelling catheterization.[2] The patient can assist in prevention by drinking 2000 to 2500 ml of fluids daily. This helps flush invading

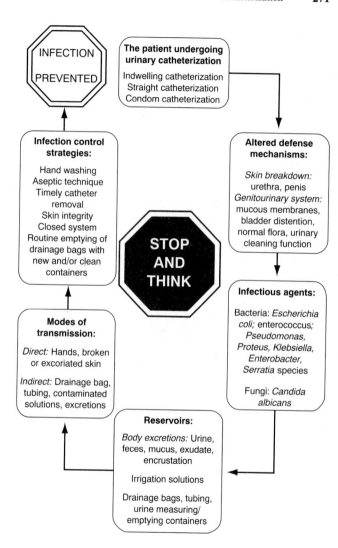

Figure 14-1.
Factors affecting the patient undergoing urinary catheterization leading to the selection of the strategies to prevent infectious complications.

organisms out of the urinary tract.[5] Standard precautions should be followed to decrease the risk of contact with blood and body fluids during these procedures. (See Chapter 7.) The box on p. 270 outlines further specific strategies.

Summary

UTI caused by catheterization causes 40% of all nosocomial infections each year. The procedure alters the normal body defense mechanisms and provides easy access for invading microorganisms. Prevention of infection is of the utmost importance. Microorganisms causing UTI may originate from endogenous sources such as the patient's bowel flora or skin breakdown or from exogenous sources such as contaminated solutions, breaks in aseptic technique, skin breakdown, use of nonsterile equipment, or organisms carried on the hands of personnel. Figure 14-1 summarizes the factors that cause infection and the strategies to prevent it.

References

1. Axnick K, Yarbrough M, editors: *Infection control: an integrated approach,* St Louis, 1984, Mosby.
2. Soule B, editor: *The APIC curriculum for infection control practice,* vol. 2, Dubuque, Iowa, 1983, Kendall/Hunt.
3. Palmer M: *Infection control: a policy and procedure manual,* Philadelphia, 1984, WB Saunders.
4. Grimes D, Grimes R, Hamelink M: *Infectious disease: Mosby's clinical nursing series,* St Louis, 1991, Mosby.
5. Potter P, Perry A: *Fundamentals of nursing: concepts, process and practice,* St Louis, 1993, Mosby.
6. Garibaldi R: Hospital acquired urinary tract infections. In Wenzel R, editor: *Prevention and control of nosocomial infections,* Baltimore, 1993, Williams & Wilkins.
7. Tucker S et al: *Patient care standards,* St Louis, 1992, Mosby.

Wound and Ostomy Management 15

Until the 20th century, wound care was serendipitous, based on necessity and individual philosophy, without benefit of research. Herbs, cotton, sawdust, and other items were used to cover and treat wounds. Following Pasteur's germ theory in the late 19th century, wound care consisted of covering and protecting an area of skin loss to promote a dry wound environment. Between 1958 and 1975, however, a revolution occurred that fostered the concept of moist wound healing. With intensive research into molecular and cell biology, scientists began developing tissue repair methods to enable clinicians to have direct, active control over a wound healing environment.

Nurses understand the physiological process of wound healing and are challenged to provide assessment of wounds based on knowledge of skin integrity and prevention of infection. Effective wound care management must be based on scientific research with a multidisciplinary approach.

Infection

Approximately 10% of patients with wounds acquire nosocomial wound infections, including surgical and trauma wounds, burns, neuropathic ulcers, and pressure ulcers.[1] Infection-causing bacteria may be transmitted to a patient from a health care worker or from visitors. Patients and staff must be educated on infection control practices, such as proper hand washing technique and proper dressing change procedures to reduce the incidence of wound contamination or cross infection.

Infection versus Colonization

Infection occurs when wound tissue is invaded by bacterial concentration greater than 10^5 organisms per gram of tissue.[2] Localized wound infection is clinically characterized by one or more of the following: increase in erythema, edema, and warmth of the surrounding tissue and malodorous, purulent exudate and localized pain at the wound site. Systemic characteristics of infection are fever, leukocytosis, lymphangitis, lymphedema, tachycardia, and, in some patients, hypertension and confusion.[1] Infection may develop from an imbalance in the number of bacteria, tissue hypoxia, necrosis, presence of a foreign body, or susceptibility of the client.

Staphylococcus aureus and *Pseudomonas aeruginosa* are the most common organisms found in wounds.[3] They usually are evidenced by green or gray purulent and malodorous drainage, with necrotic tissue in the wound. Differentiation must be made between an infected wound and a colonized wound.

Colonization is defined by Crowe as the presence of microbes without infection. Colonization of a wound with bacteria can be found without the presence of infection and does not necessarily stop the wound healing process.[4] These wounds may appear pale, with serous, pale white or yellow wound drainage, but generally they have no odor after the wound is cleaned.[1]

Physiology of Wound Healing

All wound repair begins at the cellular level with the inflammatory phase and progresses to the proliferative phase with manifestation of red granulation tissue and shrinkage of the wound. Final closing of the wound occurs in the maturation stage, which includes collagen remodeling, capillary regression, and scar tissue formation.[5] Surgical wounds or sharply demarcated lacerations with minimal tissue loss may be closed by primary closure with sutures, staples, or tape. Delayed wound closing allows for cleansing and observation to ensure that granulation tissue has started to bud without occurrence of infection. These wounds can then be closed with sutures after 4 to 5 days with approximation of the wound edges and minimal tissue loss.[3]

Partial Thickness versus Full Thickness Wounds

Partial thickness wounds involve the epidermis and nerve endings and may extend into the top layer of the dermal matrix. Repair is by regeneration, with epithelial proliferation and reestablishment of normal skin layers and function. Infection seldom develops in these wounds.[6]

Full thickness wounds involve total loss of the epidermal and dermal layers, may extend to subcutaneous tissue, and involve deep muscle and bone. Healing occurs by connective tissue repair mediated by the macrophages for scar formation.[2] Infection, necrosis, and extensive tissue damage with sinus tract formation may occur. Critical observation is necessary to assess for development of osteomyelitis. If osteomyelitis is suspected, a bone scan, biopsy, or both, must be considered.

Specific Infection Risks

The state of a healing wound is a mirror of the client's overall systemic health status. Every aspect of the client's condition may affect the healing process.[7] Research has identified many factors that may impede wound healing in an individual (see box on p. 276).

Oxygenation

Hypoxic conditions that impair wound healing result from either inadequate blood supply to the wound or decreased blood oxygen. Hypoxic cells are unable to continue adequate tissue defense and wound healing. Patients with compromised blood vasculature from pulmonary, cardiac, or diabetic conditions; external pressure on the capillary bed; edema; or hypovolemia are at high risk for delayed wound healing and infection.[8]

Nutrition

Adequate nutrition supports wound healing and repair and is the body's main defense against infection. A well-nourished individual has adequate stores to meet the increased physiological and metabolic demands of tissue repair. Protein metabolism is altered in the presence of deep wounds, and higher amounts of protein are needed for elderly patients and for patients with extensive wounds.[9]

Wound Assessment and Management Guidelines

Assess

Risk Factors	Causative Factors	Awareness
Age	Pressure	Patient and
Nutritional	Shear	family
status	Friction	knowledge
Mobility	Moisture	of wound
Continence	Circulatory im-	care
Sensory status	pairment	Infection
Previous skin	Neuropathy	control
loss		techniques
Presence of		
disease or		
infection		

Manage

Systemic Support	Elimination of Causative Factors	Other Interventions
Nutritional	Reduction	Appropriate
support	relief of	topical
Fluid intake	pressure	therapy
Oxygenation	Turning sched-	Patient edu-
Temperature	ules	cation
changes	Use of turn	Family edu-
Edema	sheets	cation
Cardiovascular	Heel elevation	Infection
function		control
Pulmonary		strategies
function	Prevention,	
	identification	
	and elimina-	
	tion of in-	
	fection	
	Manage	
	incontinence	
	with prompted	
	voiding pro-	
	grams, bowel	
	training pro-	
	grams, col-	
	lection devices	
	and appropriate	
	skin care	

Increased urinary excretion of nitrogen occurs in the presence of deep wounds and severe trauma, resulting in a negative nitrogen balance.[8] Protein, vitamin A, vitamin C, thiamine, iron, copper, and zinc are all vital for tissue regeneration and prevention of infection. An adult with a major wound requires 1500 to 5000 calories per day to meet the demands of an impaired system.[10]

Aging

Epidermal repair is decreased in the elderly. Cell fragility, decreased wound tensile strength, and decreased collagen fiber crosslinking affect the rate of wound repair. The geriatric population is at increased risk for malnutrition, immobility, and impaired respiratory, cardiovascular, and immune systems. These conditions impede oxygen transport to the underlying tissues and provide opportunistic sites for infection.[11] Optimal nutritional and wound bed support must be provided to allow for adequate granulation and epithelialization of the wound.

Systemic Disease

Diabetes mellitus, bleeding abnormalities (thrombocytopenia, anemia, or neutropenia), immunosuppression caused by disease or medication, and renal failure are all factors affecting the wound healing process. Wounds in patients with these problems frequently involve delayed cellular response, increased rate of infection, and slow wound proliferation. Measures to ensure maximal tissue perfusion are vital to establish the integrity of the open wound.[1] To promote adequate repair and prevent infection, the systemic disease process must be managed at the same time wound care is provided.

Wound Management
Topical Wound Dressings

Dressings optimize the healing environment, protect the wound from contamination and trauma, apply medications if indicated, absorb drainage, and debride necrotic tissue.[8] Ideally, the proper dressing keeps the wound surface moist and prevents bacterial growth in the wound. Selection of the proper dressing for wound care involves knowledge of the different types of dressings, amount of exudate present, frequency of dressing changes required, ease or difficulty in changing the dressing, and cost of dressings. The

Table 15-1 Topical wound dressings

Dressing Type	Wound Type	Examples
Gauze Plain Impregnated	Partial thickness Full thickness	All acute and chronic wounds
Semipermeable membrane dressing	Partial thickness Noninfected Low exudate	Intravenous sites Superficial abrasions Blisters Minor burns Donor sites Stages I and II pressure ulcers
Hydrocolloids	Partial thickness Shallow full thickness Low to moderate exudate Necrotic Noninfected	Lacerations Donor sites Second-degree burns Abrasions Blisters Stages I, II, and III pressure ulcers Shallow stage IV ulcers
Hydrogels	Partial thickness Full thickness	All acute and chronic wounds

patient setting (i.e., acute care, ambulatory care, or home care) and care provider also influence the selection of dressings. Changes in types of dressings are indicated as wound characteristics change. A complete patient assessment may indicate that wound healing is not progressing and dressings may need to be modified. Table 15-1 summarizes the different types of topical dressings, lists indications for use, and gives examples.

Gauze

Gauze dressings are used in wounds to absorb fluid, to protect from trauma and infection, and to provide mechanical debridement. Moist gauze should not be allowed to dry out between dressing changes because healthy tissue growth may be damaged when the dry gauze is removed. Moisten gauze with normal saline, if the gauze is dry, before removing it from the wound. Gauze impregnated with hydrogels, petroleum, or other moistening agents may be used to provide moisture to the wound for a longer period of time and may decrease the number of dressing changes required per day.

Indications for use

Moist gauze can be used on all partial and full thickness wounds and on both acute and chronic wounds. Intact skin around the wound must be protected from the moist gauze to prevent maceration.

Frequency of dressing changes

Dry gauze moistened with saline or isotonic solutions should be changed every 8 hours or before moisture evaporates. Impregnated gauze should be changed every 8 to 48 hours, depending on the type of wound and the manufacturers' directions.

Semipermeable membrane dressings

Semipermeable membrane film dressings are used to provide a moist wound environment and allow a free flow of oxygen through the dressing. They are impermeable to bacteria and environmental microorganisms. The mechanism of action includes the attraction of white blood cells to the occluded wound surface and the facilitation of migration and proliferation of epithelial cells in the wound. These dressings also facilitate autolytic debridement. Semipermeable membrane dressings are most suited for small, partial thickness, noninfected wounds with minimal drainage located on flat body surface areas. Semipermeable membrane dressings allow for visibility of the wound bed.

Indications for use

Semipermeable membrane dressings can be used on intravenous sites; superficial abrasions; blisters; minor burns; donor sites; partial thickness, nonexudating wounds; and pressure ulcers (stages I and II). They should not be used on infected wounds. When removing them from aging, thin skin, caution should be used to prevent skin tears. Semipermeable membrane dressings should always be removed in the direction of hair growth to prevent tissue trauma.

Frequency of dressing changes

Semipermeable wound dressings should be assessed daily and changed every 3 to 7 days or when wound drainage reaches 1 inch of the dressing border.

Hydrocolloids

Hydrocolloids are occlusive dressings that create a moist environment, provide a barrier to external bacteria, protect from reinjury, foster autolytic debridement, reduce pain, and absorb wound exudate. They are best suited for dry wounds or those with low to moderate drainage. They can be molded around body curves, but they remain in place best on flat body surface areas.

Indications for use

Use hydrocolloids for partial thickness wounds; shallow, full thickness wounds; lacerations; donor sites; second-degree burns; abrasions; blisters; and stages I, II, and III pressure ulcers. They are not recommended for use on wounds with suspected or known anaerobic infections.

Frequency of dressing changes

Hydrocolloid wound dressings should be assessed daily and changed every 3 to 7 days or when the wound drainage softens the dressing to within 1 inch of the dressing border or when all edges of the dressing are lifted. Dressings placed in body crevices, such as gluteal folds, may require more frequent changes. They should be secured with paper tape on the border to prevent migration of the dressing. Hydrocolloids must be at least 2 inches larger than the diameter of the wound to allow for sufficient absorption of wound fluid.

Topical therapy with the use of semipermeable membrane dressings and hydrocolloids prevents bacterial invasion of the open wound by occluding the surface of the wound, maintaining a moist wound surface, and facilitating cellular migration. The patient should be assessed for underlying pathologic conditions or host deficiencies that may delay healing or provide an environment for infection.

Hydrogels

Hydrogels generally consist of 96% water and 4% polyethylene oxide, and they maintain a moist wound environment. They support autolytic debridement by hydrating dry eschar and may increase fibrolytic activities in the wound.[6]

Indications for use

Partial thickness wounds are best managed with the sheet form of hydrogels. The hydrogel is applied directly to the wound surface and secured with paper tape or netting. Full thickness wounds are managed with the gel form to maintain wound moisture from 8 to 24 hours. This is followed with a slightly moist saline gauze dressing and then covered with a dry gauze or transparent film dressing. Patients suffering from wound pain may benefit from the use of hydrogels because of their cooling and soothing effect on the wound.

Frequency of dressing changes

Hydrogel dressings are to be changed every 8 to 24 hours, depending on the amount of wound exudate and also the type of hydrogel used. These dressings are only moderately absorptive. Therefore, hydrogel dressings should not be used in heavily draining wounds except to maintain wound moisture. Transparent film dressings may be used as a secondary dressing over hydrogels to prevent drying of the wound bed to protect from bacterial invasion and to decrease the frequency of dressing changes to every 12 to 24 hours.

Procedure Preparation

To prevent microbial transfer to the wound, sterile technique is always employed when dressing acute, full thickness wounds that extend to the dermis, muscle, or bone. Clean technique is usually employed for chronic wounds. This method is usually sufficient for local wound care of partial thickness wounds and is useful in home care when the patient or family members are providing care.

Purposeful prevention of the transfer of microbes (asepsis) is essential in all aspects of wound care. Good hand washing by the care provider with soap, water, and vigorous friction before and after contact with the wound is essential. (See Chapter 6.) Clean gloves must be worn when handling body fluids but may not provide a 100% barrier. Research has demonstrated that minute tears can occur, allowing bacteria to penetrate latex glove material. Therefore, good hand washing before and after glove use is the best defense against bacterial contamination.[1]

Clean technique for chronic wound care

1. Use a gown, gloves, goggles or eyeglasses, and a mask if splashing of body fluids may occur.
2. Wash hands vigorously with soap and water for 10 to 15 seconds. (See Chapter 6.)
3. Apply clean disposable gloves to remove the contaminated dressing from the wound, and discard the dressing in an appropriate container according to agency policy. Discard gloves with dressing. Wash hands.
4. Prepare clean area for wound care by removing all nonessential items from the area, and place wound dressing supplies where they are accessible.
5. Protect the patient area with a clean dry towel or plastic-backed pad.
6. Apply clean gloves.
7. Apply dressings to the wound by touching only the outside edges or back of the dressing with clean gloves.
8. Discard gloves and all contaminated wound equipment in an appropriate container according to agency policy.
9. Wash hands vigorously with soap and water.

Sterile technique for full thickness wound care

1. Wash hands vigorously with soap and water for 10 to 15 seconds. (See Chapter 6.)

2. Apply clean gloves to remove the contaminated dressing from the wound, and discard the dressing and gloves in an appropriate container according to agency policy. Wash hands.

3. Apply sterile gloves (and gown and face protection if splashing of body fluids may occur).

4. Irrigate wound (see wound cleansing section) using caution and barrier protection to reduce the risk of splashing body fluids.

5. Discard gloves with old dressing in an appropriate container according to agency policy.

6. Wash hands vigorously with soap and water, and prepare sterile field.

7. Apply sterile gloves, then apply wound dressing according to treatment recommendations (see topical wound dressings section).

8. Discard gloves and all contaminated wound equipment in the appropriate container according to agency policy.

9. Wash hands vigorously with soap and water.

Wound Cleansing

Cleansing a wound decreases the bacterial count and removes surface contaminants while protecting new and delicate epithelial and granulation tissue. Cleansing all open wounds with each dressing change promotes removal of wound debris and bacteria from the wound surface. Protection of the wound bed is a primary factor in planning care. Selection of nontoxic, wound-irrigating solutions is vital to maintaining a healthy, healing wound.

Chemical cleansing agents may delay healing, despite their antimicrobial or cleansing actions.[10] The active chemical ingredients interact with the cell membrane, inhibiting wound healing or actually causing cell death. Common cleansing agents that may impair wound healing include hexachlorophene, chlorhexidene, Dakin's solution, povidone-iodine scrubs, soaps, detergents, and hydrogen peroxide. Wound irrigation with normal saline or a nonionic surfactant is reported to be the most beneficial method of cleaning a wound.[12]

Health care workers must use standard precautions whenever they provide care to any body orifice or wound because of the possibility of contamination with blood or body fluids. These precautions include the use of gloves, gowns, masks, or goggles if the risk of contamination by spray or splashing is possible. (See Chapter 7.)

Procedure: wound irrigation (clean technique)

Equipment

1. #18 or #19 angiocatheter (without needle)
2. 30-cc or 35-cc syringe
3. Normal saline or nonionic surfactant
4. Nonsterile gloves
5. Emesis basin (reusable or disposable) and plastic backed pads
6. Face protection (goggles and masks)
7. Disposable gowns when splashing is anticipated

Nursing technique

1. Protect the patient's surroundings with plastic-backed pads. Place patient on side or sitting up, depending on location of the wound.
2. Wash hands vigorously with soap and water. Apply clean gloves and put on protective equipment (i.e., gown, goggles, mask). Place emesis basin at bottom of wound to collect irrigation fluid and residue.
3. Fill syringe with normal saline or nonionic solution. Apply full-force hand pressure to the plunger of the syringe while irrigating the entire wound bed. Continue the irrigation until the wound bed is clean and free of debris and drainage.
4. Pat edges of wound dry with clean, dry gauze.
5. Dispose of wound irrigation fluid in the commode, using caution not to splash fluid. Place plastic pads and gauze in an appropriate container according to agency policy.
6. Dispose of the syringe and angiocatheter in the needle disposal container.
7. Clean the reusable emesis basin with a soap and water, and send it to Central Service for sterilization. Alternately, discard the disposable basin in the trash.
8. Remove gloves. Wash hands vigorously with soap and water.
9. In home settings, discard dressings in double plastic bags and place them in a garbage can.

   The hand pressure on the syringe keeps the pressure safely at 8 psi while the user applies full force to the plunger of the syringe. This pressure adequately cleanses the wound but protects the fragile wound bed. This method also protects the surrounding skin, which may be at risk for contamination from wound drainage. High-pressure irrigation with water devices and mechanical scrubs are contraindicated because they destroy fragile granulation tissue.

Home Care Considerations

Dressing procedures at home should be performed using the same techniques as in the hospital. However, modifications may be necessary based on the knowledge and availablity of a caretaker.[13] Dressings that retain moisture in the wound may decrease the need for more than daily dressing changes (reducing the frequency of visits by the health care provider). These dressings also protect the wound from exposures to contaminants by caregivers.

When the patient is discharged from an acute or skilled care facility, he or she should be given sufficient supplies to continue care at home for 48 hours, written instructions on specific wound care and supplies, and information on the location of the medical suppliers in the area. Reimbursement of wound care products by insurance carriers should be considered in discharge planning so that the family or patient can afford and obtain the proper supplies after discharge. Medicare now provides coverage for most wound care supplies. A prescription for these supplies must be obtained from the practitioner overseeing the wound care. If visiting nurses are involved, they should be given specific written instructions.

Ostomy Management

Management of the patient with an ostomy ideally begins preoperatively with marking of the optimal stoma site and evaluation of the physical, psychological, educational, and psychosocial status of the patient.[14] Assessment of the patient immediately after surgery is necessary to evaluate the stoma for viability and security of the ostomy pouch, to check the incision, and to locate drains. Prevention of urine or stool leakage into the incision or onto drain sites is necessary to prevent localized or systemic infection. Assess the stoma every 4 to 8 hours to ensure viability of the stoma. If stomal changes occur, notify the physician immediately. Inadequate blood flow to the area may result in obstruction, hemorrhage, or peritonitis.

Ostomy Care

After the immediate postoperative period, ostomy care is focused on urine or stool containment, parastomal skin protection and care, and patient and family education, which is aimed at promoting self-care. Ostomy appliances may be in one or two pieces and are designed with either flexible or rigid backings to fit the contours of the abdomen. Each patient is individually fit with an appropriate appliance that accommodates that client's abdominal contours, mobility, budget, clothing, and lifestyle. Discharge planning includes a 1-month supply of pouches and supplies for stoma care. Instruction before discharge includes care in emptying, changing, and cleaning the pouch and guidelines for diet and activity. Each patient should be provided with written instructions on obtaining supplies from local medical suppliers and given a list of all needed supplies. Medicare and some private insurers provide partial coverage for ostomy supplies, but the patient should be instructed to contact his or her provider for individual coverage limitations. At discharge, a follow-up appointment for outpatient assessment should be scheduled by the physician or ostomy nursing specialist.

Fungal Infections

Containment of urine or stool prevents leakage into the surrounding incision and drains. The parastomal infection that most commonly occurs is *Candida albicans.* This fungus usually grows under the wafer or faceplate of the pouch within the first two weeks after surgery because of systemic antibiotic treatment, but it may occur at any time. The initial lesion is a pustule, leading to papules and erythema, usually with satellite lesions outside the plaque.

Nursing interventions

If fungal infections occur, an antifungal powder (Nystatin) is applied to the parastomal skin after cleansing the area thoroughly with warm water. The powder is sealed in with a copolymer skin sealant (wipes, sprays, gels, liquids) to allow for adhesion of the faceplate or wafer around the stoma.[14] The pouch is applied and left in place for 3 to 5 days, unless leakage occurs. Treatment is continued with each pouch change until the skin is clear or free of fungal infection.

Bacterial Infections

Bacterial infections may appear as large, erythematous crusty areas with plaques occurring around the stoma. These can be identified by culture of the infected site after removal of the pouch. Specific systemic antibiotics should be initiated to treat the bacteria. Cellulitis, abscesses, or ulcers may occur under the appliance, leading to pain and frequent appliance leakage.

Nursing interventions

Nursing care is directed to prevention of pouch leakage and maintenance of parastomal skin integrity. Frequent leakage of the pouch may aggravate the bacterial infection. A change in type of pouch may be indicated. Occasionally, a nonadhesive pouch may be used as a temporary measure during treatment. Topical ointments are usually contraindicated under ostomy pouches because the oily surface prevents the wafer or faceplate from adhering to the skin. A pouch with the faceplate or wafer that is trimmed to allow treatment of the parastomal skin may be necessary until the skin is clear. After the infection is clear, the pouching system is evaluated so that the bacterial infection does not recur because of an improper fit.

Leakage of urine or stool into the healing incision or nearby drains requires a complete assessment of stoma size, abdominal contours and skin folds, pouching system, and skin reaction to prevent further contamination of the area. Flushing the incision with normal saline until it runs clear is essential. If fecal drainage remains in the incision, a mixture of equal parts 3% H_2O_2 and normal saline applied to the incision can be used to cleanse the area. Follow with a normal saline flush.

Other Common Complications

Some of the more common complications may occur at the stomal site, including hyperplasia or pseudoverrucous lesions (identified by white-gray or brown wartlike papules or firm nodules that develop at the mucocutaneous border and protrude above the skin level).[15] These lesions usually occur on skin that is constantly exposed to effluent under a large wafer or faceplate.[14] Treatment includes correction of the skin exposure with a change in size or type of pouching system to prevent further exposure to effluent and an evaluation of urine pH to ensure acidic urine pH of 6.

Herpesvirus infection in the parastomal area is manifested by erythema and uniformly shaped vesicles with crust formation. Treatment includes systemic (intravenous or oral) and topical antiviral medication. The pouching system must allow for protection of the lesions from effluent and access to the site. A one-piece, nonadhering pouch may be used until the parastomal skin is clear.

Folliculitis may occur under a pouching system when hair follicles become inflamed. The skin appears erythematous, with pustular lesions. This is usually caused by careless removal of the ostomy pouch or traumatic hair removal in the parastomal region. If *Staphylococcus aureus* is cultured, an antibacterial powder may be applied to the lesions and covered with a skin sealant before applying the wafer or faceplate.

Parastomal skin infections occur less frequently now with the improvement of pouching systems and surgical technique. Many problems such as weight gain, weight loss, or parastomal hernias may trigger skin conditions that result in infections from improper sizing and fitting of the pouching system. The nurse needs to be alert to recognize complications. Referrals for care should be initiated to the patient's physician or ostomy nurse specialist when a nonhealing lesion occurs or the patient suffers frequent pouch leakage or pain around the stoma.

Home Care Considerations

Home care for the patient with an ostomy should be designed to allow for easy access to toilet facilities and should include a pouch that the patient or family can manage self-sufficiently. Home care should also be cost effective. Follow-up nursing care includes evaluation of the home, toilet facilities, and plumbing and review of the client's understanding of the procedure, self-care practices, infection control practices, pouch fitting, and financial resources. If the patient or family is unable to afford or to obtain the necessary supplies, complications of stoma care may develop quickly. Assessment of both physical and psychosocial adjustments to the stoma is necessary. Recognition of the patient's coping mechanisms for a changed body image, ability to accept these changes, and self-care practices is a major challenge facing the home care nurse, who must facilitate the process of recovery without infection.

Infection Prevention

A primary goal among staff members must be the prevention of infections to reduce morbidity and mortality of patients. Prevention techniques should be addressed in the initial plan of care. Monitoring of wound healing and infection rates in the acute,

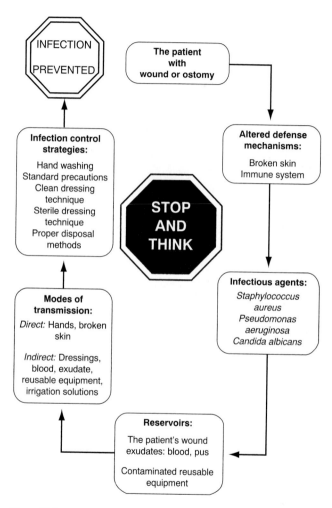

Figure 15-1.
Factors affecting the patient with a wound or ostomy leading to the selection of the strategies to prevent infectious complications.

skilled, and home care settings should be a priority. Patients with high risk factors for infections should be monitored by nutritional and wound assessments daily. Wounds with necrotic tissue must be closely observed for signs of infection. Indications of wound infection in a necrotic wound bed include gray, purulent drainage from the wound, erythema and crepitus extending around the periphery of the wound, and fever. Debris must be removed by surgical excision, chemical enzyme debriding agents, mechanical debridement, or autolysis.[10]

Standard precautions must be followed during wound care (see Chapter 7). In most settings the use of clean gloves and appropriate disposal of contaminated materials is sufficient for small, non-draining wounds. Mask, gown, and individual eyeglasses or goggles should be worn during any wound care procedure that involves wound or body fluids and in which there may be risk of contamination to the health care worker. These practices reduce transmission of nosocomial infections, hepatitis B and C, and human immunodeficiency virus.[16]

Summary

Wound and ostomy management must include the proper infection prevention techniques. Altered defense mechanisms and infectious agents may combine with patient exudate, contaminated equipment, and lack of proper infection control measures by the caregiver to allow for transmission of infection. Nursing interventions using proper infection control strategies reduce the likelihood of contamination and infection and allow wound healing and ostomy containment with optimal patient outcomes.

References

1. Corum, G: Characteristics and prevention of wound infection, *J ET Nurs* 20(1):21, 1993.
2. Bryant R: *Acute and chronic wounds: nursing management,* St Louis, 1992, Mosby.
3. Eaglestein WH: *New directions in wound healing, a wound care manual,* Princeton, 1990, ER Squibb & Sons.
4. Kravitz R et al: Dermal ulcer cultures: frequency and associated symptoms, *JWOCN* 21(1):21, 1994.
5. Gogia P: The biology of wound healing, *Ostomy Wound Manage* 1(9):18, 1992.

6. Lawrence JC: *International forum on wound microbiology,* Barcelona, 1989, Excerpta Medica.

7. Alvarez O et al: Moist environment for healing; matching the dressing to the wound, *Wounds* 1(1):35, 1989.

8. Maklebust J, Sieggreen M: *Pressure ulcers: guidelines for prevention and nursing management,* St Louis, 1991, S-N Publications.

9. Pinchofsky-Devin G et al: Why won't this wound heal? *Ostomy Wound Manage* 24:42, 1989.

10. Rodeheaver G et al: Wound healing and wound management: focus on debridement, *Adv Wound Care* 7(1):22, 1994.

11. Blaylock B: The aging immune system and common infections in elderly patients, *J ET Nurs* 20:63, 1993.

12. Lineweaver W et al: Topical antimicrobial toxicity, *Arch Surg* 120: 267, 1987.

13. Baharestani MM: The lived experience of wives caring for their frail, homebound, elderly husbands with pressure ulcers, *Adv Wound Care* 7(3):40, 1994.

14. Hampton BG, Bryant R: Ostomies and continent diversions. In *Nursing Management,* St Louis, 1992, Mosby.

15. Nordstrom GM, Borglund E, Nyman CR: Local status of the urinary stoma: the relation to peristomal skin complications, *Scand J Urol Nephrol* 24:117, 1990.

16. Crow S: Infection control perspectives. In Krasner D, editor: *Chronic wound care,* Philadelphia, 1990, Health Management Publications.

Burn Care

16

Burn injuries present a unique set of nursing management problems and are among the greatest challenges in infection control and prevention. Despite advances in the physiological and metabolic management of these patients, sepsis remains a leading cause of morbidity and mortality.[1] In burn patients 40% of deaths are a result of infection.[2]

Burn wounds are treated by applying topical antimicrobial agents to the burned site. Immersion or hydrotherapy are used to remove eschar and old dressings. Topical antimicrobial agents help prevent bacterial invasion. Common agents include sulfur sulfadiazine, sulfamylon acetate, and povidone-iodine.

To cover large exposed surface areas, surgical grafts may be done in full-thickness tissue losses. In these cases an additional donor site also must be given an optimal environment for healing. Grafting plays an important role in minimizing the risk of infection and promoting healing. Grafts are biological dressings that reduce bacterial counts and prevent water and protein losses. Previously contaminated wounds become sterile within hours of successful grafting.[1]

Debridement of necrotic areas is done to prevent further tissue loss from infection. This chapter describes this aspect of burn treatment.

Characteristics of Burn Wounds
Description

Thermal injuries may be partial- or full-thickness wounds. The factors that stimulate healing in burns are the same factors that affect healing in other types of wounds. (See Chapter 15.) Burns may cover a larger surface area than a pressure ulcer, surgical wound, or extremity ulcer, and they place the patient at greater risk

Burn Wound Characteristics

First Degree	Second Degree	Third Degree
Affects superficial epidermal layer	Affects whole epidermis and varying depths of dermis	Destroys all dermal elements
No blistering	Blistering present	No blistering
Pain and erythema	Pain	No pain
Healing by subsequent epithelial slough (peeling)	Healing by epithelial regeneration from viable dermal remnants	Healing only with skin grafting

Modified from Axnick K, Yarbrough M: *Infection control: an integrated approach,* St Louis, 1984, Mosby.

for infection and hypovolemia. Greater metabolic responses such as anemia, loss of the thermoregulatory response, and loss of lymphocyte function may cause fluid shifts, edema, and systemic circulation dysfunction. Characteristics of burn wounds are listed in the box above.

Infectious Process

A burn wound is avascular, necrotic tissue that becomes an excellent medium for the growth of microorganisms. Immunosuppression occurs. Following the burn injury few gram-negative organisms are present on the wound surface.[3] However, within 10 days, gram-negative bacteria predominate on the wound surface. When these organisms multiply, invasion into the eschar occurs with subsequent penetration into blood vessels and the lymphatic system, leading to septicemia.[4] When there is extensive skin injury, aerobic, gram-negative bacilli can be an endogenous source of infection.[1] Wound biopsy is used to diagnose a wound infection and to identify the causative organisms.[5]

The pathophysiological changes associated with burns affect the patient's ability to withstand bacterial challenges. Both humoral and cellular defense mechanisms are reduced either qualitatively or quantitatively in the first 2 weeks after the burn injury.[1,2] Decreased circulating immunoglobulins and defects in the chemotoxic, phagocytic, and killing abilities of white blood cells inhibit the inflammatory response. In addition, the avascular nature of the wound prohibits the delivery of phagocytes and antibodies and leads to colonization and infection of the burn.[1,2]

The line between colonization and actual infection is often obscure in burn wounds. After the initial injury, when aerobic, gram-positive organisms pose the greatest threat, the burn becomes ischemic and gram-negative organisms proliferate in the devitalized tissue. *Noninvasive* infection is characterized by mild to moderate systemic symptoms, including fever and leukocytosis. *Invasive* infections occur when formerly healthy granulation tissue becomes pale and edematous and fails to bleed briskly when abraded. Fever or subnormal temperatures, progressive leukocytosis, and alteration in mental status accompany the local symptoms. Failure to stem this process may cause a partial-thickness wound to develop into a full-thickness injury because of destruction of the epithelium and thrombosis, which extends necrosis into deeper subcutaneous tissues. A further insult may occur with the development of sepsis from bacterial invasion of the lymphatic system of blood vessels.[1,6]

Burn wound infections are nosocomial in origin, whether endogenous or exogenous. The most frequently isolated organism in burn wound cultures is *Staphylococcus aureus*. Direct and indirect sources of microorganisms causing burn infections include hospital personnel (hand transfer), gastrointestinal contamination (patient feces), the wound itself, and environmental objects or surfaces (tubs, medications, solutions).[2,6]

Specific Infection Risks

Susceptible Hosts

Very young and elderly burn patients suffer increased risk for complications of burns because of a compromised state of the immune system. Altered fluid status, nutrition, and temperature maintenance decrease immune function.

Altered Defense Mechanisms

The most immediate and obvious alteration of the host defense mechanisms is the destruction of the protective integument (skin).[1,2] Both the severity and the extent of the burn wound influence the patient's subsequent susceptibility to infection. Breaks in the skin or the absence of the skin as an anatomical barrier expose underlying tissues to microorganisms, which may result in local infections or infections of underlying tissue or structures (bone infection, bacteremia). Loss of the protective skin also increases fluid loss.[2]

The wound is rapidly colonized with bacteria because of direct access through an open wound and because the damaged vascular system at the wound site prevents the humoral elements of the immune system from reaching the burned tissues. The risk to the patient is the spread of bacteria from personnel and cross-contamination.

Devices and Procedures

Wounds may be inoculated with exogenous microorganisms if wound care is performed with contaminated equipment or materials. Large, shared multidose containers may be sources of contamination.[2]

Maintenance of percutaneous devices is a particular problem with burn patients because of decreased amounts of intact skin. Devices placed through burn eschar present an infection hazard. Purulent intravenous (IV)-associated phlebitis may occur. During hydrotherapy, the IV cannula placed through intact skin may be contaminated with microorganisms from the perineal areas of the burn wound.[2,5]

Personnel

Risks to personnel are associated with failure to observe standard precautions during exposure to blood and body fluids. (See Chapter 7.) Personnel also pose a risk to the patient by direct inoculation of the wound from the hands of personnel.

Wound Care Procedures
Description

The burn wound contains a large amount of eschar or scar tissue and is rapidly colonized with bacteria. Wound care involves cleaning and debridement of the wound and application of topical antimicrobial ointments or creams and dressings on the wound. Hydrotherapy loosens and helps remove the eschar. The procedure may be done by total or partial immersion using tap water, normal saline, antiseptic solutions, or a combination of these agents. Plastic liners may be used in tubs to reduce the risk of cross-contamination.

Preparation

1. For pain management, medicate the patient 30 minutes before the procedure.
2. Maintain the bath temperature at 100°F (37.8°C).
3. Limit the procedure to 20 to 30 minutes to prevent chilling.
4. Gather the following equipment:
   a. Sterile and nonsterile gloves
   b. Waterproof apron or gowns (masks, caps according to agency policy)
   c. Plastic liner for tub (optional according to agency policy)
   d. Antiseptic solutions or normal saline as ordered
   e. Debridement brushes
   f. Sterile towels or gauze pads
   g. Sterile tongue blades
   h. Antimicrobial ointment or cream
   i. Sterile dressing materials as ordered or needed

Procedure

1. Wash and dry hands. Put on nonsterile gloves and waterproof apron or gown.
2. Immerse the patient or the affected body part.
   a. Cleanse large body surface burns using hydrotherapy tanks, whirlpools, or tubs.
   b. Cleanse small burn sites with sterile gauze pads saturated with warm normal saline, or soak the affected area in a clean or sterile basin.
3. Remove the eschar by gently brushing the burn site.
4. Remove the patient from the bath. Remove wet gloves, and wash and dry hands. Gently pat wounds dry with sterile towels or gauze pads, or allow the patient to dry himself or herself. Examine all burn areas for signs of infection. Warming lights may be used after hydrotherapy to maintain the patient's body temperature.
5. Gather and open antimicrobial ointment and sterile tongue blades. Prepare the dressing field. Put on sterile gloves.
6. Using a sterile tongue blade, apply a thin layer of the topical

antimicrobial ointment to the entire burn area. To prevent contamination of the ointment, *do not* reenter the ointment with a tongue blade that has touched the wound.

7. Apply dressings as ordered; cover the burn area with fluffed sterile gauze moistened with normal saline, and cover with dry sterile gauze.

8. Remove and discard gloves; wash and dry hands.

9. Observe and document the color, odor, size, exudate, progress in healing, and character of the eschar with each wound intervention. Assess and document the patient's response to the procedure.

Home Care Considerations

In the home setting, the wound care should be the same as in the hospital. However, some modifications may be necessary based on the knowledge and availability of a caregiver as well as the availability of tub equipment.[7] Discharge planning includes teaching the family or the caregiver proper care of the patient's wounds to ensure healing.[8] Give the patient written instructions about wound care procedures, a list of supplies, and the location of medical suppliers in the area. Acquaint the patient and family with resources, including support groups and community resources for recovering burn victims.[5] Home care guidelines are listed in the box on pp. 298-299.

Infection Prevention

Prevention is directed at eliminating potential risks for wound infection, systemic infection, or both. Infection prevention goals include the maintenance of adequate respiration, fluid and electrolyte balance, body temperature, nutrition, and appropriate wound care.

Provide the nutritional support necessary for the high metabolic demands of wound healing. For example, increase protein and calories; add vitamins and mineral supplements to the diet; or use parenteral hyperalimentation, supplementary nutrition, or liquid tube feedings.[2] Initiate adequate nutrition or the skin surface will lack growth nutrients and will provide a host environment for microbial invasion. Monitor the levels of albumin, vitamins A, C, and D, thiamine, magnesium, and zinc. The patient may need

Home Care Guidelines for the Caregivers of the Burn Patient

Before discharge, the patient and family or other caregiver must be taught proper care of the patient and his or her wounds to ensure proper healing and to help the patient begin readjustment into society.

General Care

Notify the physician if any of the following occurs:

1. Change in wound status (open, draining, enlarging, blisters, redness, swelling)
2. Signs of infection (temperature > 99°F, foul smelling or copious wound drainage)
3. Difficulty with dressings

Skin Care

Daily skin care includes the following:

1. Gentle bathing with a mild soap
2. Moisturizer applied to healed burn areas (as ordered by physician)
3. Dressing change procedure for open areas as follows:
   a. Wash hands.
   b. Wear gloves.
   c. Remove and dispose of old dressing.
   d. Use a clean wash cloth with mild soap and water to clean area.
   e. Apply dressing as specified.
   f. Clean and disinfect basin or tub.

Daily Living

Resume activities according to the patient's abilities and the physician's orders.

1. Take protective measures in sunlight because skin is much more sensitive.
   a. Avoid direct, intense sunlight.
   b. Wear long-sleeved shirts, pants, and hat.
   c. Use a sunscreen with a sun protective factor greater than 15.

Home Care Guidelines for the Caregivers of the Burn Patient—cont'd

2. Avoid shearing of the skin.
   a. Wear soft clothing; wash new clothing before wearing.
   b. Use caution when cleaning, cooking, or ironing or any instance when potential damage to the skin can occur.
3. Eat a well-balanced diet.
4. Avoid excess weight gain or loss because it will affect the pressure of garments on the skin.
5. Drink ample fluids (64 ounces or more per day).
6. Exercise injured limbs and joints at least four times a day.
7. Increase endurance with aerobic activity.
8. Take medications as prescribed (review side effects, indications, and dosages before discharge).
9. Clean pressure garments daily in mild soap.
10. Keep appointments with the clinic or physician.

Modified from Beare P, Myers J: *Adult health nursing,* ed 2, St Louis, 1994, Mosby.

supplements until he or she is able to eat adequately. To prevent contractures and loss of function, mobilize the affected areas as soon as the burn is stabilized and shows signs of healing. Give tetanus prophylaxis because burns are considered contaminated wounds.[5]

Use aggressive debridement accompanied by topical antimicrobial agents to minimize the proliferation of microorganisms on the burn surface.[1] Remove foreign material and dead or damaged tissue to reduce the reservoir for bacterial growth.[2,5]

Maintain exercise, ambulation, and appropriate positioning to decrease the possibility of circulatory and respiratory complications. Provide adequate rest to enhance the release of growth hormone, which influences the rate of protein synthesis. Provide pain control. Pain may have a hemodynamic effect, resulting in increased metabolic activity, which is detrimental to wound repair.[2,5]

Maintain the healthy skin with regular cleansing or bathing to preserve future donor sites. Provide mouth care to preserve the function of the oral cavity and to prevent infection of the oral structures. Maintain normal bowel pattern; diarrhea increases the potential for burn wound contamination.[2] Provide special care to face, eyes, ears, nares, and mouth to remove eschar and ointments. Cleanse perineal and genital areas to prevent deposits of urine and feces on the burned areas. Keep exposed tendon and bone moist with sterile supplies to avoid tissue death and infection.[2,5]

Ironically, the burn wound places the patient at high risk for infection while serving as a reservoir for potential cross-infection to others. The patient's endogenous fecal flora give rise to colonization and infection.[1] Observe the mouth and perineal areas for signs of candidiasis and changes in bowel function that may indicate *Clostridium difficile* invasion. Monitor and observe vital signs and urinary output to watch for hypovolemia or tissue anoxia.

Measures to control or reduce cross-infection include isolation or barrier techniques, personnel practices, and environmental control. Isolation or barrier techniques vary in complexity from the use of a single room or open ward to laminar flow units.[1]

Personnel may serve as both the source and the transmitter of infection. Strict adherence to hand washing cannot be overemphasized as a basic control measure. (See Chapter 6.) Any staff member with an active infection should be excluded from direct patient care.[1,5] Gowns, gloves, and masks are recommended when caring for an infected patient. Cover gowns should be worn during wound care and hydrotherapy. Impervious gowns or aprons are preferable.[2] When providing hydrotherapy treatments, personnel should wear waterproof aprons and elbow-length gloves for both patient and employee protection.[1] Aseptic technique should be used in all aspects of patient care:

1. Wash hands carefully with antibiotic cleansing agent before and after caring for the patient.
2. Wear cap and mask when wound is exposed.
3. Change IV tubing and perform site care according to agency policy.
4. Wear gowns when in contact with the patient.
5. Wear sterile gloves in patient care with exposure to wound.
6. Wear clean gloves in other patient care activities.[9]

Minimizing potential environmental reservoirs requires the

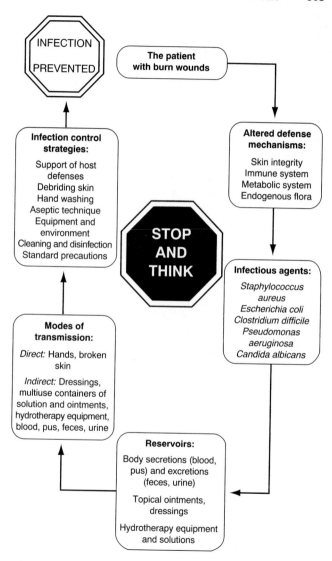

Figure 16-1.
Factors affecting the patient with burn wounds leading to
the selection of the strategies to prevent infectious complications.

development of regular, effective cleaning procedures. Particular attention must be given to disinfection of equipment used in the treatment of multiple patients. The most critical area is the hydrotherapy area. The design of the equipment poses a major infection control problem; agitators and filling hoses are extremely difficult to adequately disinfect. The tub surfaces should be mechanically cleaned and disinfected between patient treatments; however, disinfection is not a substitute for sound, aseptic technique by personnel.[1] Remove reservoirs of gram-negative organisms such as open containers of water or saline and irrigating solutions.[2]

Summary

Treatment of burns requires consideration of infection until all burned areas heal. A multidisciplinary approach to the treatment of these patients is recommended to encompass all phases of care. By understanding the complications and optional treatment modalities, health care workers can help the patient recover in an optimal healing environment.

Infection is the cause of 40% of deaths in burn patients. These injuries alter the normal body defense mechanisms drastically, making infection prevention critical for burn patients. Microorganisms arise from both endogenous and exogenous sources. Figure 16-1 summarizes the factors that cause infection and the strategies to prevent it.

References

1. Axnick K, Yarbrough M: *Infection control: an integrated approach,* St Louis, 1984, Mosby.
2. Soule B, editor: *The APIC curriculum for infection control practice,* vol 2, Dubuque, Iowa, 1983, Kendall/Hunt.
3. Pruitt B et al: Current approach to prevention and treatment of *Pseudomonas aeruginosa* infections in burned patients, *Rev Infect Dis* 5:889, 1989.
4. McManus et al: Burn wound infection, *J Trauma* 21:753, 1981.
5. Suddarth D: *The Lippincott manual of nursing practice,* Philadelphia, 1991, JB Lippincott.
6. Mayhill G: Surgical infections including burns. In Wenzel R, editor: *Prevention and control of nosocomial infections,* Baltimore, 1993, Williams & Wilkins.

7. Baharestani M: The lived experience of wives caring for their frail, homebound, elderly husbands with pressure ulcers, *Adv Wound Care* 7(3):40, 1994.

8. Beare P, Myers J: *Adult health nursing,* ed 2, St Louis, 1994, Mosby.

9. Brunner D, Suddarth A: *Medical-surgical nursing,* Philadelphia, 1992, JB Lippincott.

Intravenous Techniques

17

Of all patients admitted to hospitals each year, 50% receive intravenous (IV) therapy. However, IV therapy occurs in all health care settings: acute care, emergency care, ambulatory care, and home health. This provides a large population at risk for IV-related infections. IV-related infections occur from skin colonization, IV access port colonization, and contaminated solutions.[1,2]

IV devices are used for administration of fluids or medications, for hemodynamic monitoring, for diagnostic testing, and for maintenance of cardiac and renal function. The cardiovascular (CV) system is normally sterile, so all devices with access to or direct contact with the CV system must be sterile.[2]

The risk of infection associated with these IV procedures is reduced by specific prevention strategies related to device insertion and maintenance, attached equipment, and fluids.[2] Guidelines for preparation, insertions, maintenance, and infection prevention measures for intravascular access, arterial access, and blood administration are summarized in this chapter.

Specific Infection Risks

Devices inserted into the CV system bypass the normal skin defense mechanism and provide a portal of entry for microorganisms from the device at the time of insertion, from subsequent device contamination, or from the insertion site. Microorganisms cause infections at the point of entry, in the blood, or at remote sites. The devices or infusion fluids most commonly become contaminated during use, but they may be intrinsically contaminated as well at the place of manufacture or when mixed in the pharmacy.[2]

Host Factors

The critically ill or immunosuppressed patient has the greatest risk for bacteremia caused by intravascular devices.[3] A number of additional host factors increase the risk of infection associated with intravascular devices[2,3]:

1. Trauma, burns, or surgical wounds
2. Immunosuppression such as granulocytopenia, corticosteroid suppression, or other immunosuppressive therapy
3. Cardiovascular implants or structural defects, including congenital anomalies and valvular diseases
4. Preexisting infection at remote sites, which can contaminate IV devices via endogenous spread
5. Severe malnutrition
6. Underlying phlebitis (increases risk 18-fold)
7. Prolonged placement of an IV device (catheter/needle, tubing, solution container)

Device and Solution Factors

Contaminated equipment and solutions provide microorganisms with a portal of entry into the CV system. The following device-related factors increase the risk of infection associated with intravascular devices.[3]

1. Intrinsic risk factors (before use)
   a. Cracks in glass bottles
   b. Punctures in plastic containers
   c. Contaminated infusion fluid or additives
   d. Leaky bottle closure system
   e. Administration equipment with multiple points of access (and potential contamination)
   f. Antiseptics or ointments
   g. Cannulas
2. Extrinsic risk factors (during use)
   a. Additives (at pharmacy or on nursing unit)
   b. Container changes (multiple entries and manipulations)
   c. Attachment of administration equipment (multiple entries and manipulations)
   d. Injections and irrigations
   e. Central venous pressure measurements
   f. Cannula insertion and manipulations

Person-to-Person Factors

Health care worker (HCW) and patient factors also increase the risk of infection associated with intravascular devices[3]:

1. Cross-contamination with other infected areas of the patient's

body either by the patient or on the hands of the HCW
2. Cross-contamination from another infected patient's body on the hands of the HCW
3. Cross-contamination from the patient when the HCW comes in contact with the patient's blood
4. Nonaseptic IV insertion or dressing change

IV Insertion
Description

Using a sharp, rigid stylet partially covered by a plastic catheter or attached to a syringe, the HCW can access a vein, generally on the patient's hands, arms, or feet. This procedure is done to collect blood samples, begin an IV line, or administer medications. Site selection requires careful assessment of vein condition, site mobility, previous trauma to veins, hydration and nutrition status, and signs of thrombosis or infection.[4]

Procedure

The procedure for IV cannula insertion is outlined in Table 17-1.

Follow Up

The patient should be assessed to determine if the vascular access is patent. Also, the HCW should observe the site for signs of infection or infiltration (swelling, redness, pain, warmth), check the flow rate, and determine if the correct solution is infusing. The patient's response to therapy should be evaluated. The patient should be assessed hourly to ensure desired outcomes, and the integrity of the IV line should be maintained.

Arterial Puncture
Description

Arterial blood sampling involves puncturing an artery, usually the radial artery, using a heparinized syringe. The HCW can then collect blood samples to assess oxygenation status.

Procedure

The procedure for arterial puncture is outlined in Table 17-2.

Text continued on p. 328.

Table 17-1 Venipuncture with an over-the-needle plastic catheter

Steps	Rationale
1. Observe for signs and symptoms indicating fluid or electrolyte imbalances: a. Sunken eyes b. Periorbital edema c. Greater than 2% increase or decrease in body weight d. Dry mucous membranes e. Flattened or distended neck veins f. Change from baseline vital signs g. Irregular pulse rhythm h. Auscultation for crackles in lungs i. Poor skin turgor j. Increased or decreased bowel sounds k. Decreased urine output l. Behavioral changes m. Confusion	Because fluid and electrolyte disturbances can affect every system in body, nurse must systematically assess client to identify abnormalities related to fluid or electrolyte imbalance. Daily weight measurements document fluid retention or loss. Change in body weight of 1 kg corresponds to 1 L of fluid retention or loss.
2. Review physician's fluid replacement orders.	Venipuncture before IV therapy is an invasive technique requiring a physician's order. IV fluids are medications and require an order.

Modified from Potter P, Perry A: *Fundamentals of nursing*, St Louis, 1993, Mosby.
IV, intravenous; *ONC,* over-the-needle catheter; *HIV,* human immunodeficiency virus.

Continued.

Table 17-1 Venipuncture with an over-the-needle plastic catheter—cont'd

Steps	Rationale
3. Assemble necessary equipment for initiating IV line (see illustration):	Correct solution and preparation of equipment assist in safe and quick placement of IV line.
a. Correct solution	
b. Proper needle for venipuncture	
c. Infusion set (infants and children require a 60 drop/ml [gtt/ml] drip and often a volume control device)	
d. IV tubing	
e. Alcohol or povidone-iodine cleansing swabs	
f. Tourniquet	
g. Arm board	
h. Gauze or transparent dressing and povidone-iodine solution or ointment	
i. Tape	
j. Towel to place under client's hand	
k. IV pole	
l. Disposable gloves	
4. Identify client and explain procedure.	Explanation reduces anxiety and promotes cooperation.
5. Organize equipment on clutter-free bedside stand or overbed table.	Organization reduces risk of contamination and accidents.

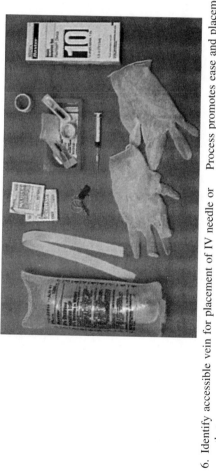

6. Identify accessible vein for placement of IV needle or catheter:

Process promotes ease and placement of IV catheter and needle.

a. Avoid bony prominences.
b. Use most distal portion of vein first.
c. Avoid placing IV line over patient's wrist.
d. Avoid placing IV line in patient's dominant hand.

Continued.

Table 17-1 Venipuncture with an over-the-needle plastic catheter—cont'd

Steps	Rationale
7. Wash hands.	Hand washing reduces transmission of microorganisms.
8. Open sterile packages using aseptic technique.	Technique maintains sterility of equipment and reduces spread of microorganisms.
9. Check solution, using five rights of drug administration. Make sure prescribed additives, such as potassium and vitamins, have been added.	IV solutions are medications and should be double-checked to reduce risk of error.
NOTE: When using bottled IV solution, remove metal cap and metal and rubber disks beneath cap.	This permits entry of infusion tubing into solution.
10. Open infusion set, maintaining sterility of both ends.	Sterile technique prevents bacteria from entering infusion equipment and thus bloodstream.
11. Place roller clamp (see illustration) about 2-4 cm (1-2 inches) below drip chamber, and move roller clamp to *off* position.	Close proximity of roller clamp to drip chamber allows more accurate regulation of flow rate and prevents accidental spillage of fluid on patient, nurse, bed, or floor.
12. Insert infusion set into fluid bag:	
a. Remove protective cover from IV bag without touching opening.	Technique maintains sterility of solution.
b. Remove protector cap from tubing insertion spike, not touching spike, and insert spike into opening of IV bag (see illustration). Or insert spike into black rubber stopper of IV bottle.	This permits entry of infusion solution into tubing and prevents contamination of solution from contaminated insertion spike.

Continued.

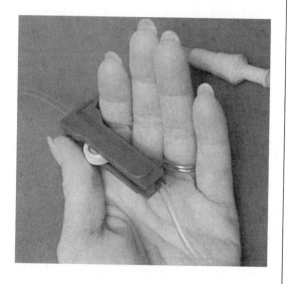

Table 17-1 Venipuncture with an over-the-needle plastic catheter—cont'd

Steps	Rationale
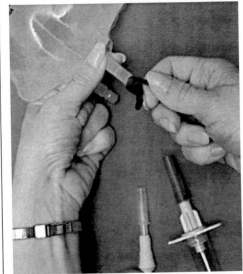	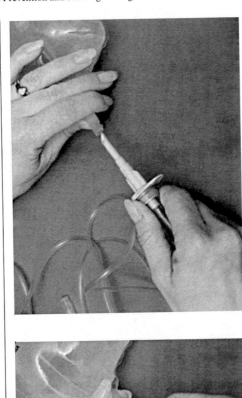

13. Fill infusion tubing:

    a. Compress drip chamber and release.

Compression and release creates suction effect; fluid enters drip chamber.

    b. Remove needle protector and release roller clamp to allow fluid to travel from drip chamber through tubing to needle adapter. Return roller clamp to *off* position after tube is filled.

This removes air from tubing and permits tubing to fill with solution.

    c. Be certain tubing is clear of air and air bubbles.

Large air bubbles can act as emboli.

    d. Replace needle protector.

This maintains system sterility.

14. Select appropriate IV needle or ONC.

Needle or ONC is necessary to puncture vein and instill IV fluid.

15. Select distal site of vein to be used.

If sclerosing or damage to vein has occurred, proximal site of same vein is still usable.

16. If large amount of body hair is present at needle insertion site, clip it.

Clipping reduces risk of contamination from bacteria on hair, assists in maintaining intactness of IV dressing, and makes removal of adhesive tape less painful. Shaving may cause microabrasions and predispose to infection.

17. If possible, place extremity in dependent position.

Position permits venous dilation and visibility.

18. Place tourniquet 10-12 cm (5-6 inches) above insertion site. Tourniquet should obstruct venous, not arterial, flow (see illustration). Check distal pulse.

Diminished arterial flow prevents venous filling.

Continued.

Table 17-1   Venipuncture with an over-the-needle plastic catheter—cont'd

Steps	Rationale
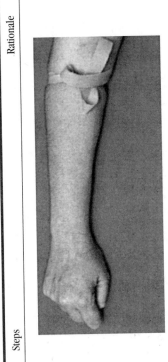	
19. Select well-dilated vein (see illustration). Methods to foster vein dilation include stroking extremity from proximal to distal, opening and closing fist, lightly tapping over vein, and applying warmth. NOTE: Be sure needle adapter end of infusion set is nearby and on sterile gauze or towel.	Methods increase venous dilation and permit smooth, quick connection of infusion to needle after vein is punctured.

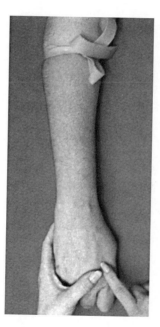

20. Apply disposable gloves.

    Gloves decrease exposure to HIV, hepatitis, and other bloodborne organisms.

21. Cleanse insertion site with firm, concentric, circular motion outward from insertion site using povidone-iodine solution. Allow to dry (see illustration). If patient is allergic to iodine, use 70% alcohol for 30 seconds.

    Povidone-iodine is topical antiinfective that reduces skin surface bacteria. It must dry to be effective.

Continued.

Table 17-1 Venipuncture with an over-the-needle plastic catheter—cont'd

Steps	Rationale

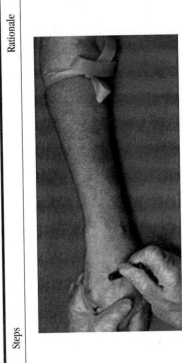

22. Perform venipuncture. Anchor vein by placing thumb over vein and by stretching skin against direction of insertion 2-3 inches distal to site.

a. *ONC:* Insert bevel at 20- to 30-degree angle in direction of venous blood return distal to actual site of venipuncture.

Nurse must place needle parallel with vein. Thus, when vein is punctured, risk of puncturing both sides is reduced.

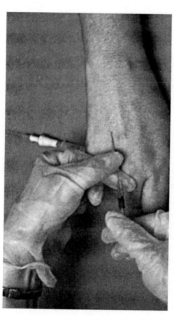

b. *Butterfly needle:* Place needle at 20- to 30-degree angle with bevel up, about 1 cm (½ inch) distal to site of venipuncture.

23. Look for blood return through tubing of butterfly needle or flashback chamber on ONC, indicating that needle has entered vein. Lower needle until almost flush with skin. Advance catheter approximately ¼ inch into vein and then loosen stylet (see illustration). Continue advancing flexible catheter or butterfly needle until hub rests at venipuncture site.

Increased venous pressure from tourniquet increases backflow of blood into catheter or tubing. Stylet helps puncture skin and advance catheter but must be removed to avoid puncture of vein.

Continued.

Table 17-1 Venipuncture with an over-the-needle plastic catheter—cont'd

Steps	Rationale

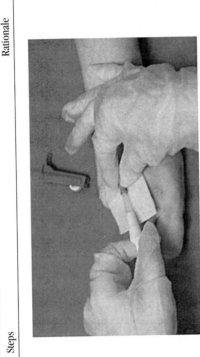

24. Stabilizing catheter with one hand, release tourniquet and remove stylet from ONC.

Technique reduces backflow of blood.

25. Connect needle adapter of infusion to hub of ONC or needle. Do not touch point of entry of needle adapter or inside hub of ONC (see illustration).

Prompt connection of infusion set maintains patency of vein. Maintains sterility.

26. Release roller clamp to begin infusion at rate to maintain patency of IV line.

This permits venous flow and prevents clotting of vein and obstruction of flow of IV solution.

27. Secure IV catheter or needle:

a. Place narrow piece (½ inch) of tape under hub of catheter with adhesive side up, and cross tape over hub.

Tape prevents accidental removal of catheter from vein.

b. Place small amount of povidone-iodine solution or ointment at venipuncture site. Allow solution to dry.

Povidone-iodine solution or ointment is topical antiseptic germicide that reduces bacteria on skin and decreases risk of local or systemic infection. When transparent dressing is used, povidone-iodine solution is recommended; ointment interferes with adherence of dressing to skin.

c. Place second piece of narrow tape directly across catheter's hub.

Tape prevents accidental disconnection of IV infusion.

d. Place transparent dressing over venipuncture site, following manufacturer's directions (see illustration). (Alternate method: place 2 × 2 gauze dressing over venipuncture site and catheter hub. Do not cover connection between IV tubing and catheter hub. Secure it with two 1-inch pieces of tape.)

Transparent dressing allows continual observation of venipuncture site. (Allows tubing changes without disturbing dressing.)

Continued.

Table 17-1   Venipuncture with an over-the-needle plastic catheter—cont'd

Steps	Rationale

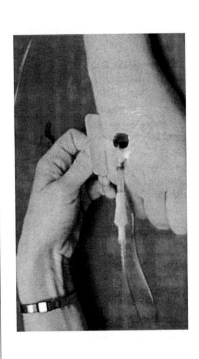

e. Secure infusion tubing to catheter with piece of 1-inch tape.

Tubing further stabilizes connection of infusion to catheter.

28. Write date, time of placement of IV line, size of needle, and nurse's initial and title on IV dressing.

This provides immediate data as to time of IV insertion and subsequent dressing changes.

29. Adjust flow rate to correct drops per minute.

Nurse must maintain correct rate of flow for IV solution.

30. Discard gloves and supplies and wash hands.

Sterile technique reduces transmission of microorganisms.

31. Observe client every hr to determine response to fluid therapy:
    a. Correct amount of solution infused as prescribed
    b. Proper flow rate (drops per minute)
    c. Patency of IV catheter or needle
    d. Absence of infiltration, phlebitis, or inflammation

Observation provides continuous evaluation of type and amount of fluid delivered to client. Hourly inspection prevents accidental fluid overload or inadequate infusion rate.

32. Record in nurses' notes type of fluid, insertion site, flow rate, size and type of IV catheter or needle, and time infusion was begun. Note response to IV fluid, amount infused, and integrity and patency of IV system (whether infusing by gravity or by pump), according to agency policy.

Documents initiation of IV fluid therapy as ordered by physician. Follow-up documentation provides data about response to therapy.

Table 17-2 Arterial puncture

Steps	Rationale
1. Collect the following equipment and bring it to bedside:	Permits quick and efficient performance
a. Heparinized 5-ml syringe	Prevents coagulation of arterial sample
b. ⅝-inch 20-gauge needle	Promotes atraumatic cannulization of artery
c. Crushed ice for arterial blood sample	Decreases oxygen metabolism of sample
d. Local anesthetic	Reduces local pain when more than one attempt is necessary and reduces likelihood of arterial spasm
e. Topical skin antibacterial scrub and alcohol wipes	Reduces entry of surface bacteria into puncture site
f. Air lock or cap for syringe	Prevents air from entering blood after sample has been obtained, thus altering results of blood gas analysis
g. 2 × 2 gauze	Allows application of pressure after arterial puncture
h. Disposable gloves	Reduces risk of exposure to HIV, hepatitis, and other bloodborne bacteria
i. Tape	
2. Check patient's identity. Explain procedure and patient's responsibility.	Ensures that correct client undergoes procedure; prevents hyperventilation that results from anxiety and resulting temporary change in blood gases

3. Palpate radial artery and perform Allen's test:	Prepares artery (Radial artery is selected because it is superficially located, has collateral circulation, and is not adjacent to large vein.)
a. Have patient make tight fist.	Determines adequate collateral flow to hand
b. Apply direct pressure to radial and ulnar arteries.	Removes as much blood from hand as possible Obstructs arterial blood flow to hand
c. Have patient open hand.	Determines if fingers and hand pale and blanched, indicating lack of arterial blood flow
d. Release pressure over ulnar artery; observe color of fingers, thumbs, and hand. Fingers and hand should flush within 15 seconds. If test is negative (no flushing), radial artery should be avoided. Check other hand.	Indicates if collateral circulation to hand is present through ulnar artery (Ulnar artery can supply blood flow to hand if radial artery is damaged or becomes occluded during procedure.)
4. Hyperextend patient's wrist over rolled towel.	Maintains radial artery in superficial position
5. Wash hands. Apply disposable gloves.	Reduces risk of exposure to HIV, hepatitis, and other bloodborne bacteria
6. Cleanse site with circular motion using povidone-iodine followed by alcohol wipe.	Reduces risk of skin bacteria entering puncture site

Continued.

Modified from Potter P, Perry A: *Fundamentals of nursing*, St Louis, 1993, Mosby.
HIV, human immunodeficiency virus.

Table 17-2   Arterial puncture—cont'd

Steps	Rationale
7. Apply local anesthetic. Xylocaine 2% is usually inject-ed subcutaneously.	Reduces pain and subsequent hyperventilation in some clients and decreases likelihood of arterial spasm
8. Flush 3-ml syringe with small amount of heparin (1000 units/ml) and then empty syringe, leaving heparin in needle and hub.	Prevents clotting of blood sample (Excess heparin in syringe affects pH value of sample blood.)
9. While palpating artery, insert needle at 45-degree angle while stabilizing patient's artery with your free hand (see illustration).	Minimizes formation of hematoma at puncture site
10. Observe for pulsating flow of blood into syringe.	Indicates puncture of artery
11. Withdraw 2 ml of blood.	Provides sufficient amount for analysis
12. Remove needle and syringe from artery. Expel any air in syringe. Cork syringe with air lock.	Prevents entry of air into syringe (If air enters syringe, blood must be discarded to avoid inaccurate blood gas results.)
13. Rotate syringe so that blood mixes with heparin.	Prevents clotting of sample
14. Submerge syringe in crushed ice.	Reduces rate of oxygen metabolism of sampled blood

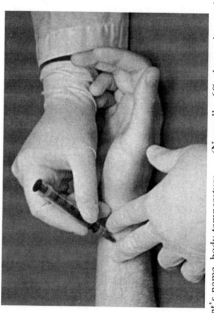

15. Label specimen with client's name, body temperature, and (for client on oxygen therapy) inspired oxygen concentration.

(Normally, 6% change in arterial PaO_2 occurs with each degree of centigrade of body temperature. Measurement of oxygen concentration is important in evaluating effectiveness of oxygen therapy.)

Continued.

Table 17-2 Arterial puncture—cont'd

Steps	Rationale

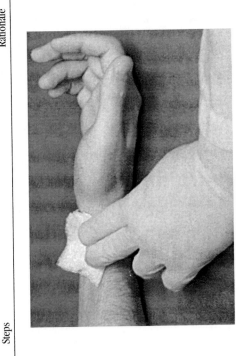

16. Have specimens transported to laboratory immediately.	Prevents alteration of blood gas values by cellular metabolism
17. Apply pressure to puncture site by applying 2 × 2 gauze over site and holding for 5 minutes. Length of time may be increased for patient receiving anticoagulants (see illustration).	Reduces risk of hematoma formation and damage to artery
18. Apply tape over gauze when bleeding stops.	Prevents bleeding as extremity is moved
19. Discard equipment in appropriate container, remove and dispose of gloves, and wash hands.	Reduces transmission of microorganisms
20. Record in nurse's notes time of arterial blood gas test and extremity from which specimen was drawn.	Documents that arterial blood gas specimen was obtained

Follow Up

Following arterial puncture, pressure is applied to the site for at least 5 minutes (or longer if the patient is on anticoagulants). The site is checked for signs of continued bleeding.

Blood Administration

Description

Blood or blood products replace lost blood or plasma, platelets, or red blood cells. Blood or blood products increase the vascular volume, increase the number of formed elements such as red blood cells, maintain the hemoglobin and hematocrit levels, and assist clotting by the administration of clotting factors.[1] Administration of the correct type of blood is vital to prevent a transfusion reaction.

Procedure

The following materials are collected, and the procedure described in Table 17-3 is followed.

1. Correct blood or blood product
2. 0.9% (normal) saline solution
3. Infusion tubing with in-line filter
4. Y-type administration set
5. Latex gloves

Follow Up

The patient is monitored for signs of transfusion reaction, with diverse symptoms ranging from rash to shock. Vital signs are monitored every 5 minutes for the first 15 to 30 minutes, then hourly. Blood-contaminated materials are then appropriately discarded.

IV Therapy Solution and Tubing Maintenance

Description

IV tubing can be a reservoir for the growth of microorganisms. All tubing should be changed every 24 to 48 hours according to agency policy. Solutions should be changed at least every 24 hours. The following procedure describes exchanging old tubing with new tubing and ensures that all solutions are changed as well.

Text continued on p. 338.

Table 17-3   Administering a blood transfusion

Steps		Rationale
1. Explain procedure to patient. Determine if there have been prior transfusions and note reactions, if any.	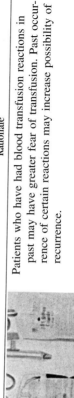	Patients who have had blood transfusion reactions in past may have greater fear of transfusion. Past occurrence of certain reactions may increase possibility of recurrence.
2. Ask patient to report chills, headaches, itching, or rash immediately.		These are signs of transfusion reaction. Prompt reporting and discontinuation of transfusion can help minimize reaction.
3. Be sure patient has signed consent forms.		Some agencies require patients to sign consent forms before receiving blood component transfusions.
4. Wash hands. Apply disposable gloves.		Gloves reduce risk for transmission of HIV, hepatitis, and other bloodborne bacteria.
5. Establish IV line with large-gauge (#18 or #19) catheter.		Large-gauge catheters permit infusion of whole blood and prevent hemolysis.
6. Use infusion tubing that has in-line filter. Tubing should also be Y-type administration set (see illustration).		Filter removes debris and tiny clots from blood. Y-type set permits administration of additional products or volume expanders easily and immediate infusion of isotonic 0.9% sodium chloride solution after completion of blood infusion.

Continued.

Modified from Potter P, Perry A: *Fundamentals of nursing*, St Louis, 1993, Mosby.
HIV, human immunodeficiency virus; *RBC,* red blood cell.

Table 17-3 Administering a blood transfusion—cont'd

Steps	Rationale
7. Hang solution container of 0.9% normal saline to be administered after blood infusion.	Solution prevents hemolysis of RBCs.
8. Follow agency protocol in obtaining blood products from blood bank. Request blood when you are ready to use it.	Whole blood or packed RBCs must remain in cold (1° to 6°C) environment.
9. With another registered nurse, correctly identify blood product and patient:	One nurse reads out loud while other nurse listens and double-checks information to reduce risk of error.
a. Check compatibility tag attached to blood bag and information on bag itself.	This verifies that ABO group, Rh type, and unit number match.
b. For whole blood, check ABO group and Rh type, which is on patient's chart.	This verifies that information matches that on compatibility tag and blood tag.
c. Double-check blood product with physician's order.	This verifies correct blood component.
d. Check expiration data on bag.	After 21 days, blood has only 70% to 80% of original number of cells and 23 mEq/L of potassium.

e. Inspect blood for clots.

Anticoagulant citrate-phosphate-dextrose (CPD) is added to blood and permits preserved blood to be stored for 21 days. Another anticoagulant, citrate-phosphate-dextrose-adenine (CPD-A), allows storage for 35 days. If clots are present, return blood to blood bank.

f. Ask patient's name, and check arm band.

Verify correct patient. Do not administer blood to patient without arm band. Identification name and number on wristband must be identical to those on blood compatibility tag.

10. Obtain baseline vital signs.

Verify pretransfusion temperature, pulse rate, blood pressure, and respirations.

11. Begin transfusion:

a. Prime infusion line with 0.9% normal saline.

Isotonic saline prevents hemolysis.

b. Begin transfusion slowly by first filling in-line filter.

If filter is not filled, transfusion will not infuse properly.

c. Adjust rate to 2 ml/min for first 15 minutes, and remain with patient. If you suspect reaction, *stop* transfusion, flush line with normal saline, infuse normal saline slowly, and notify blood bank and physician.

This allows detection of reaction while infusing smallest possible volume of blood product. Flushing line prevents further infusion of blood product.

Continued.

Table 17-3   Administering a blood transfusion—cont'd

Steps	Rationale
12. Remove and dispose of gloves. Wash hands.	Hand washing reduces transmission of microorganisms.
13. Monitor vital signs:	
a. Take vital signs every 5 minutes for 15 minutes of transfusion and every hour thereafter.	Document change in vital sign status that could indicate early warning of reaction.
b. Observe patient for flushing, itching, dyspnea, hives, and rash.	Signs may indicate reaction.
14. Maintain prescribed infusion rate using infusion pumps, if necessary.	Infusion pumps maintain prescribed rate.
15. Continually observe for adverse reactions.	Adverse reactions can occur at any point during transfusion.
16. Record administration of blood or blood product.	Record documents administration of blood component.
17. When infusion is completed, return blood bag and tubing to blood bank.	This provides material for analysis if reaction is later discovered.

Table 17-4 Changing IV solutions and tubing

Steps	Rationale
Changing IV Solution	
1. Identify patient. Review physician's orders and have next solution prepared at least 1 hour before needed. If solution is prepared in pharmacy, be sure it has been delivered to floor. Check that solution is correct and properly labeled.	Ensures that correct patient undergoes procedure (Prevents finding empty IV bag without having replacement. Checking prevents medication error. If order is written for KVO, change solution every 24 hours. Sterility of solution cannot be ensured longer than 24 hours.)
2. Prepare to change solution when less than 50 ml remains in bottle or bag.	Prevents air from entering IV tubing and maintains patency of tubing and catheter or needle
3. Be sure drip chamber is half full.	Provides IV fluid to vein while bag is being changed
4. Wash hands.	Reduces transmission of microorganisms
5. Prepare new solution for changing. If using plastic bag, remove protective cover from entry site. If using glass bottle, remove metal cap, metal disk, and rubber disk. Maintain sterility of entry site on bag or bottle.	Permits quick, smooth, and organized change from old to new solution
6. Move roller clamp to reduce flow rate.	Prevents solution remaining in drip chamber from emptying while changing solutions
7. Remove old solution from IV pole.	Brings work to nurse's eye level
8. Quickly remove spike from old IV solution, and without touching tip, spike new solution bottle.	Reduces risk of solution in drip chamber (Step 3) running dry and maintains sterility

Modified from Potter P, Perry A: *Fundamentals of nursing*, St Louis, 1993, Mosby.

IV, intravenous; *KVO*, keep vein open; *RBC*, red blood cell; *ONC*, over-the-needle catheter; *HIV*, human immunodeficiency virus.

Continued.

Table 17-4 Changing IV solutions and tubing—cont'd

Steps	Rationale
9. Hang new bag or bottle of solution. Discard empty bag or bottle according to agency policy.	Allows gravity to assist with delivery of IV fluid into drip chamber
10. Check for air in tubing.	Reduces risk of air embolus
11. Make sure drip chamber contains solution.	Reduces risk of air entering IV tubing
12. Regulate flow rate to prescribed rate.	Restores fluid balance and delivers IV fluid as ordered
13. Observe IV system for patency, absence of infiltration phlebitis, and inflammation. Observe response to IV therapy.	Provides ongoing evaluation of response to IV therapy
Changing IV Tubing	
14. Determine when new infusion set is warranted:	
a. Hanging first solution of day	Prevents contamination (Changing tubing prevents infection. Procedure is simplified by changing tubing with new solution.)
b. Puncture of infusion tubing	Results in leakage of fluid
c. Contamination of tubing	Can allow entry of bacteria into bloodstream
d. Occlusion of IV tubing (e.g., after infusion of packed RBCs, whole blood, or albumin)	Avoids contamination (Whole blood or blood component products may occlude or partially occlude IV tubing.)
e. Date on tubing indicating that tubing has been in place for 48 hours	Avoids contamination
15. Assemble the following:	Enables nurse to complete procedure efficiently and safely
a. Infusion tubing	
b. Sterile 2 × 2 gauze	

c. If new IV dressing must be applied:
   (1) Sterile 2×2 gauze or transparent dressing
   (2) Povidone-iodine ointment or solution
   (3) Adhesive remover
   (4) Alcohol swabs
   (5) Strips of tape or polyurethane film dressing
   (6) Disposable gloves

16. Explain procedure to patient.

Promotes cooperation and prevents sudden movement of extremity, which could dislodge needle or catheter

17. Wash hands.

Reduces transmission of microorganisms

18. Open new infusion set, keeping protective coverings over infusion spike and insertion site for butterfly needle or ONC.

Provides nurse with ready access to new infusion set and maintains sterility of infusion set

19. Apply nonsterile disposable gloves.

Decreases risk of exposure to HIV, hepatitis, and other bloodborne bacteria

20. Place sterile 2×2 gauze on bed near IV puncture site.

Provides sterile field for new sterile needle adapter before connection to IV needle or catheter

21. If needle or catheter hub is not visible, remove IV dressing. Do not remove tape that secures needle or catheter to skin.

Smooths process (Needle hub must be accessible to provide smooth transition when removing old tubing and inserting new tubing.)

Continued.

Table 17-4 Changing IV solutions and tubing—cont'd

Steps	Rationale
22. Take new IV tubing and move roller clamp to *off* position.	Prevents spillage of solution after new bag or bottle is spiked
23. Slow rate of infusion by regulating drip rate on old tubing.	Prevents complete infusion of solution remaining in tubing
24. With old tubing in place, compress drip chamber and fill chamber.	Provides surplus in drip chamber so that there is sufficient fluid to maintain patency while changing tubing
25. Discontinue old tubing from solution, and hang drip chamber over IV pole.	Allows fluid to continue to flow through catheter while new tubing is prepared
26. Place insertion spike of new tubing into old IV solution opening, and hang solution pole.	Permits flow of fluid from solution into new infusion tubing
27. Compress and release drip chamber on new tubing.	Allows drip chamber to fill and promotes rapid, smooth flow of solution through new tubing
28. Open roller clamp, remove protective cap from needle adapter, and flush tubing with solution.	Removes air from tubing and replaces it with fluid
29. Place needle adapter of new IV tubing, with protective cap off, between sterile 2 × 2 gauze near IV site.	Allows smooth, quick insertion of new tubing into needle hub while maintaining sterility of infusion tubing
30. Turn roller clamp on old tubing to *off* position.	Prevents spillage of fluid as tubing is removed from needle hub

31. Stabilize hub of IV catheter or needle, gently pull out old tubing, and quickly insert needle adapter of new tubing into hub.	Prevents accidental displacement of catheter or needle; prevents clot formation in catheter or needle
32. Open roller clamp on new tubing.	Permits solution to enter catheter or tubing
33. Regulate IV drip according to physician's orders, and monitor rate hourly.	Maintains infusion flow at prescribed rate
34. If necessary, apply new dressing.	Reduces risk of bacterial infection from skin
35. Discard old tubing and gloves in container for contaminated materials, and wash hands.	Reduces transmission of microorganisms
36. Evaluate flow rate, and observe connection site for leakage.	Maintains prescribed rate of flow of IV therapy and determines whether fit is secure
37. Record changing of tubing and solution on patient's record and place piece of tape with date and time below level of drip chamber. Record fluid infused on input and output form.	Documents procedure and records that measures to maintain sterility were carried out; provides visual cue to all care providers of when IV tubing was changed

The solution in a keep-vein-open IV line should be changed every 24 hours.

Procedure

The procedure for changing IV solutions and tubing is described in Table 17-4.

Follow Up

The patency of the new tubing and the IV site is monitored. The HCW should ensure that the solution is infusing and check for signs of infiltration, infection, or thrombophlebitis.

Infection Prevention

Infection control strategies interrupt the modes of transmission to prevent microbial access into the cardiovascular system. The strategies include consistently using sterile solutions and devices and using aseptic technique when starting IV or arterial lines, flushing lines, changing tubing/dressings, or administering medication or blood and blood products. Hand washing is the single most important procedure to prevent nosocomial infections. The following lists of strategies outline specific measures to prevent IV-related infections.

Interrupt Device and Solution Related Transmission

1. Wash hands before any manipulations of the system.
2. Wear gloves for insertion and dressing changes.
3. Inspect all solutions, additives, IV devices, and containers before use.
4. Ensure that solutions never hang longer than 24 hours.
5. Maintain sterility of solution and devices.
6. If large amount of body hair is present at IV insertion site, clip it to reduce the risk of contamination from bacteria on hair. It also helps in maintaining intact IV dressings and makes removal of adhesive tape less painful. Shaving may cause microabrasions in the skin, predisposing the area for microbial growth and/or entry.
7. Maintain sterility of tubing. Contamination of tubing allows entry of bacteria into bloodstream.
8. Blood and blood products:
   a. Do not permit blood to stand at room temperature longer than necessary. Warm temperatures promote bacterial growth.

Standard Precautions As They Pertain to IV Therapy

1. Wear gloves to reduce risk of exposure to blood, body fluids containing visible blood, and other fluids to which standard precautions apply. (See Chapter 7.)
2. Wash hands and other skin surfaces immediately and thoroughly if contaminated with blood or body fluids. Wash hands immediately after removing gloves.
3. To prevent needlestick injuries, do not recap, purposely bend, or break needles by hand; do not remove them from disposable syringes or otherwise manipulate them by hand.
4. Place used needles, syringes, and IV equipment in puncture-resistant disposal containers that are located as close as practical to the use area.
5. If you have exudative lesions or weeping dermatitis, refrain from all direct care and from handling invasive equipment until the condition resolves.

Modified from Centers for Disease Control and Prevention: Draft guidelines for isolation precautions in hospitals, *Federal Register* 59(214):55552, 1994.
IV, intravenous.

b. Inspect blood for gas bubbles, clotting, or abnormal color before transfusion.
c. Complete infusions within 4 hours. Change administration set after 4 hours of use. Blood or blood products may occlude or partially occlude IV tubing.[3,4]

Interrupt Person-to-Person Transmission

1. Wash hands. Adequate and frequent hand washing is the most effective means of infection prevention.
2. Wear gloves to protect both the patient and yourself from cross-contamination.
3. Use proper site preparation to reduce risk of skin bacteria entering puncture site.[4]
4. Refrain from all direct contact with IV or invasive equipment if you have exudative lesions.
5. Use standard precautions to protect yourself from potentially infectious body fluids. See the box above.

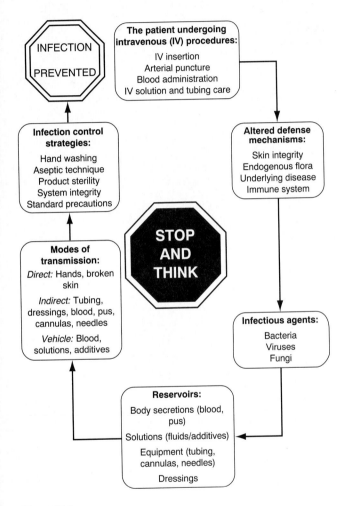

Figure 17-1.
Factors affecting the patient undergoing intravenous procedures leading to the selection of the strategies to prevent infectious complications.

Specific Prevention Measures

1. Use strict aseptic technique when inserting IV or changing IV dressing.
2. Wash hands adequately and frequently. (See Chapter 6.)
3. Anchor needle or catheter securely at insertion site.
4. Change insertion site at least every 72 hours.
5. Sufficiently dilute irritating agents before infusion.
6. Ensure that solutions never hang longer than 24 hours.
7. Use filter (preferably 0.22 micron) with infusion unless contraindicated.
8. Change insertion site at least every 48 to 72 hours.
9. Change IV administration set every 24 to 48 hours.
10. Change IV dressing every 24 to 48 hours.
11. Maintain the integrity of the infusion system.[3]

Summary

IV therapy occurs in all health care settings: acute care, ambulatory care, and home health care. Fifty percent of all patients admitted to the hospital each year receive infusion therapy. Devices inserted into the CV system bypass the normal skin defense mechanism and provide a portal of entry for microorganisms either from the device at the time of insertion, from subsequent device contamination, or from contamination at the insertion site. The risk of infection is reduced by specific prevention strategies that interrupt the modes of transmission by which microbes gain access to the CV system. Figure 17-1 summarizes the factors that cause infection and lists the prevention strategies to prevent it.

References

1. Widmer A: IV related infections. In Wenzel R, editor: *Prevention and control of nosocomial infections,* Baltimore, 1993, Williams & Wilkins.
2. Soule B, editor: *The APIC curriculum for infection control practice,* vol. 2, Dubuque, Iowa, 1983, Kendall/Hunt.
3. Suddarth D: *The Lippincott manual of nursing practice,* ed 5, Philadelphia, 1991, JB Lippincott.
4. Potter P, Perry A, *Fundamentals of nursing,* St Louis, 1993, Mosby.

Gastrointestinal Procedures 18

Procedures involving the gastrointestinal (GI) tract require precautions to prevent transmission of organisms that may cause a nosocomial GI infection and to prevent transmission of infection to health care workers (HCWs). There are limited data on the magnitude of nosocomial gastroenteritis, although a nosocomial GI infection rate of 10.5 per 10,000 hospital discharges has been reported. The highest infection rates are among medicine, surgery, and pediatric patients. Within the subspecialty services, rates are highest with burn, trauma, surgery, high-risk nursery, and oncology patients. Patients 60 years and older account for 64% of all infections.[1]

Specific Infection Risks

The most frequently reported organisms are *Clostridium difficile,* rotavirus, *Candida albicans,* and staphylococcus.[2] Bacteria are reported in 93% of the cases of nosocomial infections. The organisms that cause gastroenteritis are transmitted by fecal/oral transfer. The spread of the infection occurs by person-to-person direct contact but may also be spread by indirect or vehicle contact. Organisms within fecal matter survive for long periods, so feces are a reservoir for transmission.[1] Feeding formulas also act as reservoirs for infection. Inadequate hand washing and disinfection of equipment are culprits in transmission and colonization of patients with nosocomial gastroenteritis.[3]

Risk of infection is highest for neonates, elderly patients, and patients with burn or trauma injuries. Intrinsic risk factors include skin breakdown, aspiration, impaired immunity, decreased gastric acidity, decreased intestinal motility, and altered normal flora, as occurs with antibiotic administration.[1,4] Extrinsic risk factors are frequent nasogastric or jejunal feedings, treatment with cimetidine, and stay in an intensive care unit.[5] The risk to HCWs from gastric and jejunal procedures is unclear. Tube feedings carry little risk for HCW exposure to infectious disease.[6] The risks of exposure to blood with GI procedures are greater with a GI bleed than with tube feedings.

Home Care Considerations

Home care of the elderly or disabled often involves feeding by nasogastric, gastrostomy, or jejunal tubes. Vigorous hand washing to prevent transmission of organisms to the patient or the caregiver is also required of all persons who provide care in the home. (See Chapter 6.) Hand washing is required before and after any patient care activity. It also prevents transmission of infection from the patient to the family caregiver.

Nasogastric Tube Placement

A tube inserted nasally into the stomach or small intestine delivers feedings or medications. Problems with large-bore rubber tubes led to the development of more pliable, small-bore tubes. The size of the nasogastric (NG) tube selected varies by age and size of the patient. Usually, adults require 8 to 12 French tubes that are 36 to 43 inches long.[7] Children require a tube suitable to the size of the child and the viscosity of the fluid.[8]

Procedure Preparation

Before inserting the NG tube, the patient is assessed for bleeding, difficulty in swallowing, head or neck injury or surgery, decreased level of consciousness, and facial injury. The patency of each nostril and the presence of a normal gag reflex is also assessed. The patient's medical history is checked for evidence of nasal surgery or a deviated septum. The following equipment is assembled:

1. Small-bore NG tube (8-12 French)
2. Large syringe (30-ml irrigation syringe)
3. Tape
4. pH test strips
5. Water
6. Emesis basin
7. Tongue blade
8. Penlight
9. Towel and tissues

10. Clean disposable latex gloves
11. Face protection and gown

Procedure

1. Wash hands vigorously. Adequate hand washing is the most effective method of decreasing disease transmission to both the HCW and the patient. (See Chapter 6.)
2. Explain the procedure to the patient and stand on the side of the bed that corresponds to your dominant hand (i.e., right side if right-handed).
3. Place the patient in high Fowler's or semi-Fowler's position if decreased level of consciousness.
4. Place a towel over patient's chest.
5. Guide the patient in relaxing and breathing.
6. Determine the length of tube to be inserted by measuring the distance from the tip of the nose to the ear to the xiphoid process (traditional), or mark the 50-mm point on the tube and then do the traditional method. Insert the tube to the point midway between 50 mm and the traditional mark.
7. Inject 10 ml of water into the NG tube.
8. Dip the tip into water (do not ice plastic tubes).
9. Cut a 10-cm piece of tape, and split one end 5 cm.
10. Put on clean disposable latex gloves.
11. Insert the tube through a nostril to the back of the throat and down toward the ear.
12. Flex the patient's head to his or her chest after the tube passes through the nasopharynx.
13. Have the patient swallow to advance the tube (do not force the tube).
14. Check the position in the back of the throat using a penlight and tongue blade.
15. Check the placement of the tube by aspirating gastric contents and measuring the pH of the aspirate (acidic if gastric).
16. Tape the tube in place or fasten it to the patient's gown with a pin and rubber band; position the patient on the right side.
17. Remove gloves, and discard them according to agency policy.
18. Wash hands vigorously.
19. Talk with the patient and instruct him or her on care and maintenance of the tube.
20. Provide oral hygiene frequently.

21. Record the type of tube placed, the aspirate obtained, and the patient's tolerance of the procedure.[9]

Nasogastric Feedings

Verify the physician's orders for feeding, including tube size, length of time in place, feeding, and schedule of feedings. Determine the patient's tolerance of the previous feedings, including residuals before the feedings. Proceed as follows:

1. Place the patient in high Fowler's position.
2. Wash hands.
3. Assemble equipment as follows:
   a. Disposable feeding bag and tubing
   b. Irrigation syringe (60 ml)
   c. Feeding in ordered amount
   d. Water
   e. Emesis basin
   f. Infusion pump for feeding tubes
   g. Disposable latex gloves
4. Determine the placement of the tube.
5. Auscultate the patient's bowel sounds.
6. Wash hands vigorously, and put on gloves.
7. Administer feeding using bolus/intermittent method or continuous-drip method with infusion pump.
8. Administer additional water as ordered or needed.
9. Remove and dispose of gloves according to agency policy.
10. Wash hands thoroughly.
11. Record the type and amount of feeding and the patient's tolerance.[9]

Follow Up

The placement and patency of the tube should be checked frequently. The position of the tube should be checked before feedings and medication administration. Skin integrity is also checked.

Gastrostomy/Jejunostomy Feedings
Procedure Preparation

1. Check the physician's order for the method, amount, and type of feeding.

2. Gather the following equipment:
   a. Disposable latex gloves
   b. Disposable feeding bag and tubing
   c. Irrigation syringe (60 ml)
   d. Stethoscope
   e. Feeding and water
   f. Infusion pump for feeding tubes

Procedure

1. Explain the procedure to the patient and assist the patient in relaxing during the procedure.
2. Place the patient in high Fowler's position.
3. Verify gastrostomy tube placement as follows:
   a. Aspirate gastric secretions.
   b. Check pH.
   c. Auscultate the gastric area.
   d. Inject 15 ml of air.
4. Verify jejunostomy tube placement as follows:
   a. Aspirate intestinal secretions.
   b. Check for residuals.
5. For a gastrostomy tube, feed by intermittent (bolus) or continuous methods.
6. For jejunal tubes, feed by the intermittent method.[9]

Follow Up

The HCW washes hands, puts on gloves, and changes the exit site dressing after the feeding. The site is cleaned with warm water and mild soap each day. Gloves and used supplies are disposed of. The patient's tolerance of the feeding is assessed, and the type and amount of feeding is recorded.[9]

Flexible Endoscopy
Specific Infectious Risks

Flexible endoscopy allows visualization of the GI tract and early diagnosis and treatment of disease. Complications include bleeding and perforations. Very low rates of infection have been reported, but nosocomial transmission of microorganisms by endoscopes has been reported. Organisms from the endoscoped patient include normal flora (*Escherichia coli* and *Klebsiella* species), colonizing organisms (*Serratia* organisms), acute infections (salmonella and *Mycobacterium tuberculosis*), and chronic carrier states (salmonella, hepatitis B, and *M. tuberculosis*). The inanimate environment may contribute organisms from irrigating solutions (*Pseudomonas* species and atypical *Mycobacteria* organisms) and washing solutions (*Enterobacter, Citrobacter,* and *Pseudomonas* species). Parasitic cross-infections from a single endoscope have been reported. Viral transmission of hepatitis A, hepatitis C, and human immunodeficiency virus by means of endoscope has not been reported.[10]

Recommendations for Care of Equipment

Organic soil on endoscopes contributes to failure of the disinfectant solution. Vigorous cleaning to remove matter from the equipment is necessary before disinfection or sterilization. Equipment is cleaned using a nonabrasive, manufacturer recommended enzymatic detergent. The insertion tube is washed and rinsed and the channels are scrubbed to remove organic matter.

Endoscopes come into contact with mucous membranes and are considered semicritical equipment needing high-level disinfection (see Chapter 9). All internal and external surfaces and channels must be in contact with the disinfectant agent for at least 20 minutes. Agents recommended for all levels of disinfection are discussed in the Association for Practitioners of Infection Control guideline for selection and use of disinfectants.[11] Recommended disinfectants include the following:
1. 2% glutaraldehyde preparations
   a. Alkaline glutaraldehyde
   b. Acid glutaraldehyde
2. 6% hydrogen peroxide/0.85% phosphoric acid solution
3. 0.2% peracetic acid.

Agents not recommended for disinfection of endoscopes are glutaraldehyde with phenol preparations, iodophors, hypochlorite (bleach), quaternary ammonium compounds, and phenolics.[10]

Infection Prevention

Interventions by the HCW can decrease the risk of infection transmission.

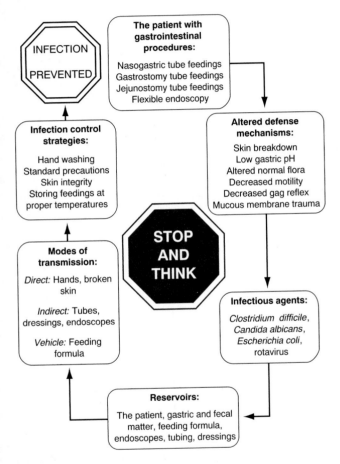

Figure 18-1.
Factors affecting the patient undergoing gastrointestinal procedures leading to the selection of the strategies to prevent infectious complications.

1. *Endoscopy:* Risks of infection are low, although mucous membranes may be broken. To reduce the risk of transmission, clean instruments completely, then use high-level disinfection or sterilization.

2. *Nasogastric and feeding tubes:* Risks arise from trauma to the mucous membrane from pressure on membranes and tissue anoxia. Suctioning and movement of the tube can injure tissue. There is increased exposure to microorganisms. To reduce the risks of infection, tissues should not be traumatized during tube insertion, atraumatic suction and irrigation should be provided, nostril care should be provided to decrease irritation, the patient should be assessed for adequate hydration, feeding equipment should be rinsed and cleaned, and feeding solutions should be stored at the recommended temperature.[12] Feedings should be hung for no more than 4 hours, and stomach capacity should not be exceeded. Tube placement must be checked before each feeding.

3. *Gastrostomy:* Infection risk is associated with wound or skin excoriation by gastric secretions. To reduce the risks of infection, dressings should be changed immediately if they are wet or soiled. Skin protective agents, such as karaya gum, should be used.

Summary

Procedures involving the GI tract require precautions to prevent the transmission of harmful organisms. Defense mechanisms are altered, including skin breakdown, low gastric pH, altered normal flora, decreased motility and gag reflex, and trauma to the mucous membrane. Infectious agents can enter from reservoirs by hands, broken skin, tubes, dressings, feeding formula, and endoscopes. To control infection, the HCW must wash hands, use standard precautions, maintain skin integrity, and store feedings at proper temperatures (Fig. 18-1).

References

1. Jarvis W, Hughes J: Nosocomial gastrointestinal infections. In Wenzel R, editor: *Prevention and control of nosocomial infections,* ed 2, Baltimore, 1993, Williams & Wilkins.

2. Garner J et al: The Centers for Disease Control definition for nosocomial infections, 1988, *Am J Infect Control* 138:131, 1988.

3. Henderson D: Human immunodeficiency virus infection in patients and providers. In Wenzel R, editor: *Prevention and control of nosocomial infections,* ed 2, Baltimore, 1993, Williams & Wilkins.

4. Yolken R et al: Infectious gastroenteritis in bone marrow transplant recipients, *N Engl J Med* 306:1010, 1982.

5. Gurevich I: *Infectious diseases in critical care nursing,* Rockville, 1989, Aspen Publishers.

6. Lettau L, Blackhurst D, Steed C: Human immunodeficiency virus testing experience and hepatitis B vaccination and testing status of healthcare workers in South Carolina: implications for compliance with US Public Health Service Guidelines, *Infect Control Hosp Epidemiol* 13:336, 1992.

7. Potter P, Perry A: *Fundamentals of nursing: concepts, process & practice,* St Louis, 1993, Mosby.

8. Scipien G et al: *Pediatric nursing care,* St Louis, 1990, Mosby.

9. Kozier B et al: *Techniques in clinical nursing,* Redwood City, Calif, 1993, Addison-Wesley.

10. Martin M, Reichelderfer M: APIC guidelines for infection control practice: APIC guideline for infection prevention and control in flexible endoscopy, *Am J Infect Control* 22:19, 1994.

11. Rutala W: APIC guideline for selection and use of disinfectants, *Am J Infect Control* 19:99, 1990.

12. Soule B, editor: *The APIC curriculum for infection control and practice,* vol 2, Dubuque, Iowa, 1983, Kendall/Hunt.

Dialysis

19

In 1973 Medicare began reimbursement for the treatment of end-stage renal disease. Now, thousands of people undergo treatment via peritoneal dialysis or hemodialysis. Both types of dialysis require maintenance of an artificial access site that predisposes the patient to infection. In addition, dialysis patients experience immunosuppression related to depression of the total number of lymphocytes and impairment in cell-mediated or humoral immune responses.[1] Of all deaths in patients with renal failure, 10% result from infection.[2]

This chapter describes the two methods of dialysis. Steps to reduce the risk of access-associated infection are presented, and signs and symptoms of site infection, peritonitis, and systemic infection are described.

Dialysis Methods

Both peritoneal dialysis and hemodialysis replace normal kidney function by removing metabolic waste products and achieving electrolyte and water balance. Semipermeable membranes are used for this function. A balanced electrolyte solution (dialysate) is introduced on one side of the membrane, and blood flows to the other side. Solutes move from the blood to the dialysate by diffusing down a concentration gradient and/or by movement from introduced pressures. The membrane differs for peritoneal dialysis and hemodialysis. Peritoneal dialysis uses the peritoneum as the membrane; therefore, the dialysate is infused into the peritoneal cavity. Hemodialysis uses an artificial membrane and circulates the patient's blood through an external machine.[3]

Peritoneal Dialysis

Peritoneal dialysis is used for acute in-hospital intervention for acute renal failure or as chronic intervention for end-stage renal disease. Continuous ambulatory peritoneal dialysis (CAPD) or continuous cyclical peritoneal dialysis (CCPD) is used. Peritoneal dialysis is achieved by osmosis and diffusion. A hyperosmolar dialysate fluid is instilled into the peritoneal cavity through a peritoneal dialysis catheter. The dialysate remains in the cavity for several hours, allowing uremic toxins, fluids, and metabolic waste products to diffuse across the peritoneal membrane in a process known as *exchange*. The hyperosmolar peritoneal dialysate fluid "pulls" the toxins from the blood and is then drained out. Fresh dialysate is infused, and the process is repeated.

Specific Infection Risks

During the exchange process, there is high potential for patient infection. Microbial contamination can be introduced during initial insertion of the catheter, at the skin site where the catheter exists, or anytime during the procedure. Peritonitis is a major complication of peritoneal dialysis and can be life threatening to the patient.[4,5]

Staphylococcus aureus is the most common microorganism in exit site infection, accounting for 61% of these infections.[6-8] Other common pathogens include *Staphylococcus epidermidis* and *Pseudomonas* species. Prompt recognition of infection and early treatment with the appropriate antibiotic reduces the necessity for catheter removal and reduces patient morbidity and mortality. Endogenous or exogenous bacteria found on the skin or the perineum are the most frequent causes of pathogen infections.

Catheter Site Infections

The National Institute of Health Continuous Ambulatory Peritoneal Dialysis Registry reports an occurrence rate of 0.7 episodes of exit site and tunnel infections per patient per year.[9] Exit site and tunnel infections account for 16% of peritonitis infections and frequently result in peritoneal dialysis catheter loss.[10,11] Twardowski describes a healthy exit site as follows:

> It is mature, 6 months or longer; strong mature epithelium is present in the sinus; the sinus tract is usually dry but may be damp or contain thick drainage; crust forms no more frequently than every seven days; the exit color is natural or dark; a pale pink color is occasionally present.[11]

Peritonitis

It is estimated that peritonitis occurs in approximately 60% of CAPD patients within the first year of dialysis.[5] The development of recurrent peritonitis (20% to 30% of patients) is the most frequent reason for CAPD failure.

Signs and symptoms

One of the earliest signs of peritonitis may be cloudy dialysate. Other common signs and symptoms of peritonitis include abdominal pain, elevated temperature, nausea, vomiting, chills, and drainage problems. Because these "classic" signs and symptoms of infection may be absent, it is important to teach patients to report changes in the color of their dialysate fluid.[7]

Diagnosis and treatment

A cell count with gram stain and culture may be performed and the patient started on a broad spectrum antibiotic as soon as the causative organism is identified. Specific therapy for infection should be used because long-term antibiotic treatment is often required. However, prolonged antibiotic use can cause development of antibiotic resistance to specific organisms with subsequent severe infections.

Cultures demonstrating mixed gram-positive and gram-negative bacteria may indicate bowel perforation and may indicate the need for emergency surgical intervention. In 10% to 20% of cases, no organism can be identified.[8] Individuals with impaired renal function may have a lower threshold for development of toxicity to aminoglycosides, so with gram-negative infections, therapeutic levels must be monitored to prevent ear and vestibular toxicities.

Dialysis Catheter Procedures

Peritoneal dialysis catheters may be inserted at the bedside or in the operating room by a physician. All health care workers (HCWs) who are directly involved in the dialysis catheter insertion should complete a surgical hand scrub. The surgical hand scrub reduces the risk of infection by decreasing the number of microorganisms that can be transferred from the hands of HCWs to the patient. A sterile work field should be set up for the procedure.[5] (See Chapter 10.)

Patient preparation

The procedure and possible complications are explained to the patient. After giving appropriate explanation, the patient is asked to sign a permission form. The patient is instructed to void (a straight catheter is inserted if the patient is unable to void).

(See Chapter 14.) Additionally, preoperative antibiotics may be administered.[12]

The patient is placed in a supine position. Immediately before catheter insertion, abdominal hair is removed with an electric razor or clippers, avoiding cuts to the skin.

Catheter placement

The physician or nurse chooses the catheter exit site. The exit site should be

1. Above or below the belt line
2. Away from scars
3. Above fat folds (assess with patient in a sitting position)
4. Respectful of patient preference and easily accessed by the patient
5. Lateral on either flank in sexually active persons[12]

Equipment

Place sterile gowns, masks, and surgical tray at the patient's bedside. Place the following equipment on the sterile field:

1. Abdominal catheter (soaked in saline or antibiotic solution for 5 minutes)[12,13]
2. Suture material
3. Radiopaque dye (optional) if physician installs in the x-ray department
4. Peritoneal dialysis fluid (to be instilled once the catheter is in place)

Catheter safety

Once the catheter is inserted, peritoneal dialysis fluid (dialysate) is instilled. The fluid should easily flow into the peritoneal wall without occlusion. If no flow problems exist, the catheter is capped. A sterile or transparent dressing is applied over the insertion and exit site, and is left in place. The catheter is immobilized by taping it securely to the abdominal wall. This prevents movement of the catheter and allows tissue ingrowth into the cuff to improve healing. When a dressing change is necessary, *strict* aseptic technique should be followed. (See Chapter 10.)

Incision and catheter care procedure
Supplies

Gather the following supplies:

1. 70% isopropyl alcohol
2. Peritoneal dialysis tray (includes sterile drapes, 4×4 sponges, cotton-tipped applicators, and solution cups)
3. Masks, sterile gloves (2 pairs)
4. Package or basin of 10% povidone-iodine or swabs (if patient is allergic, 3% hydrogen peroxide may be used)
5. Medium-size transparent wound dressings
6. Soft-wick drain sponges or 4×4 sponges
7. Sterile scissors, tape

Procedure

1. Explain procedure to patient.
2. Clean area with 70% isopropyl alcohol.
3. Wash hands. (See Chapter 6.)
4. Don gloves and masks.
5. Open tray. Prepare sterile field. Pour povidone-iodine solution and hydrogen peroxide into containers. Do not touch bottle tops of containers.
6. Place transparent wound dressing and sterile scissors on sterile field.
7. Carefully remove old dressing and discard. Remove gloves and wash hands.
8. Don sterile gloves.
9. Place sterile drapes around catheter exit site and incision.
10. Gently palpate exit site and tunnel, and observe site for any signs of infection.
11. Moisten 4×4 sponge with 3% peroxide solution. Clean around catheter exit site from wound outward in a circular motion. Repeat if necessary to remove any crusting. Do not cause irritation or bleeding. Manipulate the catheter as little as possible.
12. Moisten another 4×4 sponge with povidone-iodine solution or use povidone-iodine swabs (use 3% hydrogen peroxide if patient is allergic to povidone-iodine).
13. Let area dry.
14. Clean incision area in a similar manner, repeating steps 11 through 13.

15. Dress both areas using appropriate dressing sponge trimmed to appropriate size with sterile scissors.
16. For a moisture/vapor-permeable dressing, cover with transparent wound dressing. Trim any excess dressing.
17. If necessary, reinforce transparent wound dressing with tape.
18. Remove masks and gloves. Discard in appropriate receptacle.
19. Wash hands.
20. Document procedure and observations in patient's chart.[4,5]

Infection Prevention

Specific precautions for infection prevention during peritoneal dialysis catheter care include the following steps:

1. Wash hands before performing this procedure.
2. Wash hands before handling the catheter.
3. Secure the catheter to prevent tension or trauma.
4. Avoid pressure at the catheter exit site.
5. Instruct patient to follow strict aseptic technique when performing this procedure.

Patient Education

Patients should be instructed that using a dressing is optional depending on the individual's lifestyle. Tub bathing should be discouraged, but swimming is allowed if the patient performs exit site care immediately afterward. The client is encouraged to wear loose clothing, because there is an increased incidence of exit site infection in patients who wear tight clothing.[6]

Other important teaching topics include catheter care, signs and symptoms of exit site and tunnel infections, and the importance of early intervention. The following basic exit site assessment provides an easy method for patient evaluation of the exit site:

1. Description of color of exit site
2. Measurement of any discoloration
3. Presence of pain, drainage, or scab

If patients experience any of these signs or symptoms, they should notify the nurse or physician immediately so that effective therapy can be initiated.

Any infection may cause the catheter to be removed, so prevention and early treatment of exit site and tunnel infections are of critical importance. Disinfection of the Y connector reduces the incidence of peritonitis. Patients often complete this procedure in homes, restrooms, or public toilets by using a disinfectant to flush the catheter.[8,14] Teach patients that preventing environmental contamination is just as important as catheter site care.

Hemodialysis

During hemodialysis, water and uremic toxins (by-products) are removed as the patient's blood passes across a semipermeable membrane in an external hemodialysis machine. Negative and positive pressures are applied to the membrane, with the dialysate fluid on the opposite side of the membrane. By diffusion, the membrane pulls, or draws, uremic toxins from the blood as it circulates through it. Approximately 200 to 500 cc of blood must pass over the dialyzer membranes every minute to adequately remove uremic waste products and fluid. Although the membrane draws by-products out of the blood, it does not allow the blood cells to migrate into the dialysate. Therefore, there is no direct contact between the dialysate solution and the blood. To provide for blood access to the semipermeable membrane, a circulatory access site is created surgically. The most common types of circulatory access sites are arteriovenous (AV) fistulas or grafts and circulatory access devices (CADs).

Arteriovenous Fistulas and Grafts

An AV fistula surgically creates communication between arterial and venous circulation. Arterial blood flows through the vein, causing venous engorgement and enlargement. A bruit results from the mixture of arterial flow into the venous circulation. Palpation of the bruit assesses proper functioning of the fistula. Large-bore needles are inserted into the fistula to remove and return blood for the hemodialysis procedure. For patients without adequate vessels for the creation of a fistula, a biological, semibiological, or prosthetic graft may be implanted subcutaneously and interposed between an artery and a vein.[4]

Circulatory Access

A CAD is usually a temporary venous access. Generally, a double lumen catheter is placed in the femoral artery or in a large vein such as the subclavian vein of the internal jugular. If long-term use is anticipated, a double lumen, siliconized, rubber catheter with a dacron cuff is used.

Specific Infection Risk

Rates of infection vary, depending on the type of circulatory access. The infection rate for fistulas is less than 3%; for grafts it is 5% to 25%; and for CADs it is 12% to 38%.[7] The majority of fistula infections are treated with antibiotics. Graft and CAD infections often require removal of the access as well. Infection of an AV graft is more serious than that of an AV fistula because of the secondary risk of disintegration of the synthetic material and hemorrhage.[13]

Infection Prevention

Fistula and grafts

With the fistula or graft, infection usually occurs during cannulation of the vessel for hemodialysis. Graft infection can also occur via seeding from another source. Steps to prevent fistula or graft infection include the following:

1. Restrict access to the fistula or graft to trained dialysis personnel.
2. Site preparation: Before cannulation, wash the access site with antimicrobial soap and water; follow with povidone-iodine and alcohol.
3. Wash hands with antimicrobial soap and water immediately before cannulation. Wear gloves during the procedure. Observe standard precautions. (See Chapter 7.)
4. Check materials and equipment for contamination.
5. Rotate cannula sites. Begin at the bottom of the graft and work "upward" when puncturing the site.
6. Check the cannula sites frequently for dislodgment of needles or contamination (e.g., emesis, or feces with thigh grafts) during the hemodialysis procedure.
7. If the needle becomes dislodged during the procedure, remove it without causing hemorrhage. Usually, heparin should be administered.
8. After the procedure, achieve hemostasis at the puncture site before applying a dressing. Apply careful pressure so that the graft or fistula does not clot.
9. Educate the patient in the care of the fistula or graft (e.g., washing the skin over the access site daily, or when needed; checking daily for signs and symptoms of infection or diminished blood flow).
10. Never use the fistula or graft sites to draw blood or take blood pressures.

11. Train family members to instruct nonnursing or nonmedical personnel about fistula or graft care.[3,6]

Circulatory access devices

Because infection rates in the majority of CADs are caused by *S. epidermidis* and *S. aureus,* it is important to practice good infection control techniques. Microorganisms can colonize a percutaneously placed vascular catheter by one of the following three basic mechanisms:

1. Contamination of the catheter at the time of skin puncture
2. Seeding of the catheter from a distant focus of infection
3. Seeding of the catheter from contaminated infusates[8]

Use sterile technique to place the CAD. Wash hands thoroughly. Consider skin preparation, site care, and aseptic technique in handling all equipment. When accessing CADs the procedure should include the following steps.

1. Wash hands with antimicrobial soap.
2. Use protective gear (sterile gloves, mask, eye shields, as mandated by OSHA standards).[15]
3. Clean the exit site with both povidone-iodine (allow to dry) and alcohol.
4. Apply a sterile gauze dressing with porous tape to the exit site.
5. Clean caps with alcohol and povidone-iodine before removing them. Clean ports with alcohol and povidone-iodine before connecting them to the dialysis machine.
6. Use the CAD for hemodialysis only.
7. Observe the site and the patient for any signs of infection (change in temperature, lethargy, or disorientation).
8. Teach the patient to report signs and symptoms of infection (unusual drainage, pain, fever, swelling, redness, or unusual tenderness).

Preventing Occupational Exposure

All individuals performing dialysis procedures *must* have documentation of the hepatitis B vaccine series or hepatitis B immunity. Individuals performing dialysis access must protect themselves from exposure to bloodborne pathogens (hepatitis B and C and human immunodeficiency virus). Barrier techniques *must* be used for every patient during dialysis procedures, especially in procedures involving dialysis access.

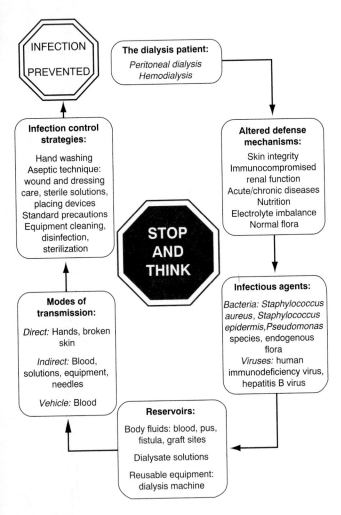

Figure 19-1.
Factors affecting the dialysis patient leading to the selection of the strategies to prevent infectious complications.

Barrier Techniques

Barrier techniques include the use of protective clothing: moisture-resistant gowns, gloves, eye protection (shields, goggles), and masks. All sharps must be disposed of in puncture-resistant, leak-proof containers. Needles must never be recapped, bent, broken, or cut, and blood spills must be immediately contained and cleaned with an Environmental Protection Agency approved germicidal agent.[3,15]

Accidental Exposure

Any HCW exposure to the blood or other body fluids of the patient requires immediate first aid. If the skin is contaminated, wash it with soap and water immediately or use a germicidal agent; flush eyes and mucous membranes with copious amounts of water or normal saline. Report all incidents to occupational health personnel (see Chapter 8).[3,15]

Summary

Infectious complications for both peritoneal dialysis and hemodialysis accesses are responsible for significant morbidity and mortality in the end-stage renal disease population. HCWs must take precautions to ensure the successful management of a dialysis access. Implementing strategies to minimize the risk of infection and ensuring rapid intervention to treat infection can greatly reduce infectious complications for this high risk population. Figure 19-1 summarizes infection risks and infection control strategies to protect patients, their families, and HCWs.

References

1. Lewis SL: Alteration of host defense mechanisms in chronic dialysis patients, *ANNA J* 17:170, 1990.
2. Anagnostou AD, Fried W: The hemopoietic system. In Eknoyan G, Knechel JP, editors: *The systematic consequences of renal failure,* Orlando, 1984, Grune & Stratton.
3. Soule B, editor: *The APIC Curriculum for infection control practice,* vol 2, Dubuque, Iowa, 1983, Kendall/Hunt.
4. Lancaster LE: *American Nephrology Nurses Association core curriculum,* ed 2, Pitman, NJ, 1991, Jannetti A.
5. Copley JB et al: Prevention of postoperative peritoneal dialysis catheter related infections, *Perit Dial Int* 8:195, 1988.

6. Prowant BF et al: A tool for nursing evaluation of the peritoneal dialysis catheter exit site, *ANNA J* 14(1):29, 1987.

7. Fan HY, Schwab SJ: Vascular access: concepts for the 1990's, *J Am Soc Nephrol* 3:1, 1992.

8. Hamory BH: Nosocomial sepsis related to intravascular access, *Crit Care Nurs Q* 11(4):58, 1989.

9. Prowant BF et al: Peritoneal dialysis catheter exit site care, *ANNA J* 15(4):219, 1988.

10. Nolph KD: Access problems plague both peritoneal dialysis and hemodialysis, *Kidney Int* 43(suppl 40):S81, 1993.

11. Twardowski AJ: Exit site infection in peritoneal dialysis, *Proceedings of the Fourth International Course on Peritoneal Dialysis*, Vicenza, Italy, 1991.

12. Han DC et al: Subcutaneously implanted catheters reduce the incidence of peritonitis during CAPD by eliminating infection by periluminal route, *Adv Perit Dialy* 8:298, 1992.

13. Nghien DD, Schulak JA, Corry RJ: Management of the infected hemodialysis access graft, *Trans Am Soc Artif Intern Organs* 29:360, 1983.

14. Levine A et al: Prevention of hemodialysis subclavian vein catheter infections by topical povidone-iodine, *Kidney Int* 40:934, 1991.

15. Department of Labor Occupational Safety and Health Administration: Occupational exposure to bloodborne pathogens: final rule, *Federal Register* 56(235):64004, 1991.

Respiratory Care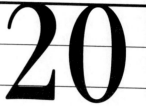

According to the Centers for Disease Control and Prevention, the respiratory tract is the second leading site for nosocomial infections (the urinary tract is the leading site). Responsible for 18% of all nosocomial infections, respiratory infections are the leading cause of death from nosocomial infection.[1] Respiratory procedures such as endotracheal intubation, suctioning, and mechanical ventilation present opportunities for the transfer of microorganisms from inanimate objects to the patient (on contaminated humidifiers, nebulizers, and ventilator components) and for transfer of microorganisms on the hands of personnel moving from patient to patient.[2]

Most nosocomial pneumonias occur by aspiration of bacteria colonizing the oropharynx or upper gastrointestinal tract of the patient. Intubation and mechanical ventilation greatly increase the risk of infection because they alter first-line body defense mechanisms—cough, sneeze, and gag reflexes and the washing actions of cilia and mucus—and provide a direct pathway into the lungs. Pneumonias caused by *Legionella* species, *Aspergillus* species, and influenza viruses are often caused by inhalation of contaminated aerosols. Respiratory syncytial virus infection usually follows viral inoculation of the conjunctival or nasal mucosa by contaminated hands. Pathogens such as gram-negative bacilli and *Staphylococcus aureus* are prevalent in the hospital, especially in intensive or critical care areas. Transmission to patients frequently occurs via the health care workers' (HCWs') hands that become contaminated or colonized with microorganisms. Procedures such as tracheal suctioning and manipulation of ventilatory circuits or endotracheal tubes increase the opportunity for cross-contamination.[3]

Procedures that may compromise the respiratory tract are oxygen administration, intermittent positive pressure breathing (IPPB) treatment, artificial airway insertion and maintenance, and endotracheal suctioning. Guidelines for infection control for these procedures are discussed in this chapter.

Infection Risks

Most of the patients who develop nosocomial pneumonia are very young or old; have severe underlying disease, immunosuppression, depressed sensorium, or cardiopulmonary disease; or have had thoracoabdominal surgery.

Devices used in the respiratory tract are potential reservoirs, or vehicles, for infectious microorganisms. Routes of transmission may be from device to patient, from one patient to another, or from one body site to the lower respiratory tract of the same patient via hands or devices. Contaminated reservoirs allow the growth of bacteria that may be subsequently released in aerosol form during device use. Gram-negative bacilli such as *Pseudomonas* species, *Legionella* species, and nontuberculous mycobacteria can multiply to substantial concentrations in fluids and increase the patient's risk of acquiring pneumonia. Aerosolization and spraying can also put the HCW at risk during device use.[3]

Oxygen Administration

Description

Oxygen is delivered by low-flow or high-flow systems. Low-flow systems include the nasal cannula, face mask, partial rebreathing mask, humidity tent, and oxygen tent. The oxygen concentrations vary with these systems. High-flow systems provide a consistent oxygen concentration, as with the Venturi mask or a ventilator. Because oxygen facilitates combustion, precautions must be taken to remove fire hazards: ban smoking, ground electrical equipment, and remove flammable materials such as oil, alcohol, and nail polish remover. Visitors and patients must be informed of the restrictions during oxygen use.

Specific Infection Risks

Humidifiers and nebulizers may become reservoirs of infection, and outbreaks of nosocomial gram-negative pneumonias have been linked to these contaminated devices. Small volume nebulizers can produce bacterial aerosols. If contaminated condensate forms in the inspiratory tubing, the patient is at increased risk for infection because the nebulizer aerosol is directed through the trachea and bypasses many of the normal host defenses.[3] There is a risk of introducing microorganisms on inadequately cleaned masks and equipment, so proper disinfection or sterilization of respiratory equipment is an important infection prevention strategy.[2]

Preparation

Gather the following equipment based on the method of oxygen administration:

1. Nasal cannula
   a. Oxygen supply with flow meter
   b. Humidifier with sterile, distilled water
   c. Nasal cannula and tubing
   d. Tape and gauzes
2. Face mask
   a. Prescribed face mask
   b. Padding for elastic band
3. Face tent of appropriate size

Procedure

1. Verify the order for oxygen therapy.
2. Explain the procedure to the patient.
3. Set up the oxygen equipment and humidifier.
4. Apply the oxygen delivery device:
   a. Cannula: Place elastic bands around the head with prongs in nares.
   b. Face mask: Fit to the contours of the patient's face and tighten the elastic band.
   c. Face tent: Place the tent over the patient's face and secure the band.

Follow-Up Assessment

The patient's response to oxygen therapy should be assessed, and the patient should be observed for signs of respiratory infection. The HCW should ensure that the oxygen equipment is clean and does not become contaminated. Condensation in the tubing may become a reservoir for the growth of organisms. Any condensate that collects in tubing must be drained and discarded, taking care not to allow fluid to drain toward the patient. After handling the tubing or fluid, hands must be washed.[3]

Home Care Considerations

Patients (and family caregivers, if appropriate) are taught to clean and safely use oxygen equipment. The oxygen equipment company is also a resource for home cleaning and maintenance.

Endotracheal Suctioning

Description

Intubation places an artificial airway in a patient to maintain a patent airway. Types of airways include oropharyngeal and na-sopharyngeal airways, endotracheal tubes, and tracheostomy. Tubes vary in size, styles, and composition to suit the type of insertion. Tubes placed in the trachea, including those for tracheostomies, are cuffed to allow for a tight seal for artificial ventilation. To maintain patent airways, effective suctioning is required. Suctioning of the lower airway through an endotracheal tube or tracheostomy requires sterile technique to avoid the introduction of microorganisms into the sterile lower respiratory tract.

Specific Infection Risks

Patients receiving continuous, mechanically assisted ventilation have 6 to 21 times the risk of developing nosocomial pneumonia than do patients who are not receiving ventilation. The increased risk is partly caused by oropharyngeal organisms that are passed during intubations and partly by depressed host defenses secondary to severe underlying illness. In addition, bacteria collects on the tube's surface over time and forms a film that protects bacteria from antimicrobial agents or host defenses. Risk is also increased by the direct access of bacteria to the lower respiratory tract, often because of leakage around the endotracheal cuff that allows pooled secretions above the cuff to enter the trachea. Microorganisms are also introduced into the respiratory tract during suctioning.[3]

The release of microbes through aerosolization with negative pressure during suctioning creates risk for the HCW.[4] Suctioning should be performed with gloves and protective face wear. HCWs should wash their hands before and after suctioning procedures or after contact with body fluids or secretions.[2,3]

Procedure

The suctioning procedure is outlined in Table 20-1.

Text continued on p. 380.

Table 20-1 Suctioning

Steps	Rationale
1. Assess for signs and symptoms indicating presence of upper airway secretions: gurgling respirations, restlessness, vomitus in mouth, drooling.	Confirms condition (Physical signs and symptoms result from decreased oxygen to tissues as well as pooling of secretions in upper airway.)
2. Explain to patient how procedure will help clear airway and relieve some breathing problems. Explain that coughing, sneezing, or gagging is normal.	Relieves patient's anxiety
3. Prepare necessary equipment and supplies:	Ensures that procedure is completed quickly and efficiently
a. Portable or wall suction unit with connecting tubing with Y connector if needed	
b. Sterile catheter	
c. Yankauer catheter (oropharyngeal)	
d. Sterile water or normal saline, sterile basin	
e. Sterile gloves, nonsterile gloves (Yankauer only)	Clears catheter of secretions
f. Drape or towel	
g. Nasal or oral airway if indicated	Protects linen and client's bedclothes
4. Close door or pull curtain.	Ensures access to airway Ensures privacy

Continued.

From Potter P, Perry A: *Fundamentals of nursing: concepts, process and practice,* St Louis, 1993, Mosby.

Table 20-1 Suctioning—cont'd

Steps	Rationale
5. Properly position patient:	
a. Place conscious patient with functional gag reflex for oral suctioning in semi-Fowler's position with head turned to one side. Place such a patient for nasal suctioning in semi-Fowler's position with neck hyperextended.	Eases insertion (Gag reflex helps prevent aspiration of gastrointestinal contents. Positioning of head to one side or hyperextending neck promotes smooth insertion of catheter into oropharynx or nasopharynx, respectively.)
b. Place unconscious patient in side-lying position facing nurse.	Prevents patient's tongue from obstructing airway, promotes drainage of pulmonary secretions, and prevents aspiration of gastrointestinal contents
6. Place towel on pillow or under patient's chin.	Prevents soiling of bed linen or bedclothes from secretions (Secretions on towel can be removed after procedure, thus reducing spread of bacteria.)
7. Select proper suction pressure for patient and type of suction unit. For wall suction units, this is 110 to 150 mm Hg in adults, 95-110 mm Hg in children, and 50-95 mm Hg in infants.	Provides safe but effective negative pressure according to patient's age; decreases possibility of damage to mucous membranes and hypoxemia
8. Wash hands.	Reduces transmission of microorganisms

9. Yankauer catheter:

a. Apply nonsterile gloves.

Reduces transmission of microorganisms

b. Connect one end of connecting tubing to suction machine and other to Yankauer suction catheter. Fill cup with water.

Prepares suction apparatus

c. Check that equipment is functioning properly by suctioning small amount of water from cup or basin.

Ensures equipment function and lubricates catheter

d. Remove oxygen mask, if present.

e. Insert catheter into mouth along gum line to pharynx. Move catheter around mouth until secretions are cleared.

Provides continuous suction (Care must be taken not to allow suction tip to invaginate oral mucosal surfaces.)

f. Encourage patient to cough. Replace oxygen mask.

Moves secretions from lower airway into mouth and upper airway

g. Rinse catheter with water in cup or basin until connecting tubing is cleared of secretions. Turn off suction.

Rinses catheter and reduces probability of transmission of microorganisms (Clean suction tubing enhances delivery of set suction pressure.)

h. Reassess patient's respiratory status.

Directs nurse to initiate or cease intervention

i. Remove towel and place in laundry. Remove gloves and dispose in receptacle.

Reduces transmission of microorganisms

Continued.

Table 20-1   Suctioning—cont'd

Steps	Rationale
j. Reposition patient; Sims' position encourages drainage and should be used if patient has decreased level of consciousness.	Facilitates drainage of oral secretions.
k. Discard remainder of water into appropriate receptacle.	Reduces transmission of microorganisms and maintains medical asepsis
l. Rinse basin in warm soapy water and dry with paper towels. Discard disposable cup in appropriate receptacle.	
m. Place catheter in clean dry area.	
n. Wash hands.	Reduces transmission of microorganisms to other patients
10. Nasopharyngeal or nasotracheal suction:	
a. Turn suction device on, and set vacuum regulator to appropriate negative pressure.	Prevents excessive negative pressure from damaging nasal pharyngeal and tracheal mucosa and from reducing greater hypoxia
b. If indicated, increase supplemental oxygen to 100% or as ordered by physician.	Reduces suction-induced hypoxemia (The literature is inconclusive as to the necessity of hyperoxygenation.)
c. Connect one end of connecting tubing to suction machine and place other end in convenient location.	Prepares for connection of suction catheter to suction apparatus

d. If using suction kit:

(1) Open package. If sterile drape is available, place it across client's chest or use towel.

Reduces transmission of microorganisms

(2) Open suction catheter package. Do not allow suction catheter to touch any surface other than inside of its package.

Maintains medical asepsis

(3) Unwrap or open sterile basin and place on bedside table. Be careful not to touch inside of basin. Fill with about 100 ml sterile normal saline.

Saline is used to clear tubing after each suction pass

e. Open lubricant. Squeeze onto open sterile catheter package without touching package.

Prepares lubricant while maintaining sterility (Water-soluble lubricant is used to avoid lipoid aspiration pneumonia.)

f. Apply sterile glove to each hand or apply nonsterile glove to nondominant hand and sterile glove to dominant hand.

Reduces transmission of microorganisms and allows nurse to maintain sterility of suction catheter

g. Pick up suction catheter with dominant hand without touching nonsterile surfaces. Pick up connection tubing with nondominant hand. Secure catheter to connector tubing (see illustration).

Maintains catheter sterility; connects catheter to suction

Continued.

Table 20-1 Suctioning—cont'd

Steps	Rationale

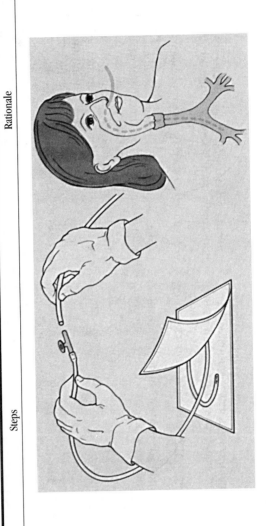

h. Check that equipment is functioning properly by suctioning small amount of normal saline from basin.

Ensures equipment function; lubricates internal catheter and tubing

i. Coat distal 6 to 8 cm of catheter with water-soluble lubricant.

Lubricates catheter for easier insertion

j. Remove oxygen-delivery device, if applicable, with nondominant hand. Without applying suction, gently but quickly insert catheter (with dominant thumb and forefinger) into naris using slight downward slant or through mouth when patient breathes in. Do not force through naris (see illustration).

Prevents injury to patient (Application of suction pressure while introducing catheter into trachea increases risk of damage to mucosa, as well as increasing the risk of hypoxia from removal of oxygen present in airways. Epiglottis is open on inspiration and facilitates insertion into trachea. Patient should cough. If patient gags or becomes nauseated, catheter is most likely in esophagus.)

(1) *Pharyngeal suctioning:* In adults, insert catheter about 16 cm; in older children, 8 to 12 cm; in infants and young children, 4 to 8 cm. Rule of thumb is to insert catheter distance from tip of nose to base of ear lobe.

(2) *Trachea suctioning:* In adults, insert catheter 20 to 24 cm; in older children, 14 to 20 cm; and in young children and infants, 8 to 14 cm.

Continued.

Table 20-1 Suctioning—cont'd

Steps	Rationale
(3) *Positioning:* In some instances, turning patient's head to right helps nurse suction left mainstem bronchus; turning head to left helps nurse suction right mainstem bronchus.	
If resistance is felt after insertion of catheter for recommended distance, nurse has probably hit carina. Pull catheter back 1 cm before applying suction.	
k. Apply intermittent suction for up to 10 sec by placing and releasing nondominant thumb over vent of catheter and slowly withdrawing catheter while rotating it back and forth between dominant thumb and forefinger. Encourage patient to cough. Replace oxygen device, if applicable.	Prevents injury to mucosa (If catheter "grabs" mucosa, remove thumb to release suction. Suctioning longer than 10 seconds can cause cardiopulmonary compromise.)
l. Rinse catheter and connecting tubing with normal saline until cleared.	Removes secretions from catheter
m. Remove gloves. Wash hands. Discard or remove suction equipment appropriately.	Reduces transmission of microorganisms
11. Artificial airway:	
a. Wash hands.	Reduces transmission of microorganisms

b. Turn suction device on and set vacuum regulator to appropriate negative pressure (see Step 7).	Prevents damage (Excessive negative pressure damages tracheal mucosa and can induce greater hypoxia.)
c. Connect one end of connecting tubing to suction machine and place other end in convenient location.	Prepares suction apparatus
d. If using sterile suction kit:	
(1) Open package. If sterile drape is available, place it across client's chest.	Prevents contamination of clothing
(2) Open suction catheter package. Do not allow suction catheter to touch any nonsterile surface.	Prepares catheter and prevents transmission of micro-organisms
(3) Unwrap or open sterile basin and place on bedside table. Be careful not to touch inside basin. Fill with about 100 ml sterile normal saline.	Prepares catheter and prevents transmission of micro-organisms
e. If indicated, open lubricant. Squeeze onto sterile catheter package without touching package.	Prepares lubricant for use while maintaining sterility
f. Appy one sterile glove to each hand or apply non-sterile glove to nondominant hand and sterile glove to dominant hand.	Reduces transmission of microorganisms and allows nurse to maintain sterility of suction catheter

Continued.

Table 20-1 Suctioning—cont'd

Steps	Rationale
g. Pick up suction catheter with dominant hand without touching nonsterile surfaces. Pick up connecting tubing with nondominant hand. Secure catheter to tubing.	Maintains catheter sterility
h. Check that equipment is functioning properly by suctioning small amount of saline from basin.	Ensures equipment function; lubricates catheter and tubing
i. Coat distal 6 to 8 cm of catheter with water-soluble lubricant. In some situations, catheter is lubricated only with normal saline. Nursing assessment indicates need for lubrication.	Promotes easier catheter insertion (If lubricant is needed, it must be water soluble to prevent petroleum-based aspiration pneumonia. Excessive lubricant can adhere to artificial airway.)
j. Remove oxygen- or humidity-delivery device with nondominant hand.	Exposes artificial airway
k. Hyperinflate and/or oxygenate patient before suctioning or using manual resuscitation (Ambu) bag or sigh mechanism on mechanical ventilator.	Decreases atelectasis caused by negative pressure (Preoxygenation converts large proportion of resident lung gas to 100% oxygen to offset amount used in metabolic consumption while ventilator or oxygenation is interrupted, as well as to offset volume lost out of suction catheter.[*])

l. Without applying suction, gently but quickly insert catheter (with dominant thumb and forefinger) into artifical airway (best to time catheter insertion with inspiration).

Places catheter in tracheobronchial tree (Application of suction pressure while introducing catheter into trachea increases risk of damage to tracheal mucosa and risk of hypoxia from removal of oxygen present in airways.)

m. Insert catheter until resistance is met, then pull back 1 cm.

Stimulates cough and removes catheter from mucosal wall

n. Apply intermittent suction by placing and releasing nondominant thumb over vent of catheter and slowly withdraw catheter while rotating it back and forth between dominant thumb and forefinger. Encourage patient to cough.

Prevents injury to tracheal mucosa lining (If catheter "grabs" mucosa, remove thumb to release suction.)

o. Replace oxygen-delivery service. Encourage patient to deep breathe.

Reoxygenates and reexpands alveoli (Suctioning can cause hypoxemia and atelectasis.)

p. Rinse catheter and connecting tubing with normal saline until clear. Use continuous suction.

Removes catheter secretions (Secretions left in tubing decrease suction and provide environment for microorganism growth.)

q. Repeat Steps k–p as needed to clear secretions. Allow adequate time (at least 1 full minute) between suction passes for ventilation and reoxygenation.

Clears airway of excessive secretions and promotes improved oxygenation

Continued.

---

*Luce J, Tyler M, Pierson D: *Intensive Respiratory Care*, Philadelphia, 1984, Saunders.

Table 20-1 Suctioning—cont'd

Steps	Rationale
r. Assess patient's cardiopulmonary status between suction passes.	Verifies health status (Suctioning can induce arrhythmias, hypoxia, and bronchospasm.)
s. When artificial airway and tracheobronchial tree are sufficiently cleared of secretions, perform nasal and oral pharyngeal suctioning to clear upper airway of secretions. After this suctioning is performed, catheter is contaminated; do not reinsert into endotracheal or tracheostomy tube.	Removes upper airway secretions (Upper airway is considered clean, whereas lower airway is considered sterile. Therefore, same catheter can be used to suction from sterile to clean areas but not from clean to sterile areas.)
t. Disconnect catheter from connecting tubing. Roll catheter around fingers of dominant hand. Pull glove off inside out so that catheter remains in glove. Pull off other glove in same way. Discard into appropriate receptacle. Turn off suction device.	Reduces transmission of microorganisms
u. Remove towel and place in laundry, or remove drape and discard in appropriate receptacle.	Reduces transmission of microorganisms

v. Reposition patient.

Promotes comfort (Sims' position encourages drainage and reduces risk of aspiration.)

w. Discard remainder of normal saline into appropriate receptacle. If basin is disposable, discard into appropriate receptacle. If basin is reusable, place it in soiled utility room.

Reduces transmission of microorganisms

x. Wash hands.

Reduces transmission of microorganisms

12. Prepare equipment for next suctioning.

Provides ready access to suction equipment, especially if patient is experiencing respiratory distress

13. Observe patient for absence of airway secretions, restlessness, and oral secretions.

Indicates that secretions have been removed from oral and pharyngeal areas

14. Record the amount, consistency, color, and odor of secretions and patient's response to procedure; document patient's presuctioning and postsuctioning respiratory status.

Records completion of procedure and patient's status before and after the procedure

Follow-Up Assessment

The patient's response to the procedure should be assessed. Auscultation should be performed to determine effective respirations and clear breath sounds. Difficult breathing or lack of bilateral breath sounds may indicate a blocked airway or the need for additional suctioning. These are urgent situations that require immediate attention. Suctioning is performed as needed, based on assessment of respiratory function. The color, consistency, and odor of the secretions are documented.

Home Care Considerations

Suctioning of the lower airway requires aseptic technique when it is performed in the home setting. Adequate caregiver training and proper suction equipment must be available in the home.

Special Respiratory Equipment
Ventilator Tubing

When warm air flows through cooler ventilator tubing, it causes condensation of moisture in the tube. The accumulation of moisture may serve as a reservoir for organism growth. Any condensate that collects in tubing must be drained and discarded, taking care not to allow fluid to drain toward the patient. After handling the tubing or fluid, hands must be washed. Ventilator tubing should be changed at least every 48 hours.[3,5,6] Totally closed or heated systems may be left in place longer.

Manual Ventilation (Resuscitation) Bags

Manual resuscitation (Ambu) bags ventilate a patient in an emergency or during suctioning of an intubated patient. Inadequately disinfected bags have been associated with infections from *Acinetobacter*, *Staphylococcus*, and *Candida* organisms.[2] The exterior surface and exhalation port should be sterilized between uses with patients. Bags should not be shared between patients if contaminated; a sterile replacement should be obtained. Reusable resuscitation bags are particularly difficult to clean and dry between uses. Microorganisms in secretions or fluid left in the bag may be aerosolized or sprayed into the lower respiratory tract of the patient on whom the bag is used. In addition, contaminating microorganisms may be transmitted from one patient to another on the hands of HCWs. Oxygen analyzers and ventilatory spirometers have been associated with outbreaks of gram-negative respiratory tract colonization and pneumonia resulting from patient-to-patient transmission of organisms via hands of personnel. These devices require sterilization or high-level disinfection between uses on different patients.[3] See Chapter 9 for specific guidelines on choosing the correct level of disinfectant.

Ventilators and Filters

The internal components of ventilators and IPPB and continuous positive airway pressure (CPAP) machines have not been identified as major sources of nosocomial infections. External components should be cleaned and disinfected regularly. Filters on ventilators have not been proven effective in reducing nosocomial respiratory infections.[7]

Respiratory care equipment should be manually cleaned and then disinfected or sterilized before use. HCWs should put on gloves and protective face wear when breaking down and cleaning this equipment after use.

Infection Prevention Strategies

The most important way to prevent nosocomial infections is to interrupt the modes of transmission as related to respiratory care procedures. The following list of strategies comes from the current 1994 Centers for Disease Control and Prevention guidelines.[3]

Interruption of Device-Related Transmission

1. Thoroughly clean all equipment and devices to be sterilized or disinfected. (See Chapter 9.)
2. Sterilize or use high-level disinfection for semicritical equipment or devices (e.g., items that come into direct or indirect contact with mucous membranes of the lower respiratory tract). Follow disinfection with appropriate rinsing, drying, and packaging, taking care not to contaminate the items in the process. The following are some examples of semicritical devices:
   a. Breathing circuits of mechanical ventilators
   b. Endotracheal and endobronchial tubes
   c. Laryngoscope blades
   d. Mouthpieces and tubing of pulmonary function testing equipment

e. Nebulizers and their reservoirs

f. Oral and nasal airways

g. Resuscitation bags

h. Suction catheters

3. After chemically disinfecting the items, use sterile solution (not distilled, nonsterile water) to rinse reusable, semicritical equipment or devices used for the respiratory tract.

4. Maintain mechanical ventilators, breathing circuits, and humidifiers as follows:

   a. The internal machinery of ventilators does not need routine sterilization or disinfection.

   b. Change breathing circuits, including the tubing and exhalation valve, and the attached humidifier of a ventilator every 48 hours when it is in use on a patient.

   c. Periodically drain and discard any condensate that collects in the tubing, taking care not to allow fluid to drain toward the patient. Wash hands after performing the procedure or handling the fluid.

   d. Use sterile water to fill bubbling humidifiers.

5. Maintain wall humidifiers as follows:

   a. Follow manufacturers' instructions for use and maintenance of wall oxygen humidifiers.

   b. Between patients, change the tubing, including any nasal prongs or mask, used to deliver oxygen from a wall outlet.

6. Other devices should be maintained as follows:

   a. Between patients, sterilize or use high-level disinfection for portable respirometers, oxygen sensors, and other respiratory devices used on multiple patients.

   b. Between patients, sterilize or use high-level disinfection for reusable, manual resuscitation bags.

   c. Between patients, sterilize or use high-level disinfection for reusable mouthpieces and tubing or connectors or follow device manufacturer's instructions for their reprocessing.[3]

Interruption of Person-to-Person Transmission

1. Wash hands after contact with mucous membranes, respiratory secretions, or objects contaminated with respiratory secretions, whether or not gloves are worn. Wash hands before and after contact with a patient with an endotracheal or tracheostomy tube in place and before and after contact with any respiratory device used on a patient, whether or not gloves are worn.

Table 20-2   Risk factors and infection control strategies for prevention of nosocomial pneumonia

Risk Factors	Infection Control Strategies
Host-Related Risk Factors	
■ Age > 65 years ■ Underlying illness or immunosuppression	Avoid exposure to potential nosocomial pathogens.
■ Postoperative status	Properly position patients; promote early ambulation; control pain.
Device-Related Risk Factors	Properly clean, sterilize or disinfect, and handle devices; remove devices as soon as the indication for their use ceases.
■ Endotracheal intubation and mechanical ventilation	Gently suction secretions; place patient in semirecumbent position (i.e., 30 degrees to 45 degrees head elevation); use non-alkalinizing gastric agents for patients at risk for stress bleeding; change ventilator circuits at 48 hours; drain and discard inspiratory tubing condensate, or use heat-moisture exchanger if indicated.
■ NG tube and enteral feedings	Routinely verify tube placement; remove when no longer needed; drain residual; place patient in semirecumbent position as previously described.
Personnel or Procedure Related Risk Factors	Educate and train personnel.
■ Cross-contamination by hands	Wash hands adequately; wear gloves appropriately.

Modified from Centers for Disease Control, Guideline for prevention of nosocomial pneumonia, *Infect Control Hosp Epidemiol* 15:587, 1994.
NG, nasogastric.

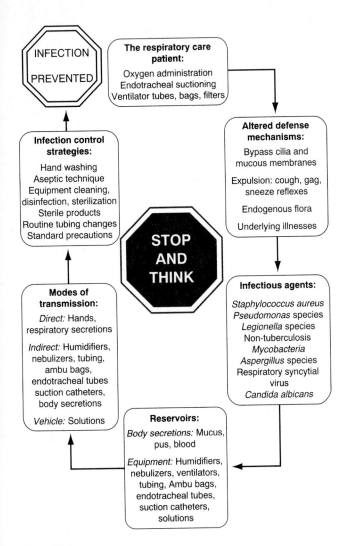

Figure 20-1.
Factors affecting the patient needing respiratory care leading to the selection of the strategies to prevent infectious complications.

2. Use barrier precautions. Wear gloves for handling respiratory secretions or objects contaminated with respiratory secretions of any patient. Wear a gown and face protection when soiling with respiratory secretions is anticipated.

3. When changing a tracheostomy tube, use aseptic technique and replace the tube with a sterile or disinfected tube.

4. Use only sterile fluid to remove secretions from the suction catheter if the catheter is used for reentry into the patient's lower respiratory tract.

5. Change suction collection tubing (up to the canister) between patients.

6. Change suction collection canisters between uses on different patients except when used in short-term care units.[3]

Table 20-2 lists some of the risk factors for pneumonia and their respective prevention strategies.

Summary

Pneumonia is the second most common nosocomial infection and is associated with substantial morbidity and mortality. Most patients with nosocomial pneumonia are characterized by extremes of age, severe underlying disease, immunosuppression, depressed sensorium, or cardiopulmonary disease, or are patients who have had thoracicabdominal surgery. Nosocomial infections caused by respiratory therapy procedures account for 18% of nosocomial infections each year. These procedures effectively bypass normal body defense mechanisms, providing easy access for invading microorganisms. Prevention strategies are of the utmost importance. Microorganisms causing these infections may originate from endogenous sources (the patient) or from exogenous sources such as contaminated equipment or solutions, lack of aseptic technique, or organisms carried on the hands of personnel. Figure 20-1 summarizes the factors that cause infection and lists the strategies to prevent it.

References

1. Horan T, Culver D, Jarvis W: Pathogens causing nosocomial pneumonia. *CDC: Antimicrobial Newsletter* 5:65-7, 1988.

2. Martin M: Nosocomial infections related to patient care support services: dietetic services, central services department, laundry, respiratory care, dialysis and endoscopy. In Wenzel R, editor: *Prevention and control of nosocomial infections,* Baltimore, 1993, Williams & Wilkins.

3. Centers for Disease Control: Guideline for prevention of nosocomial pneumonia, *Infect Control Hosp Epidemiol* 15:587, 1994.
4. Resso T: Bacteria in suction machines, *Lancet* 1970:240, 1970.
5. Potter P, Perry A: *Fundamentals of nursing: concepts, process and practice,* St Louis, 1993, Mosby.
6. Craven D, Goularte T, Make B: Contaminated condensate in mechanical ventilator circuits: a risk factor for nosocomial pneumonia, *Am Rev Resp Dis* 129:625, 1984.
7. Garibaldi et al: Failure of bacterial filters to reduce the incidence of pneumonia after inhalation anesthesia, *Anesthesiology* 54:364, 1981.

Obstetrical Procedures
21

Alterations in immunological function in both pregnant women and their neonates may predispose them to mycotic, fungal, and bacterial infections. These alterations include decreased T helper cells, altered T cell function, and decreased IgG in the pregnant woman and decreased IgG, IgM, and IgA, supressed B cell function, and decreased total complement in the neonate.[1]

Risks of transmission of infection from mother to fetus or newborn, from mother to health care worker (HCW), and from HCW to mother and fetus or newborn call for careful attention to infection prevention during procedures in obstetrical and gynecological settings. The care of the pregnant woman involves potential HCW exposure to blood and body fluids during prepartal, intrapartum, and postpartum care. HCWs may be exposed to body fluids while performing pelvic and vaginal examinations and particularly while performing invasive procedures during labor and delivery. Breast milk is a body fluid that is a potential source of infection transmission. This chapter focuses on prevention of infection during fetal and intrauterine monitoring.

Specific Infection Risks

It is estimated that 20% of all laboring women have intrauterine pressure catheters and fetal spiral electrodes placed.[2] Risks to patients from these invasive devices include intraamniotic infection, maternal endometritis, and fetal site placement infection. A high postprocedure infection rate has been reported, although most researchers find that there is no significant risk of infection from these procedures.[3-5] Waterborne contamination of obstetrical pressure transducers has been reported and may be associated with nosocomial bacteremia.[5-7] Risks of patient nosocomial infection are increased when procedures have risks or complications that result in bleeding and body fluid exposure. Examples include the following:

Procedure	Potential Complication
External version (turning the fetus)	Abruption, premature rupture of membranes
Internal version (turning the fetus)	Uterine trauma, lacerations
Induction of labor	Umbilical cord prolapse
Forceps delivery	Trauma
Vacuum extraction	Lacerations and abrasions
Vaginal birth after cesarean section	Uterine rupture
Episiotomy	Infection, bleeding
Cesarean delivery	Hemorrhage, infection[5]

Risks to the HCW stem from failure to observe standard precautions or from exposure to infected fluids from a break in barrier protection. Human immunodeficiency virus (HIV) and hepatitis B virus may be transferred by exposure to blood and body fluids.[2]

Internal Monitoring
Internal Fetal Heart Rate Monitoring
Description

Internal fetal heart rate monitoring is accomplished by placement of a spiral electrode on the fetus after the cervix is partially dilated. The presenting part of the fetus (the head is the recommended placement site) must be determined before electrode placement. The internal fetal electrode provides a reliable tracing of the fetal heart rate as well as fetal heart rate variability, periodic and nonperiodic changes, and accelerations and decelerations, which may be caused by head compression, uteroplacental insufficiency, or umbilical cord compression. Patterns of rate changes may also indicate fetal health status. A sinusoidal pattern with undulations about the baseline may indicate a severely anemic or asphyxiated fetus. The findings from internal fetal heart rate tracings may significantly alter the course of delivery.[2]

Equipment

The equipment needed for insertion of the fetal spiral electrode includes the following:

1. Gloves that fit well (properly sized latex gloves) for all participants who may be exposed to body fluids
2. Impervious gowns or protective covering
3. Face shield (or goggles and mask)
4. Internal fetal spiral electrode
5. Grounding circuit
6. Electrographic gel
7. Adequate lighting
8. Fetal monitor

Procedure

The cervix must be dilated at least 3 cm and the membranes ruptured before the spiral electrode is placed.

1. Wash hands and put on gloves, impervious gown, and face shield or goggles and mask.
2. Attach the internal fetal spiral electrode to the subcutaneous tissue of the presenting part.
3. Attach the grounding plate to a small metal leg plate after applying electrographic gel.
4. Obtain a direct tracing of the fetus's heart rate.
5. Dispose of materials, including the guide and wire, according to agency infection control policy.
6. Wash hands thoroughly.

Intrauterine Pressure Monitoring
Description

Evaluation of the relative strength of maternal contractions during labor is best accomplished by placement of an internal intrauterine pressure catheter. Placement requires that the cervix be dilated and membranes be ruptured to enter the intrauterine space. The system may consist of a fluid-filled catheter, a port for flushing the catheter, a flexible diaphragm, and a gauge (depending on the equipment and system available within the practice site). A woman on labor-augmenting medications requires monitoring of uterine contractions to determine the effectiveness of the medication. Continuous pressure monitoring offers an effective measure of the relative strength of contractions.[2]

Equipment

The equipment needed for placement of an intrauterine pressure catheter includes the following:

1. Properly sized latex gloves for all participants at risk for exposure
2. Impervious gowns and protective barriers if rupture of membranes may cause spray of amniotic fluid
3. Face shield (or goggles and mask)
4. Catheter with micropressure transducer
5. Uterine monitor

Procedure

The cervix must be dilated and the membranes ruptured before insertion of pressure catheter.

1. Wash hands and put on gloves, impervious gown, and face shield. (All contact with moist body substances or mucous membranes requires the use of gloves and standard precautions. See box on pp. 391-392.)
2. Prepare the catheter with micropressure transducer.
3. Pass the catheter through the cervix and between the fetus and uterine walls into the uterus.
4. Attach the pressure catheter to the measurement system available in the practice site.
5. Dispose of all materials according to the agency infection control policy.
6. Wash hands thoroughly.

Follow Up

The patient should be assessed for signs of infection during nursing assessments. The neonate should be assessed after birth for signs of infection and trauma from insertion.

Infection Prevention
Prevention of Communicable Disease Transmission

Measles immunity among HCWs reduces the nosocomial transmission that may cause severe fetal anomalies. However, studies have shown that up to 35% of HCWs are nonimmune.[8,9] Screening and vaccination of all HCWs are recommended.[9,10]

Although HIV transmission may occur early in pregnancy,

Standard Precautions to Reduce Risk of HIV-HBV and Other Pathogen Transmission in Obstetrical Care

Body Fluid Classifications

- Use appropriate barrier precautions to prevent skin and mucous membrane exposure when contact with blood or bodily fluid from *any* client is anticipated.

    When caring for all clients, wear gloves for these cases:

    Contact with blood (venipuncture; finger stick; intravenous insertion; changing perineal pads, chux, linen)

    Contact with bodily fluids (changing saturated pads, chux, linen, clothing after rupture of membranes)

    Contact with mucous membranes (vaginal examination)

    Contact with nonintact skin

    Handling of items soiled with blood or bodily fluids (soiled pads, chux, bedding, clothing)

    Change gloves after contact with each client and between client contacts.

    Medical gloves (vinyl or latex sterile surgical or nonsterile examination gloves) should not be washed and reused. Washing with surfactants may enhance penetration of liquids through undetected holes in gloves.

- Masks, protective eyewear, or face shields should be worn during procedures that commonly cause splashes of blood or bodily fluids onto mucous membranes of mouth, nose, or eyes.

    Vaginal or cesarean birth

    Cutting umbilical cord between infant and placenta

    Possible artificial rupture of membranes under pressure

- Fluid-resistant gowns or aprons and boots should be worn during procedures likely to cause splashes of bodily fluids.

    Persons performing or assisting with vaginal or cesarean births

    Possible artificial rupture of membranes

Modified from Centers for Disease Control and Prevention: Draft guidelines for isolation precautions in hospitals, *Federal Register* 59(214):55552, 1994; Dickason E, Schult M, Silverman B: *Maternal-infant nursing care,* St Louis, 1990, Mosby. *HIV,* human immunodeficiency virus; *HBV,* hepatitis B virus.

Continued.

Standard Precautions to Reduce Risk of HIV-HBV and Other Pathogen Transmission in Obstetrical Care—cont'd

- Gowns and gloves should be worn by health care workers handling placenta or infant until blood and amniotic fluid have been removed from infant's skin.

  Gloves should be worn for care of umbilical cord after delivery
- Use mechanical suction for removal of infant nasopharyngeal secretion at delivery (do not use for mouth suctioning).

  Use resuscitation bags or other ventilation equipment for resuscitation.
- Remove and replace gloves torn or punctured by needle stick or other injury as promptly as possible.
- Take precautions to prevent injury from needles and surgical instruments.

  Needles should not be recapped, bent, broken, or removed from disposable syringes by hand.

  After use, needles, scalpel blades, and other sharp items should be placed in puncture-resistant containers for disposal.

  Surgical instruments should be carefully cleaned to avoid injury.
- Health care workers having frequent exposures to breast milk may wear gloves.

specific rates of transmission by trimester, at delivery, and postpartally have not been reported. Reports of vertical transmission of HIV (from mother to fetus) have varied from 14% to 39%.[11-13] Every effort should be made to protect uninfected children. Of HIV infected children, 50% acquire the virus during delivery or in the postdelivery period. Maintenance of the skin barrier and protection of the infant from exposure to infected maternal fluids help reduce transmission. Episiotomy, spiral electrode placement, and fetal blood sampling may increase the risks of exposure. Postdelivery concerns include transmission in breast milk, which occurs at a reported overall risk of 29%.[13]

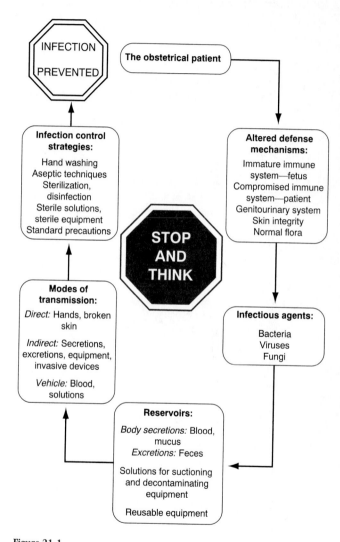

Figure 21-1.
Factors effecting the obstetrical patient leading to the selection of strategies to prevent infectious complications.

Infection Prevention in Ambulatory Care Settings

Infection control in women's ambulatory health care settings presents risk for transmission of infection similar to those in nonambulatory settings. Recommended infection control policies for these settings are as follows:

1. Disposable well-fitting latex examination gloves should be used during pelvic examinations and procedures in which body fluid exposure is expected.
2. Disposable instruments and specula should be used when possible.
3. Cryocautery probe tips should be cleaned, disinfected in glutaraldehyde (10 to 45 minutes), and then rinsed in tap water. Follow label directions for appropriate contact time.
4. Vaginal ultrasound probes should be covered with a condom during use, cleaned with soap and water, then disinfected in 2% glutaraldehyde.
5. Agency infection control policies must be in effect and followed.[5]

Standard Precautions

Guidelines for use of standard precautions to reduce risk of HIV, hepatitis B virus, and other bloodborne pathogen transmission in obstetrical care are depicted in the box on pp. 391-392.

Summary

The care of obstetrical patients presents special challenges in the prevention of infection. Altered immunological function and procedures involving breaches of body defenses and potential HCW exposure to blood and body fluid dictate careful adherence to standard precautions. Figure 21-1 outlines specific risks and infection prevention strategies for obstetrical patients undergoing internal monitoring.

References

1. Blackburn S, Loper D: *Maternal, fetal and neonatal physiology,* Philadelphia, 1993, WB Saunders.
2. Dickason E, Schult M, Silverman B: *Maternal-infant nursing care,* St Louis, 1990, Mosby.
3. Gibbs R, Listwa H, Read J: The effect of internal fetal monitoring on

maternal infection following cesarean section, *Obstet Gynecol* 48:653, 1976.

4. Newton E, Prihoda T, Gibbs R: Logistic regression analysis of risk factors for intraamniotic infection, *Obstet Gynecol* 73:571, 1989.

5. Mead P: Prevention and control of nosocomial infections in obstetrics and gynecology. In Wenzel R, editor: *Prevention and control of nosocomial infections,* Baltimore, 1993, Williams & Wilkins.

6. Baker D et al: Water-borne contamination of intrauterine pressure transducers, *Am J Obstet Gynecol* 133:923, 1979.

7. Strong T, Paul R: Intrapartum uterine activity: evaluation of an intrauterine pressure transducer, *Obstet Gynecol* 73:432, 1989.

8. Wright L, Carlquist J: Measles immunity in employees of a multihospital healthcare provider, *Infect Control Hosp Epidemiol* 15(1):8, 1994.

9. Willy M et al: Measles immunity in a population of healthcare workers, *Infect Control Hosp Epidemiol* 15(1):12, 1994.

10. Krause P et al: Quality standard for assurance of measles immunity among health care workers, *Infect Control Hosp Epidemiol* 15(1):193, 1994.

11. European Collaborative Study: Risk factors for mother-to-child transmission of HIV-1, *Lancet* 339:1007, 1992.

12. Hira S, Kamang J, Bhat G: Perinatal transmission of HIV-1 in Zambia, *Br Med J* 299:1250, 1989.

13. Craven D, Steger K, Jarek, C: Human immunodeficiency virus infection in pregnancy: epidemiology and prevention of vertical transmission, *Infect Control Hosp Epidemiol* 15(1):36, 1994.

Neonatal Procedures

22

Infection control has been a long-standing problem in neonatal nursing units. Technological advances have increased the survival of very small infants, but the invasive procedures necessary for their survival also increase their risk for infection. This chapter discusses protection of newborns from infection during common medical procedures.

Specific Infection Risks

In utero the fetus is protected from many microorganisms by the mother's immune system. It isn't until the infant is born that exposure to some microorganisms occurs. Although the immune system develops during early gestation, it does not operate as effectively in the newborn as it does in older children and adults. As a consequence, newborns (particularly preterm infants) are easily overwhelmed by infection.[1]

It is important to remember that symptoms of infection in newborns may be different from those in adults and older children. In adults and older children, febrile reaction occurs from the increased metabolic activity and from the release of endogenous pyrogens. This febrile reaction may not be seen in newborns because of the immaturity of the immune system.[1] Symptoms in newborns may be nonspecific, including changes in behavior, changes in activity level, and changes in appetite. It takes an alert nurse who is continuously aware of subtle changes to recognize an infection early on in a newborn. Often the nurse will "just know" that something is wrong.

Skin is the first line of defense against invading organisms in the human. An infant's skin is extremely fragile, especially if the infant is premature. In the case of premature infants, the skin is thin and transparent. Any physical pressure, monitoring device, or tape can easily tear the skin. A tear is moist, can be large relative to the size of the infant, and is painful to the infant. It also leaves an area for entry of organisms commonly found in a hospital or on the caretaker's or infant's skin. Although these organisms are often nonpathogenic to adults, they can be devastating to an already compromised infant. Therefore, care should be taken to maintain the skin integrity.

Smaller infants should have their heart rate and blood pressure monitored by central lines. Temperatures on transcutaneous monitors should be set at the lowest possible point to provide accurate oxygen and carbon dioxide correlations. These transcutaneous leads are to be changed more frequently than the 4-hour interval recommended for older patients. When taping intravenous therapy lines (IVs) in place, the tape should be double backed whenever possible so that the IV is secure but the skin integrity is maintained when the tape is removed. Baths are given as needed, but mild, nonabrasive, nondrying soaps should be used.

Infants born to mothers who abused alcohol and other drugs during their pregnancy tend to be very active. With the increased activity, they rub the skin off prominent surfaces such as their knees, cheeks, and nares. To help alleviate this behavior and decrease the chance of infection from skin breakdown, swaddling technique is useful. Parents should also be taught to swaddle their infants with soft blankets and linens because the behavior may continue for several weeks to months once the infant is discharged.

Infants diagnosed with bronchopulmonary dysplasia are at an increased risk for infection. The increased risk occurs secondary to prematurity, poor nutrition, prolonged need for intubation or tracheotomy, and generally debilitated health state. Because of this risk, aseptic technique should be used at all times. All equipment should be cleared according to institutional policies before it comes in contact with an infant. Toys or items brought in from home must also be cleaned in compliance with institutional policies. Preventing infection in these infants poses a challenge for the nurses involved in their care.

Infection Prevention

Just as it is the nurse who first recognizes the subtle signs of infection, it is also the nurse who holds the key to infection control and prevention. Nurses have always been on the forefront of prevention secondary to their interest in education of the client, the family, and the community.[2] Hand washing is the first line of defense in the prevention and control of infection. (See Chapter 6.) Adherence to hand washing times specified by individual institutions and use of an appropriate soap (antimicrobial for intensive care units and regular soap for newborn nurseries) is critical in the prevention of infection. Hand washing should precede all contacts with neonates.[3,4]

The following sections discuss infection control strategies for procedures specific to newborns and young children.

Umbilical Artery and Vein Catheterization

Catheterization is used most often in premature infants for infusion of fluids, frequent or continuous monitoring of blood gases, central monitoring, and resuscitation. This procedure involves threading a small sterile catheter through the umbilical artery or vein located in the remnant of the infant's umbilical cord.

Specific Infection Risks

Infection risk to the infant includes introduction of microorganisms into the central circulation and introduction of air into the central circulation. Infants need special attention to the lower extremities and the buttocks to ensure that the catheter is not impairing circulation to these areas and increasing the risk of infection from skin breakdown. Because catheterization involves the handling of blood, standard precautions should be followed. (See Chapter 7.)

Procedure

The infant is placed under the radiant warmer during the procedure. The infant is connected to a cardiorespiratory monitor to enhance assessment of the infant's condition because little of the infant is visible during the procedure. If at all possible, the infant's head should be visible to assess color and maintain adequate respiratory support.

Catheterization procedure

Most institutions have umbilical and venous catheter insertion trays. The tray, sterile gown, gloves, and mask are gathered for the practitioner performing the procedure, and gloves and a mask are gathered for the assistant. Care is taken to decrease traffic around the bedside during the procedure. Masks should be worn by any personnel at the bedside. Antiseptic solution, such as povidone-iodine, is needed to cleanse the area. Once the practitioner has dressed in the sterile garb, the assistant should do the following:

1. Hold the umbilical stump up with hemostats from the tray while the practitioner cleanses around and up the stump of the umbilical cord in a circular motion. The practitioner will also tie a sterile umbilical tie around the base of the cord.

2. After cleansing the area, the practitioner drapes the infant and will cut the cord. After slowly dilating the vessel, the practitioner threads the sterile catheter carefully into the artery or vein and sutures it in place. A predetermined length—according to the infant's length—is used for the correct arterial placement.

3. The practitioner orders abdominal x-rays to document proper placement (low position: lumbar vertebrae 3-4; high position: thoracic vertebrae 6-9) to prevent damage to vital organs.[5]

4. Once proper placement is documented, secure the catheter using thin pieces of tape in a bridge or football goal post fashion over the umbilicus. If the infant is extremely premature, protect the skin with a semipermeable membrane dressing under the tape to decrease skin breakdown and infection. Remove the povidone-iodine from the infant's skin because it is irritating and can increase the risk for infection secondary to skin breakdown.

5. On completion of the procedure, resterilize the reusable catheterization trays. Clean blood contaminated articles, using standard precautions, before sending trays for sterilization. Clean work areas contaminated with blood according to institutional policy.

The catheter should be treated as a central line. Fluids are ordered to infuse at a rate appropriate for the fluid requirements of a premature infant and to maintain line patency.

Blood sampling

After umbilical artery or vein catheterization, blood samples may be obtained through this line. To obtain blood samples, health care workers (HCWs) should use aseptic technique and standard precautions to minimize the stress to the vessel and potential for infant infection and HCW infection. A two-stopcock system is recommended in which the port from the patient is not opened to

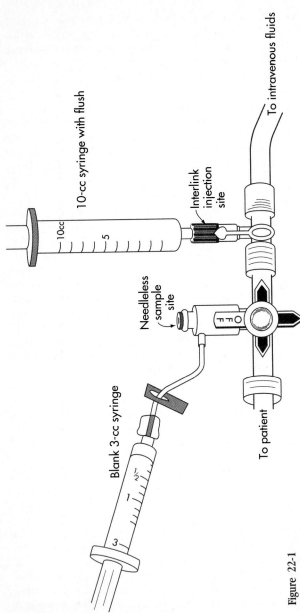

Figure 22-1
A two-stopcock system.

air. Open ports allow a backflow of blood from the patient secondary to arterial pressure that is greater than atmospheric pressure. Open ports are thus avenues for entrance of microorganisms. A needleless system is recommended to minimize the risk of needle sticks to HCWs. A technique using a needleless two-stopcock system is described here. Other techniques are appropriate according to unit policies.

1. Wash hands and apply sterile gloves.[5]
2. Place a double stopcock with a three-way stopcock proximal to the infant, and place a two-way stopcock distal to the infant.
3. Place a T-connector on the proximal three-way stopcock with a 3-cc syringe luer-locked on the end (Figure 22-1).
4. To obtain a sample, turn both stopcocks off to the IV fluids.
5. Unclamp the slide-clamp on the T-connector.
6. Draw back on the 3-cc syringe until approximately 2 cc of blood has been collected. (This 2-cc sample is the blank that clears all IV fluid from the sample to be drawn so the sample is not contaminated by IV fluid.)
7. Reclamp the T-connector.
8. After prepping the port with alcohol, spike into the needleless port of the T-connector with the appropriate sized needleless adapter and draw off the specimen.
9. Remove the syringe, which is the specimen. Unclamp the T-connector and give back the blank to minimize the amount of blood taken from the infant.
10. Turn the proximal stopcock off to the patient, and draw up 0.5 cc of heparin flush from the 10-cc syringe into the 3-cc syringe.
11. Turn the distal stopcock off to the flush, turn the proximal stopcock off to the IV fluid, and flush the line.
12. Once the 10-cc heparin flush syringe is emptied, record the entire 10-cc amount on the infant's records where indicated.[6] All blood removed and volume used for flushing the catheter should be recorded on the infant's record.
13. Dispose of gloves in an appropriate receptacle, and discard needles and syringes in an impervious, biohazard-labeled container.
14. Wash hands.

Exchange Transfusions

Umbilical and venous catheter lines are used for a procedure that is used only with newborns, known as an exchange transfusion.

Exchange transfusions are done on infants to regulate antibody-antigen levels, to remove toxins significantly concentrated in the blood and not otherwise removable, to correct life-threatening fluid and electrolyte imbalance, and to treat coagulation defects not remedied by single component replacement.[4] The incidence of exchange transfusion is decreasing secondary to technological advances in treatment of hemolytic diseases.

Specific Infection Risks

The risk of infection to the infant is great. Before 1985 the risk of human immunodeficiency virus transmission was a consideration, although with new screening methods this risk has been minimized. Viral infections carried in the blood are easily transmitted. Because of this, standard blood bank screening, including screening for sickle cell, human immunodeficiency virus, hepatitis B and hepatitis C virus, and cytomegalovirus, should be conducted. The spread of infection can be limited by the use of irradiated blood. Finally, because blood products are involved, standard precautions must be followed by all HCWs involved with the handling of the blood.

The infant will require both an umbilical arterial catheter and a venous catheter. The blood type needed is determined, and appropriate irradiated and screened whole blood is ordered. Preliminary laboratory blood samples are collected using aseptic technique. It is important to maintain a peripheral line for fluids to ensure homeostasis during the procedure.

Isometric Exchange Procedure

In an isometric exchange (volume in simultaneously equals the volume out), both the umbilical vein and artery lines are used. A stopcock with a syringe port connected to a handle is used. The handle points to the port that is open to the syringe.

1. Gather gowns, sterile gloves, masks, protective eye covering, and a prepackaged exchange transfusion tray.
2. Wash hands.
3. Open the tray using aseptic technique.
4. Apply protective equipment and sterile gloves.
5. Using sterile technique, place the stopcock with a syringe port on the venous catheter, and connect the other port to prewarmed blood.

6. The arterial line stopcock should have an empty sterile syringe attached to one port. Attach the second port to an empty sterile plastic bag fastened securely to the infant's bed.

7. The third port of both lines can remain sterile with caps instead of IV fluids, which have been turned off during the procedure.

8. As one practitioner is turning the handle of the stopcock to draw blood from the donor bag, which has been connected to the special controlled-volume administration set and blood warmer (venous line), the second practitioner is ready to pull blood from the arterial line. Once the donor blood is in the syringe, the practitioner turns the stopcock to open the port to the venous line. While the practitioner is slowly (2 to 3 cc/kg/min) pushing the blood into the venous line, the second practitioner is pulling blood from the arterial line at the same rate. While the first practitioner draws more blood from the donor bag, the second practitioner can turn the stopcock to open the port to the disposal bag and dispose of the infant's blood. This process continues until the ordered amount of whole blood has been exchanged.

Single Line Procedure

If only one line is available, the same equipment is used, but the donor blood, syringe, and disposal bag are connected to the same stopcock. One practitioner pulls blood from the infant, disposes of it, and replaces the same amount from the donor bag.

Follow-Up Procedure

Every 5 minutes, the vital signs, the amount of blood removed and given, the times of each exchange, and important data are recorded as indicated throughout the procedure. Using sterile technique, both lines of blood are cleared, and the stopcocks are changed. IV fluid may then be restarted in the arterial and venous lines.[5]

The exchange trays are disposable. Sharp objects are disposed of in an impervious biohazard-labeled receptacle before disposing of the tray. Individual institutions will have specified areas that have appropriate receptacles for materials that have come in contact with blood. The blood bag is handled according to institutional policy and disposed of in an appropriate receptacle in accordance with state regulations. Gloves should be worn by the HCW during the entire cleaning procedure. After glove removal, hands should be washed.

Percutaneous Central Venous Catheters

Percutaneous central venous catheters or percutaneous intravenous central catheters (PICCs) may also be used to secure vascular access in newborns and children. These lines are used for long-term IV access and medication administration and for administration of hyperosmolar fluids to increase calories and nutrients to a premature infant. PICC lines can be placed sterilely at the infant's bedside, reducing the risks involved with movement, reintubation (should the infant have reached the extubation stage), extubation, or general anesthesia. PICC lines are placed by physicians, nurse practitioners, or specially trained nurse IV therapist teams, depending on the institution and state regulations. Special manufactured trays are used that contain all the equipment and supplies needed. Infection risk once again includes contamination of the catheter during insertion and administration of fluids.

Procedure

1. Gather equipment.
2. Wash hands and apply gloves.
3. Using sterile technique, clean the insertion site with an antiseptic.
4. Insert the catheter into the appropriate vein.
5. Secure the catheter to the skin distal to the insertion site with 2-cm sterile strips. Antibiotic ointment can be used over the insertion site, but it is not required.
6. Use a transparent semipermeable dressing to cover the insertion site and sterile strips (but not on the hub).
7. Coil the rest of the catheter, and secure it to the skin using the same type of transparent semipermeable dressing that covers the entire catheter.
8. Secure the hub of the catheter by criss-crossing tape under the hub and over the wings of the hub. This prevents the catheter and hub from separating, which would allow contaminants to enter the venous line, causing infection.[7-9] Place gauze under the hub, and tape across it and around the extremity to further secure the line.

The transparent dressing allows for continuous inspection of the catheter insertion site; however, some research suggests increased risk of infection with a transparent semipermeable dressing.[5] This dressing should not envelop the entire circumference of the limb.

As the infant grows or venous stasis sets in, it can impede circulation and become a tourniquet.

Inspect the hub area every 8 hours for constriction and skin breakdown. Also, check the site at least every 8 hours for redness, tenderness, moisture, or signs of infiltration. The dressing need not be changed for the duration of the life of the PICC line, unless the transparent dressing comes loose. The infant's record should indicate the condition of the PICC at least at the beginning and end of each shift or according to individual institution's policy.[7,9] Intake should be recorded hourly.

Circumcision

Newborn circumcision is controversial.[10] It is a simple procedure but is not without complications. Therefore, the risk of complication must be weighed against the evidence that uncircumcised boys are at greater risk for ascending infection of the urinary tract than are circumcised boys.[11]

Procedure

Circumcisions are performed before discharge by the physician. A specially designed clamp is used, with sterile procedure. Dispose of the tissue as regulated waste, according to Occupational Safety and Health Administration standards. Apply a tight diaper for 1 hour. For 24 hours, check the penis for bleeding, excessive swelling, and difficulty voiding. Urinary retention leads to urinary tract infections. Until the area is completely healed, the infant should not be immersed for a bath.

If the area becomes infected, use wet to dry dressings and sitz baths. Although these infections are generally mild, some fatalities have been reported.[5,11] Bleeding or oozing is also a complication, but it usually can be controlled with manual pressure for 5 to 10 minutes.

Extracorporeal Membrane Oxygenation

The last procedure to be discussed is the procedure for venoarterial extracorporeal membrane oxygenation (ECMO). ECMO is used for infants with reversible respiratory failure who do not respond to maximal conventional ventilation. Requiring advanced technology, this procedure is done only at special centers across the country.

Placement of the cannulas in the carotid artery and internal jugular vein requires a team with a surgical specialist, a medical specialist, and a circuit specialist.

Procedure

The infant is paralyzed, and under sterile conditions, the team surgically places two cannulas. To prevent infection, the area is initially cleaned with iodophor iodine solution. The complete procedure is beyond the scope of this chapter.

The nurse's responsibility is to identify breaks of sterile technique and monitor the infant during the procedure. Once the procedure is complete and the infant is placed on the ECMO circuit, the two cannulas are tied together. Povidone-iodine ointment is placed on the site, and the area is covered with a transparent semipermeable membrane dressing. The site is checked frequently during the nursing shift. The condition of the cannulas, the color of the site, and drainage on the infant's chart is recorded. The infant is at risk for infection secondary to the introduction of a foreign material into the central circulation of an already compromised infant.[5]

Once the infant improves and decannulation is possible, apply the same dressing and ointment used for cannulation. At this time special attention is needed at the wound area. Because of its location in the folds of the infant's neck, the wound area is prone to bacterial growth. The condition of the cannulization site is recorded each shift. If the wound becomes reddened or drains, wound care is indicated. The area is cleaned with sterile water, and an antibiotic ointment is applied as ordered. Systemic antibiotics may also be indicated.

Summary

Avoiding infection in neonates who require invasive procedures requires vigilance by all HCWs involved in their care. HCWs must stop and think about the altered defense mechanisms of these patients, reservoirs of infectious agents, modes of infection transmission, and infection control strategies (Figure 22-2). The nurse plays an important and leading role in reducing the transmission of neonatal infections.

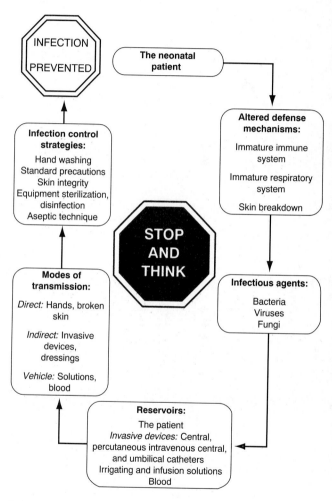

Figure 22-2
Factors affecting the neonatal patient leading to the selection
of the strategies to prevent infectious complications.

References

1. Lott J et al: Assessment and management of immunologic dysfunction. In Kerner C, editor: *Comprehensive neonatal nursing,* Philadelphia, 1993, WB Saunders.
2. Turner J: Communicable disease and infection control practice in community health nursing. In Stanhope M, Lancaster J, editors: *Community health nursing process and practice promoting health,* St Louis, 1988, Mosby.
3. Derschewitz RA: Bacteremia. In Dershewitz RA, editor: *Ambulatory pediatric care,* Philadelphia, 1988, JB Lippincott.
4. Smith D: *Comprehensive child and family nursing skills,* St Louis, 1991, Mosby.
5. Fletcher MA, *Atlas of procedure in neonatology,* Philadelphia, 1993, JB Lippincott.
6. Merenstein G, Gardner S, *Handbook of neonatal care*, St Louis, 1993, Mosby.
7. Chates MK: Percutaneous central venous catheters in neonates, *JOGNN* July/August 1986.
8. Gladman G et al: Staphylococcus epidermitis and retention of neonatal percutaneous central catheters, *Arch Dis Child* 65:234, 1990.
9. Leick-Rude MK: Use of percutaneous silastic intravascular catheters in high-risk neonates, *Neonat Netw* 9(1), 1990.
10. Poland RL: The question of routine circumcision, *N Engl J Med* 322:1312, 1990.
11. Gerhart JP, Callan NA: Complications of circumcisions, *Contemp OB GYN* 27(57), 1986.

Postmortem Care

23

The care of a patient after the patient's death and the care of the patient's family are best accomplished by the nurse who has developed a relationship with the family and who has specific knowledge of the medical history of the patient. After the patient's death, the physician certifies death in the medical record. A description of the diagnosis, treatments, and care is included to alert the postmortem caregiver of potential hazards. An autopsy may be requested or, in cases of unusual death or death within 24 hours of hospitalization, may be required. This ruling varies by state, so familiarity with state regulations is advised.

Some states require hospital staff to identify and refer potential organ donors at the time of hospital admission. Patients or families who have elected organ donation will have been informed that the organs will be removed after the patient is pronounced clinically dead, even though cardiorespiratory support may be maintained. Tissues and organs that may be used for transplant include corneas, skin, long bones, middle ear bones, heart, liver, lungs, kidneys, and pancreas.[1]

It is important to offer the family an opportunity to view the patient's body and to give the family time to remain with the body alone or with the nurse, as requested. Preparation of the body before the visit helps the family through this stressful experience.

Procedure Description

Physical changes occurring after death include stiffening of the body (rigor mortis), which develops 2 hours after death, decrease in body temperature (algor mortis), decrease in skin elasticity, softening of body tissues, and discoloration of the skin (liver mortis). These changes occur within hours after death and require early intervention in care of the patient's body.

Postmortem care of the patient involves physical preparation of the body for viewing by the family, for examination or autopsy, for retrieval of donated organs, and for transportation to the mortuary. In addition to completing the mechanics of postmortem care, care providers must protect themselves from exposure to potentially infectious body fluids and wastes during care of the body.

Specific Infection Risks

The risks for health care providers and family members are exposure to infected body fluids and substances. Contact with urine, feces, or other body fluids may occur when sphincter muscles relax following death and oozing occurs. Exposure to mucous secretions may occur when the body is rolled or bent double and mucus is expulsed. Accidental puncture wounds or mucous membrane exposure may occur as intravenous lines and tubes are removed, clamped, or cut to within 2.5 cm of the skin, depending on agency policy.[2] The body now becomes a reservoir, and the care provider becomes the susceptible host (Figure 23-1). Use of standard precautions interrupts the modes of transmission, providing adequate protection for the susceptible hosts. (See Chapter 7.)

Procedure Preparation

Preparation for care of the body includes knowing the cause of death and the potential for exposure to infected blood or body fluids. Review plans for organ donation. If the family plans to view the body, delay preparation of the body to allow the family time with the deceased.

The physical care of the body requires a morgue pack that may be available in the institution. If not, collect the following materials:

1. Latex gloves for all participants
2. Plastic shroud or a body container approved by the institution
3. Gowns
4. Washcloths
5. Towels
6. Basin with water and soap
7. Clean spread to cover the body for viewing by the family
8. Clamps and scissors
9. Tape
10. Cotton balls
11. Absorbent pads

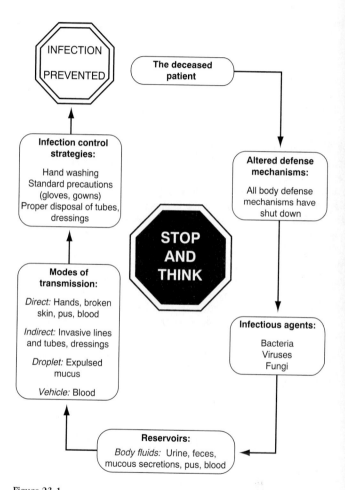

Figure 23-1
Factors affecting postmortem care of the patient leading to the selection of strategies to prevent infection transmission to the care provider.

12. Denture holder
13. Comb or brush
14. Deodorizer
15. Valuables container
16. Morgue stretcher

The assistance of a colleague is needed to complete postmortem activities to prevent injury when lifting and transferring the body.

Procedure

1. Wash hands.
2. Wear gloves and gowns if soiling is likely.
3. Wear mask and eye protection if splashes of body fluids are likely.
4. Remove tubes from the body, or clamp or cut them within 2.5 cm of the skin, according to agency policy.
5. Gently tape cut tubes in place to avoid tissue injury.
6. Remove soiled clothing, dressings, and padding, and place them in appropriate disposal containers.
7. Place all wastes and contaminated articles in plastic bags.
8. Remove and dispose of dressings, lines, tubes, and padding in bags identified by the agency for infectious material.[3]
9. Place absorbent pads under the perineal area.
10. Place the body in a supine position, with arms at side or on chest.
11. Place a small rolled towel under the head to prevent discoloration by pooling blood.
12. Gently hold the eyelids down, or place moistened cotton balls on them.
13. Insert dentures to maintain facial features, or place them in a denture cup and send them with the body, depending on agency policy.
14. Clean and dress the body in a clean gown for family viewing.
15. Following the family visit, remove the gown.
16. Apply tags to the ankle or toe and wrist that identify the body, and document the presence of any infectious disease.[1]
17. Place the body in a plastic shroud or agency-approved body container, and transport it to the morgue.

Infection Prevention

Pay special attention to the use of standard precautions—namely barrier techniques—including the following steps:

1. Wash hands vigorously before and after gloving. (See Chapter 6.)
2. Wear gowns and gloves.
3. Wash hands and other skin surfaces immediately if contaminated with blood or body fluids.
4. Do not recap or manipulate needles; discard them in a sharps container.
5. Place all wastes and contaminated materials in plastic bags.[2]
6. Dispose of materials contaminated with blood and body fluids in accordance with agency policy.[3]
7. Promptly clean blood or body fluids on surfaces with a bleach solution (1 part bleach to 10 parts water) or an EPA-approved hospital-grade disinfectant.[4]
8. Clean reusable equipment with soap and water in preparation for disinfection or sterilization. (See Chapter 9.)

Special Populations

Care of the family experiencing the death of a loved one is always difficult. When it is a child or infant who dies, the care of the family takes on special significance. Take care to prepare the child for viewing to prevent unnecessary trauma to the parents and family. Placing a loved toy by the side of the child and covering the child with a blanket may help the family. Parents of the child or infant may wish to hold, rock, or talk to the child. Time should be available for this grieving to occur. The transportation of a newborn or fetus from the morgue to a mother's room may be done in a basket carrier with blankets covering the newborn. Allow the body of the baby to warm slightly before carrying it to the parents for viewing. Apply diapers and pads to prevent body fluid exposure.[5]

Home Care Considerations

Preparation of the body at home must conform to the guidelines previously discussed. Give special consideration to the needs of the family members who are present. Follow standard precautions in care of the body to avoid exposure to potentially infectious substances. Explain these precautions and procedures to the family. Place contaminated disposables in plastic bags, and discard them with household waste.

Summary

Prevention of infection in the care of the deceased patient requires the care provider to consider the specific altered defense mechanisms, infectious agents, reservoirs for infection, and modes of transmission. Infection control strategies are employed, including hand washing, universal precautions, and proper disposal of materials. Figure 23-1 describes this process.

References

1. Potter PA, Perry AG: *Fundamentals of nursing: concepts, process and practice,* St Louis, 1993, Mosby.
2. Soule B, editor: *The APIC curriculum for infection control practice, vol 2,* Dubuque, Iowa, 1983, Kendall/Hunt.
3. Soule B, editor: *The APIC curriculum for infection control practice, vol 1,* Dubuque, Iowa, 1983, Kendall/Hunt.
4. Berg R, editor: *The APIC curriculum for infection control practice, vol 3,* Dubuque, Iowa, 1988, Kendall/Hunt.
5. Whaley L, Wong D: *Nursing care of infants and children,* St Louis, 1991, Mosby.

Index

Abscess
  temporary isolation precautions
    for, 93
  type and duration of precautions, 95
Acinetobacter
  ambu bags and, 380
  in environment, 152, 155, 157
Acquired immunodeficiency syndrome
    (AIDS); *see also* Human immu-
    nodeficiency virus;
    Immunocompromised patient
  clinical description, 21
  comments on, 21
  laboratory criteria for diagnosis, 21
Adenovirus, type and duration of
    precautions, 104
Aerobic, 75
Aerobic gram negative rods, in envi-
    ronment, 158
Age, wound care and, 277
Agenda for Change, 8
Airborne, as mode of transmission, 68
Airborne precautions
  patient placement, 88
  patient transport, 88
  respiratory protection, 88
Ambu bags, 380-381
Amebiasis
  laboratory criteria for diagnosis, 21
  case classification, 21
  clinical description, 21
  comments on, 21
American Academy of Pediatrics Infec-
    tious Disease, 52-53
American Journal Infection Control
    (Larson), 53
American Journal Infection Control
    (Martin & Reichelderfer), 53
American Journal Infection Control
    (Rutala), 53
Amoeba histolytica, 21
Anaerobic, 75
Animal bites, as reportable disease in
    some states, 49

Anthrax
  case classification, 21
  clinical description, 22
  comments on, 22
  laboratory criteria for diagnosis, 22
  type and duration of precautions, 95
Antibiotics, overusage and
    antibiotic-resistant bacteria, 58
Antimicrobial soap, 75-78
  guidelines for use of and proce-
    dures, 76-77
Antiretroviral chemoprophylaxis, 132,
    136-137
Antiseptics, defined, 140
*APIC curriculum for infection control
    practice, The* (Olmstead), 53
Arterial blood samples, 182, 185
  specific considerations for, 186
Arterial puncture
  description, 306
  follow up, 328
  procedure, 322-327
Arteriovenous fistulas and grafts, infec-
    tion prevention, 358-359
Ascariasis, type and duration of pre-
    cautions, 95
Aseptic meningitis
  case classification, 22
  clinical description, 22
  comments on, 22
  laboratory criteria for diagnosis, 22
Aspergillosis, type and duration of pre-
    cautions, 95
Aspergillus
  in environment, 152
  mode of transmission, 68
Association for Practitioners in Infec-
    tion Control (APIC) and Epide-
    miology
  as infection control resource, 51-52
  role of, 51-52
Association of Operating Room
    Nurses', standards for practice,
    176

Babesiosis, type and duration of precautions, 95
Bacilli, 31
  in environment, 155
Bacteria, 62
Benenson, A. S., 52
Bilharziasis, type and duration of precautions, 107
Biological defense mechanism, 59, 61
  bypassing, 61-63
  lymphocytes, 59, 61
Blastomycosis
  as reportable disease in some states, 49
  type and duration of precautions, 95
Block, S. S., 53
Bloodborne Pathogens Standards, 3, 11-13
  engineering controls, 12
  establishment of, 11
  exposure control plan, 12
  Hepatitis B vaccination, 13
  housekeeping, 13
  labels and signs, 13
  methods of compliance, 12-13
  orientation and training, 13
  personal protective equipment, 12-13
  post-exposure plans, 13
  regulated waste, 13
  scope and application, 12
  universal precautions, 12
  work practice controls, 12
Blood specimens, 182-186, 189
  arterial samples, 182, 185, 186
  blood for culture, 186
  capillary samples, 182
  children and, 185
  finger puncture, 186
  home care and, 186, 189
  infants, 185
  intravascular catheters, 185-186
  step-by-step guide for, 183-184
  venous samples, 185
Blood transfusion
  description, 328
  follow up, 328
  procedure, 328-332
B-lymphocytes, 59
Body defense mechanisms, 58-61
  biological, 59, 61
  bypassing, 61-63
  chemical, 61
  mechanical, 58-60
Body substance isolation (BSI), 82, 84

Bone marrow biopsy, 236-237
  description, 236
  follow up assessment, 237
  preparation, 236
  procedure for infection prevention, 236-237
  specific infection risks, 236
Bordetella pertussis, 36
  temporary isolation precautions for, 92
Borrelia burgdorferi, 32
Botulism, foodborne
  case classification, 23
  clinical description, 23
  comments on, 23
  laboratory criteria for diagnosis, 23
  type and duration of precautions, 95, 99
Botulism, infant
  case classification, 23
  clinical description, 23
  comments on, 23
  laboratory criteria for diagnosis, 23
  type and duration of precautions, 95, 99
Botulism, other
  case classification, 24
  clinical description, 24
  comments on, 24
  laboratory criteria for diagnosis, 24
  type and duration of precautions, 95, 99
Botulism, wound
  case classification, 23
  clinical description, 23
  comments on, 23
  laboratory criteria for diagnosis, 23
  type and duration of precautions, 95, 99
Bronchiolitis, type and duration of precautions, 95
Brucella, 24
Brucellosis
  case classification, 24
  clinical description, 24
  laboratory criteria for diagnosis, 24
  type and duration of precautions, 96
Bubonic plague, type and duration of precautions, 104
Burn care, 292-302
  background on, 292
  care procedures, 295-297
    description, 295-296
    preparation, 296
    steps in, 296-297

Burn care—cont'd
  characteristics of, 292-293
  first degree, 293
  home care consideration, 297-299
  infection prevention, 297, 299-300,
      302
  infectious process of, 293-294
  invasive infection, 294
  noninvasive infection, 294
  second degree, 293
  specific infection risks, 294
    altered defense mechanisms, 294-
        295
    devices and procedures, 295
    personnel, 295
    susceptible hosts, 294
  third degree, 293
Campylobacteriosis, as reportable dis-
    ease in some states, 49
Campylobacter sp., type and duration
    of precautions, 99
Candida, ambu bags and, 380
Candida albicans
  blood specimens, 183
  gastrointestinal procedures, 342
  ostomy care, 286
  urinary tract infection, 242
Candidiasis, type and duration of pre-
    cautions, 96
Capillary blood samples, 182
Category-specific isolation precau-
    tions, 81
Catheterization, 241-272
  condom
    follow up assessment, 269
    procedure, 261, 265-269
    risks, 243
  follow up assessment, 261
  home care considerations, 269-270
  indwelling
    care of, 261-264
    follow up assessment, 261
    procedure for inserting, 244-260
    risks, 242-243
  infection prevention strategies, 270,
      272
  procedure risks, 242
  specific infection risks, 241-242
  straight
    follow up assessment, 261
    procedure for inserting, 244-260
    risks, 243
Catheters,
  for dialysis, 353-356
  method of disinfecting, 141-142

Catscratch fever, type and duration of
    precautions, 96
Centers for Disease Control and Pre-
    vention
  evolution of isolation practices,
      81-82
  guidelines for infection control
      in hospital personnel,
      14, 17
  as infection control resource, 52
  National Notifiable Diseases
      Surveillance System, 19
  optimum tuberculosis control pro-
      gram for health care facilities,
      14-17
Cerebral spinal fluid (CSF), 196-197
  specific considerations, 197
  step-by-step guide for collection,
      197
Chancroid
  case classification, 25
  clinical description, 25
  laboratory criteria for diagnosis, 25
Chemical defense mechanisms, 61
  bypassing, 62-63
Chest tubes, 224-231
  description of, 224
  follow up assessment, 231
  preparation, 225
  procedure for insertion and infection
      prevention, 225-230
  specific infection risks, 225
Chickenpox
  HCW work exclusion for, 128
  mode of transmission, 67
  as reportable disease in some
      states, 49
  type and duration of precautions,
      109
Children
  blood specimens and, 185
  sputum specimens and 195
  stool specimens and, 190
  urine specimens and, 189
Chlamydia, type and duration of pre-
    cautions, 104
Chlamydia pneumoniae, 37
Chlamydia psittaci, 37
Chlamydia trachomatis, 33, 37
  as reportable disease in some
      states, 49
  type and duration of precautions, 96
Chlorhexidine, 163
Chlorine, dilution, properties and cost,
    147

Cholera
case classification, 25
clinical description, 25
comments on, 25
laboratory criteria for diagnosis, 25
mode of transmission, 68
Circulatory access, infection prevention, 359
Circumcision, 405
Cleaning, defined, 139
Clean-voided (midstream) procedure,
187-190
Closed-cavity infection, type and duration of precautions, 96
Clostridia
in environment, 155, 157
Clostridium, type and duration of
precautions, 96
Clostridium botulinum, type and duration of precautions, 96
Clostridium difficile
burns and, 300
contamination of surface equipment, 57
diarrhea, stool softeners, GI stimu-
lant, enemas and, 57
in environment, 154
gastrointestinal procedures, 342
increase risk of with antibiotics, 57
temporary isolation precautions
for, 91
type and duration of precautions, 95,
96, 98, 99
Clostridium perfringens, type and
duration of precautions,
96, 99
Clostridium welchii, type and duration
of precautions, 99
Cytomegalovirus, mode of transmission, 68
Coccidioidomycosis
as reportable disease in some
states, 49
type and duration of precautions, 97
Code for Nurses, 4
Colitis, type and duration of precautions, 95
Colonization, 62
defined, 274
vs. infection, 274
Colorado tick fever, type and duration
of precautions, 97
Colostomy, stool specimens and, 190
Communicable diseases, reference
books, 52-53

Condom catheterization
follow up assessment, 269
home care considerations, 269-270
procedure, 261, 265-269
risks of, 243
tips for preventing infection, 270,
272
Congenital rubella, type and duration
of precautions, 97
Conjunctivitis
HCW work exclusion for, 128
as reportable disease in some
states, 49
type and duration of precautions, 97
Contact, as mode of transmission
direct, 67
droplet, 67
indirect, 67
Contact precautions, 89-90
environmental control, 90
gloves, 89
gowns, 90
hand washing, 90
patient care equipment, 90
patient placement, 89
patient transport, 90
Contaminated-needle injuries, percentage of occupational acquired
HIV, 5
*Control of communicable diseases in
man* (Benenson), 52
Corynebacterium, 75
blood specimens, 183
Corynebacterium diphtheriae, 26
Coxsackie virus, type and duration of
precautions, 97
Creutzfeldt-Jakob disease, type and duration of precautions, 97
Critical medical equipment, 148
Croup, type and duration of precautions, 97
Cryptococcosis, type and duration of
precautions, 97
Cryptosporidium sp., type and duration
of precautions, 99
Cunninghamella, in environment, 155
Cytomegalovirus infection, type and
duration of precautions, 97
Cytotoxic T-lymphocytes, 59
Decontamination, process of, 148-151
defined, 139-140
infection risks and prevention
strategies, 149
preparation, 149
procedure, 149-150

Decontamination—cont'd
 purposes of, 140
 reservoirs of infectious agents in
  environment, 151-160
 waste disposal, 150-151
Decubitus ulcer, type and duration of
 precautions, 98
Defense mechanism; *see* Body defense
 mechanism
Dengue
 as reportable disease in some
  states, 49
 type and duration of precautions, 98
Depilatory
 equipment for, 171-172
 procedure for wet shave, 172
Dialysis, 351-361
 exchange, 352
 hemodialysis, 357-359
  arteriovenous fistulas and grafts,
   357
  circulatory access, 357
  infection prevention, 358-359
  specific infection risk, 358
 methods of, 351-359
 peritoneal, 351-357
  catheter procedures, 353-356
  catheter site infections, 352
  infection prevention, 356
  patient education, 356-357
  peritonitis, 352-353
  specific infection risks, 352
 preventing occupational exposure,
  359-361
  accidental exposure, 361
  barrier technique, 361
Diarrhea
 HCW work exclusion for, 128
 temporary isolation precautions
  for, 91
 type and duration of precautions, 98
Diphtheria
 case classification, 26
 clinical description, 26
 comments on, 26
 laboratory criteria for diagnosis, 26
 type and duration of precautions, 98
Disease-specific isolation precautions, 81
Disinfectants/disinfection
 common disinfectants and dilutions,
  properties and costs, 146-147
 defined, 140
 factors affecting, 140
 high-level, 140

Disinfectants/disinfection—cont'd
 intermediate-level, 140
 low-level, 140
 reference books on, 53
 type of object, and methods of, 141-
  144
 types of, 145
Disinfection, process of, 148-151
 infection risks and prevention
  strategies, 149
 preparation, 149
 procedure, 150
 reservoirs of infectious agents in environment, 151-160
 waste disposal, 150-151
*Disinfection, sterilization, and preser-
 vation* (Block), 53
Dose, 64
Draft Guidelines for Isolation Precau-
 tion in Hospitals
 standard precautions, 84-87
 transmission-based precautions, 84-
  85, 88-90
Draining wounds, HCW work exclusion for, 128
Droplet precautions, 88-89
 masks, 89
 patient placement, 89
 patient transport, 89
Dust mist respirators, inadequacy of,
 11, 14
Echinococcosis, type and duration of
 precautions, 98
E-IPV vaccine, 120
Elderly patients, sputum specimens
 and, 195
Employment at Will Doctrine, 4
Encephalitis (postinfectious)
 case classification, 27
 clinical description, 27
 comments on, 27
 laboratory criteria for diagnosis, 27
Encephalitis (primary)
 case classification, 26
 clinical description, 26
 comments on, 26
 laboratory criteria for diagnosis, 26
Endemic nosocomial infections,
 mechanisms to reduce risk of, 9
Endogenous organisms, 59
 skin and, 59
Endometritis
 type and duration of precautions, 98,
  108

Endoscopy, 237, 239
care of equipment, 347
description, 237, 239
follow up assessment, 239
infection prevention, 349
preparation, 239
procedure, 239
reference books on, 53
specific infection risks and infection prevention, 237, 239, 346-347
Endotracheal suctioning, 366-380
description, 366
follow up assessment, 380
home care considerations, 380
procedure, 367-369
specific infection risks, 366
Endotracheal tubes, 366
Engineering controls, 117-118
Bloodborne Pathogens Standards, 12
needlesticks and, 117-118
resheathing/retracting syringe devices, 118
Enterobacter organisms,
in environment, 155, 157
urinary tract infection, 242
Enterobiasis, type and duration of precautions, 98
Enterococcus faecium
vancomycin-resistant, 58
Enterococcus sp., type and duration of precautions, 98
Enterocolitis, type and duration of precautions, 107
Enteroviral infections, type and duration of precautions, 99
Environmental control of infectious agents, 151-160
contact precautions, 90
Epidemic nosocomial infections, mechanisms to reduce risk of, 9
Epiglottitis, type and duration of precautions, 99
Epstein-Barr virus infection, type and duration of precautions, 99
Erythema infectiosum, type and duration of precautions, 99
Erythema marginatum, 39
Erythema migrans, 32
Escherichia coli
blood specimens, 183
mode of transmission, 67, 68
as transient organisms, 75
type and duration of precautions, 99
urinary tract infection, 242
urine specimens, 187
Ethylene oxide gas (ETO), 145

Ewingella, in environment, 154
Exchange, 352
Exchange transfusions, 401-403
follow-up procedures, 403
isometric exchange procedure, 402-403
single line procedure, 403
specific infection risks, 402
Exogenous infection, hand washing and, 57
Exogenous organisms, 59
skin and, 59
Exposures to bloodborne pathogens, 132-137
counseling, 136
first aid, 132
postexposure follow up, 132-136
zidovudine treatment, 132, 136-137
Extracorporeal membrane oxygenation, 405-406
Eye protection,
guidelines for use of, 94, 112
standard precautions, 86
Face shield,
guidelines for use of, 94, 112
standard precautions, 86
Family caregivers, need for infection control measures in, 4
Fever, as sign of infection, 69
Fingernails, nail polish and, 163
First degree burns, characteristics of 293
Flavobacteria, in environment, 155
Flexible endoscopy, 346-347
care of equipment, 347
specific infectious risks, 346-347
Flora, normal, 59, 60
Food poisoning, type and duration of precautions, 99
Francisella tularensis, 47
Full thickness wounds, 275
Fungi, 62
Furunculosis, type and duration of precautions, 99
Gangrene, type and duration of precautions, 99
Gastroenteritis
as reportable disease in some states, 49
type and duration of precautions, 99
Gastrointestinal procedures, 342-349
flexible endoscopy, 346-347
gastrostomy/jejunostomy feedings, 345-346
home care considerations, 343
infection prevention, 347, 349

Gastrointestinal procedures—cont'd
  nasogastric tube placement, 343-345
  specific infection risks, 342-343
Gastrointestinal system
  bypassing defense mechanism of,
    61-63
  mechanical body defense, 60
Gastrostomy/jejunostomy feedings,
    345-346
  follow up, 346
  infection prevention, 349
  procedure, 346
  procedure preparation, 345-346
Gauze dressings, 278, 279
  frequency of dressing changes, 279
  indications for use, 279
Generalized infections, 64
Genitourinary system
  bypassing defense mechanism of,
    61-63
  mechanical body defense, 60
German measles
  type and duration of precautions,
    100, 107
Germicides, defined, 140
Giardia,
  mode of transmission, 68
  as reportable disease in some
    states, 49
Giardia lamblia, type and duration of
    precautions, 100
Gloves
  alternative to latex, 167
  body substance isolation and, 82
  contact precautions, 89
  guidelines for use of, 94, 112
  home care isolation precautions for,
    113
  latex sensitivity and, 167
  minute tears in, 281
  standard precautions, 85
  universal precautions and, 83
Gloving, closed technique
  equipment, 167
  preparation, 167
  procedure, 167-169
  removing soiled, 169-170
Glutaraldehyde, dilution, properties and
    cost, 147
Gram-negative rods
  in environment, 153, 158
Gonococcal ophthalmia neonatorum,
    type and duration of precautions,
    100
Gonorrhea
  case classification, 27

Gonorrhea—cont'd
  clinical description, 27
  comments on, 27
  laboratory criteria for diagnosis, 27
  mode of transmission, 67
  type and duration of precautions, 100
Gowning, 165-167
  equipment, 165
  preparation, 165
  procedure, 165-167
  removing soiled, 169-170
  standard precautions, 86
Grafts, defined, 292
Granuloma inguinale
  case classification, 27
  clinical description, 27
  comments on, 27
  laboratory criteria for diagnosis, 27
  type and duration of precautions, 100
Group D streptococci, urinary tract in-
    fection, 242
Guillain-Barré syndrome
  type and duration of precautions,
    100
Haemophilus decreyi, 25
Haemophilus influenzae
  case classification, 28
  clinical description, 28
  comments on, 28
  laboratory criteria for diagnosis, 28
  mode of transmission, 67
  type and duration of precautions,
    103, 105
Hand washing, 74-79
  contact precautions, 90
  home care considerations, 79
    isolation precautions for, 113
  immunocompromised patient, 219
  indications for, 78
  lack of proper, 74
  purpose of, 74
  reference books on, 53
  resident and transient organisms,
    74-75
  routine procedure of, 78-79
  standard precautions, 85
  types of hand washing soap, 75-78
Hantavirus, as reportable disease in
    some states, 49
HBV vaccine, 118, 136
Healthcare facilities
  accreditation by JCAHO, 7-10
    infection control indicators, 9-10
    standard of surveillance,
      prevention and control of
      infection, 9

Health care worker immunity
administrative requirements for
vaccine administration, 119
tuberculosis testing, 118
vaccine use, 118, 119
Health care workers
managing significant exposures,
132-137
preventing and managing infections
in, 116-137
work exclusions for, 127-131
Hemodialysis, 357-359
arteriovenous fistulas and grafts,
357
circulatory access, 357
defined, 351
infection prevention
circulatory access devices, 359
fistula and grafts, 358-359
Hemorrhagic fevers, type and duration of precautions, 101
Hemothorax, chest tubes and, 224
Hepatitis A
case classification, 28
clinical description, 28
comments on, 28
HCW work exclusion for, 128
in environment, 157
laboratory criteria for diagnosis, 28
mode of transmission, 67
type and duration of precautions,
101
Hepatitis B
case classification, 28
clinical description, 28
comments on, 28
counseling for, 136
exposure to, 132-136
first aid, 132
HCW work exclusion for, 128
laboratory criteria for diagnosis, 28
mode of transmission, 67, 68
postexposure follow up, 132-136
type and duration of precautions,
101
Hepatitis B vaccine, 116, 121
Bloodborne Pathogens Standards, 13
Hepatitis C
case classification, 29
clinical description, 29
comments on, 29
laboratory criteria for diagnosis, 29
mode of transmission, 68
type and duration of precautions,
101

Hepatitis delta
case classification, 29
clinical description, 29
comments on, 29
laboratory criteria for diagnosis, 29
type and duration of precautions,
101
Hepatitis type E, type and duration of
precautions, 101
Hepatitis, isoniazid (INH), 123, 127
Herpangina, type and duration of precautions, 101
Herpes simplex
HCW work exclusion for, 129
as reportable disease in some
states, 49
type and duration of precautions,
101
Herpesvirus hominis, type and duration
of precautions, 101
Herpes zoster
HCW work exclusion for, 129
as reportable disease in some
states, 49
type and duration of precautions,
101
High-efficiency particulate air (HEPA)
respirators, preventing transmission of tuberculosis and, 11
High-level disinfection, defined, 140
Histoplasmosis
as reportable disease in some
states, 49
type and duration of precautions,
101
Home care considerations
blood specimens and, 186, 189
burns, 297-299
catheterization, 269
endotracheal suctioning, 380
gastrointestinal procedures, 343
gloves, 113
hand washing procedure, 79, 113
infection control practices adapted,
112-114
infection prevention for immunocompromised patients, 213,
216
laundry, 113
need for infection control measures
in, 4
needlesticks and, 216
ostomy management and, 288
oxygen administration, 366
postmortem care, 413-414

Home care considerations—cont'd
  spills, 113
  tracheostomy care, 233
  waste disposal, 113
  wound care, 285
Hookworm disease, type and duration
    of precautions, 101
Hospital Infection Control Practices Ad-
    visory Committee (HICPAC), 84
Host,
  increasing resistance, 70
  susceptible, 66, 69
Human immunodeficiency virus (HIV);
    see also Acquired immunodefi-
    ciency syndrome (AIDS); Immu-
    nocompromised patient
  contaminated-needle injuries, 5
  ethical and legal principles related
    to HIV status of employees
    and patients, 5
  exposure to
    counseling for, 136
    first aid, 132
    postexposure follow up, 132-136
    zidovudine treatment, 132,
      136-137
  as handicap, 5
  HCW work exclusion for, 129
  mode of transmission, 67, 68
  occupational transmission of, 3, 5,
    117
  PPD test and, 123
  as reportable disease in some
    states, 49
  transmission of, and obstetrical care,
    392
  type and duration of precautions, 101
Hydrocolloids, 278, 280-281
  frequency of dressing changes, 280-
    281
  indications for use, 280
Hydrogels, 279, 281
  frequency of dressing changes, 281
  indications for use, 281
Hydrogen peroxide, dilution, properties
    and cost, 146
Hymenolepis nana, type and duration
    of precautions, 108
Ileostomy, stool specimens and, 190
Immune defense mechanisms, 59, 61
  impairment of
    age, 57
    medical disorders, 57
    patient treatments, 57
  lymphocytes, 59, 61

Immune deficiency disorders
  acquired immunodeficiency syn-
    drome, 203
  disorders associated with B cells or
    antibody, 204
  disorders associated with T cells and
    cell-mediated immunity, 204-205
  organ transplantation, 204-205
  treatment of cancer, 204
Immune globulin, vaccine and, 119
Immunization; *see* Health care worker
    immunity
Immunocompetence, defined, 203
Immunocompromise, defined, 203
Immunocompromised patient, 202-223
  elimination, 211
  health maintenance strategies for,
    213, 217-223
    environmental cleaning and
      safety, 218
    factors affecting, 222
    hair care, 217
    hand washing, 219
    intravenous drug use, 219
    mouth care, 218
    nutrition, 220-221
    pet care, 218
    physical and dental examinations,
      217
    procreation, 219
    sexual practices, 218
    skin care, 217
  home care considerations, 213
  integumentary system, 210
  methods to reduce risk of nosoco-
    mial infection, 214-215
  nutrition, 210
  physiological functioning, 212
  prevention and early detection, 207-
    208
  protection from infection, 208-209
  specific infection risks, 206
  standards of nursing care for, 206-
    213
Immunosuppression, defined, 203
Immunosuppressive agents, 57
Impetigo
  as reportable disease in some
    states, 49
  type and duration of precautions,
    101
Inactivated vaccines, 119
Indicator Measurement System, 9-10
Indwelling catheter
  care of, 261-264

Indwelling catheter—cont'd
  follow up assessment, 261
  home care considerations, 269-270
  procedure for inserting, 244-260
  risks, 242-243
  tips for preventing infection, 270,
      272
  urine specimens, 189
Infants; see also Neonatal procedures
  blood specimens and, 185
  sputum specimens and, 195
  stool specimens and, 190
  urine specimens and, 189
Infection, chain of, 64-69
  infectious agents, 65
  modes of transmission, 65, 66-68
  portals of entry, 65, 66
  portals of exits, 65, 66
  reservoirs, 65-66
  susceptible hosts, 65, 66, 69
Infection control practitioner (ICP),
      50-53
  areas of concern, 51
  certification of, 50
  as infection control resource, 50-51
  responsibilities of, 19, 51
Infection control programs, skills of
      managing person, 8
Infection control resources, 50-53
  association for practitioners in infec-
      tion control and epidemiology,
      51-52
  Centers for Disease Control and
      Prevention, 52
  infection control practioner, 50-51
  state and local departments of
      health, 52
  written resources, 52-53
Infection prevention
  bone marrow biopsy, 236-237
  burns, 297, 299-300, 302
  catheterization, 270, 272
  dialysis and, 358-359
  endoscopy, 237, 239
  gastrointestinal procedures, 347, 349
  immunocompromised patients, 213
  intravenous techniques, 338, 339,
      341
  nasogastric tube placement, 343-345
  neonatal procedures, 397-398
  obstetrical care, 390-394
  ostomy management, 288, 290
  paracentesis, 233
  postmortem care, 413
  thoracentesis, 235
  tracheostomy care, 231

Infections
  vs. colonization, 62, 274
  defining, 62
    in wounds, 274
  dose, 64
  general, 64
  local, 64
  nosocomial, 64
  pathogenicity, 64
  prevention and control strategies,
      70-71
    breaking mode of transmission,
        70-71
    inactivation of infectious
        agents, 70
    increasing host resistance, 70
  recognizing
    laboratory and radiology
        studies, 70
    signs and symptoms, 69
  virulence, 64
Infectious agents, 65
  inactivation of, 70
Infectious diseases
  cost issues, 3-4
  ethical and legal principles related
      to, 4-5
  occupational transmission of, 3
  research of efficacy and cost effective-
      ness of infection control, 5-6
  role of regulatory, accreditation and
      professional agencies in con-
      trol of, 7-18
  trends in, 4
Infectious mononucleosis, type and du-
      ration of precautions, 101
Infectious process
  age and, 57
  exogenous infection, 57
  medial disorders and, 57
  patient treatment and, 57
Influenza
  HCW immunization against, 118
  HCW work exclusion for, 129
  mode of transmission, 67
  as reportable disease in some
      states, 49
  type and duration of precautions,
      101
  vaccine, 121
Integumentary system
  bypassing defense mechanism of,
      61-63
  mechanical body defense, 60
Intermediate-level disinfection, defined,
      140

Internal fetal heart rate monitoring, 388-389
  description, 388
  equipment, 389
  procedure, 389
Intrauterine pressure monitoring
  description, 389
  equipment, 390
  follow up, 390
  procedure, 390
Intravascular catheters, blood specimens and, 185-186
Intravenous techniques, 304-341
  arterial puncture
    description, 306
    follow up, 328
    procedure, 322-327
  blood administration
    description, 328
    follow up, 338
    procedure, 329-332
  changing solution and tubing maintenance
    description, 328
    follow up, 338
    procedure, 334-338
  infection prevention, 338, 339, 341
    interrupt device and solution-related transmission, 338, 339
    interrupt person-to-person transmission, 339
    specific prevention measures, 341
    standard precautions, 339
  specific infection risks, 304-306
    device and solution factors, 305
    host factors, 304-305
    person-to-person factors, 305-306
  tubing-needle assemblies, needle stick injuries, 118
  venipuncture
    description, 306
    follow up, 306
    procedure, 307-321
Invasive infection, 294
Iodophors, dilution, properties and cost, 147
IPV vaccine, 120
Isolation precautions, 81-114
  body substance isolation, 82, 84
  CDC 1994 Draft Guidelines for Isolation Precautions in Hospitals, 84-90
  evolution of, 81
  guidelines for use of personal protective equipment, 94, 112

Isolation precautions—cont'd
  lack of research on efficacy and cost effectiveness, 5
  for selected infections and conditions, 95-111
  standard precautions, 84-87
  temporary clinical syndrome precautions, 85, 91-93
  transmission-based precautions, 84-85, 88-90
  universal precautions, 81-83
Isoniazid (INH), 123, 127
Isopropyl alcohol, dilution, properties and cost, 146
Jejunostomy feedings
  follow up, 346
  procedure, 346
  procedure preparation, 345-346
Joint Commission on Accreditation of Healthcare Organizations (JCAHO), 7-10
  Agenda for Change, 8
  importance of accreditation by, 7-8
  Indicator Measurement System, 9-10
  Infection Control Expert Task Force, 8-10
  infection control indicators, 9-10
  infection control standards, 8-10
  standard for surveillance, prevention and control of infection, 9
Kawasaki syndrome
  as reportable disease in some states, 49
  type and duration of precautions, 101
Klebsiella
  blood specimens, 183
  in environment, 153, 156, 157
  mode of transmission, 67
  urinary tract infection, 242
Larson, E., 53
Lassa fever, type and duration of precautions, 102
Latex sensitivity, 167
Laundry, home care isolation precautions for, 113
Legionella, 30
  in environment, 152, 155, 157
  mode of transmission, 68
  type and duration of precautions, 105
Legionellosis
  case classification, 30
  clinical description, 30
  comments on, 30
  laboratory criteria for diagnosis, 30

Legionnaires' disease, type and duration of precautions, 102
Lensed instruments, method of disinfecting, 142
Leprosy
case classification, 31
clinical description, 31
comments on, 31
laboratory criteria for diagnosis
case, 31
type and duration of precautions, 102
Leptospirosis, 31
case classification, 31
clinical description, 31
comments on, 31
laboratory criteria for diagnosis
case, 31
type and duration of precautions, 102
Leukocytes, counts of, and infection, 70
Leukocytosis, 70
Leukopenia, 70
Lice, HCW work exclusion for, 129
Linen, standard precautions, 86
Lister, Joseph, 139
Listeria, in environment, 158
Listeria monocytogenes, type and duration of precautions, 103
Listeriosis
as reportable disease in some states, 49
type and duration of precautions, 102
Live vaccine, 119
immunosuppressed HCW and, 119
tuberculin testing and 119
Localized infection, 64
signs and symptoms of, 69
Long-term care settings, need for infection control measures in, 4
Low-level disinfection, defined, 140
Lyme disease
case classification, 32
clinical description, 32
comments on, 32
laboratory criteria for diagnosis case classification, 32
type and duration of precautions, 102
Lymphatic system, mechanical body defense, 60
Lymphocytes, 59, 61, 70
Lymphocytic choriomeningitis, type and duration of precautions, 102

Lymphogranuloma venereum
case classification, 33
clinical description, 33
comments on, 33
laboratory criteria for diagnosis, 33
type and duration of precautions, 102
Lysozymes, 61
Malaria
case classification, 33
clinical description, 33
comments on, 33
laboratory criteria for diagnosis, 33
mode of transmission, 68
type and duration of precautions, 102
Manual ventilation (resuscitation) bags, 380-381
Marburg virus disease, type and duration of precautions, 102
Martin, M. S., 53
Masks
droplet precautions, 89
guidelines for use of, 94, 112
standard precautions, 86
Measles (red/rubeola)
case classification, 34
clinical description, 34
comments on, 34
HCW immunization against, 118
HCW work exclusion for, 130
laboratory criteria for diagnosis, 34
mode of transmission, 67
type and duration of precautions, 102
Measles/mumps/rubella vaccine, 122
Mechanical body defense, 58-60
bypassing, 61-63
gastrointestinal system, 60
genitourinary system, 60
integumentary system, 60
lymphatic system, 60
respiratory system, 60
skin, 59, 60
Medical equipment
critical, 148
noncritical, 145, 148
semicritical, 148
Melioidosis, type and duration of precautions, 102
Meningitis, aseptic
case classification, 22
clinical description, 22
comments on, 22
laboratory criteria for diagnosis, 22

Meningitis
 mode of transmission, 67
 temporary isolation precautions
 for, 91
 type and duration of precautions,
 102-103
Meningococcal disease
 case classification, 35
 clinical description, 35
 comments on, 35
 laboratory criteria for diagnosis, 35
 type and duration of precautions,
 105
Meningococcal pneumonia, type and
 duration of precautions, 103
Meningococcemia, type and duration
 of precautions, 103
Modes of transmission, 65, 66-68
 airborne, 68
 breaking, 70-71
 contact
 direct, 67
 droplet, 67
 indirect, 67
 definitions and examples of, 67-68
 vector, 68
 vehicle, 68
Molluscum contagiosum, type and duration of precautions, 103
Mononucleosis,
 HCW work exclusion for, 130
 type and duration of precautions,
 101
Mucormycosis, type and duration of
 precautions, 103
Multidrug-resistant organisms
 temporary isolation precautions
 for, 92
 type and duration of precautions, 103
Mumps
 case classification, 35
 clinical description, 35
 comments on, 35
 HCW immunization against, 118
 HCW work exclusion for, 130
 laboratory criteria for diagnosis, 35
 mode of transmission, 67
 type and duration of precautions,
 103
Mycobacteria
 contamination of surface equipment, 57
 in environment, 153, 155
 as reportable disease in some
 states, 49

Mycobacteria—cont'd
 type and duration of precautions,
 103
Mycobacterium tuberculosis, 46
 CDC guidelines for preventing
 transmission, 14-17
 flexible endoscopy, 346
 guidelines for preventing transmission, 11, 14
 temporary isolation precautions
 for, 91
Mycoplasma, type and duration of precautions, 105
Mycoplasma pneumonia, type and duration of precautions, 103
Nacardiosis, type and duration of precautions, 103
Nasogastric tube placement, 343-345
 follow up, 345
 infection prevention, 349
 nasogastric feedings, 345
 procedure, 344-345
 procedures preparation, 343-344
Nasopharyngeal airways, 366
Nasopharyngeal suction, 370-374
National Notifiable Diseases Surveillance System (NNDSS), 19
National Vaccine Inquiry Compensation Program, 119
Necrotizing enterocolitis, type and duration of precautions, 103
Needle disposal, 83
 standard precautions, 87
Needleless IV connectors, 117
Needle sticks
 engineering controls and, 117-118
 exposure follow up, 132-136
 home care settings, infection
 prevention in and, 216
 IV tubing-needle assemblies, 118
 resheathing/retracting syringe
 devices, 118
Neisseria gonorrhoeae, 27
Neisseria meningitidis, 35
 temporary isolation precautions
 for, 91
 type and duration of precautions, 103
Neonatal procedures, 396-406
 circumcision, 405
 exchange transfusion, 401-403
 follow up procedure, 403
 isometric exchange procedure,
 402-403
 single line procedure, 403
 specific infection risks, 402

Neonatal procedures—cont'd
  extracorporeal membrane oxygenation, 405-406
  infection prevention, 397-398
  percutaneous central venous catheters, 404-405
  signs of infection in, 396
  specific infection risks, 396-397
  umbilical artery and vein catheterization, 398-401
    blood sampling, 399-401
    catheterization procedure, 398-399
    procedure, 398
    specific infection risks, 398
Neurosyphilis
  case classification, 43
  clinical description, 43
  comments on, 43
  laboratory criteria for diagnosis, 43
Neutropenic patients, sputum specimens and, 195
Noncritical medical equipment, 145, 148
Noninvasive infection, 294
Norwalk agent gastroenteritis, type and duration of precautions, 104
Norwalk virus, in environment, 157
Nosocomial infections
  causes of, 64
  cost issues and, 3-4
  defined, 64
  mechanisms to reduce risk of, 9
  immunocompromised patient and reducing, 214-215
  preventability of, 64
  quality and efficacy of health care services and, 4
  as reportable disease in some states, 49
  respiratory care and, 363
Nosocomial pneumonia, risk factors and infection control strategies, 383
Nutrition
  burn care and, 297
  wound care and, 275, 277
Obstetrical procedures, 387-394
  infection prevention, 390-394
    in ambulatory care settings, 394
    prevention of communicable disease transmission, 390, 392
    standard precautions to reduce HIV-HBV and other pathogens transmission, 391-392, 394

Obstetrical procedures—cont'd
  internal fetal heart rate monitoring, 388-389
  intrauterine pressure monitoring, 389-390
  specific infection risks, 387-388
Occupational Safety and Health Administration (OSHA), 10-14
  Bloodborne Pathogens Standard, 11-13
  engineering controls, 117-118
  establishment of, 10-11
  guidelines for preventing transmission of tuberculosis in health care facilities, 11, 14
  high-efficiency particulate air (HEPA) respirators, 11
  work practice controls, 116-117
Olmstead, R., 53
Oncology Nursing Society's Outcome Standards for Cancer Nursing Practice, 202, 206
OPC vaccine, 120
Operating room, considerations for surgical asepsis, 173
Opportunistic infections, defined, 203
Opportunistic tumors, defined, 203
Opthalmia neonatorum, as reportable disease in some states, 49
Orf, type and duration of precautions, 104
Organ donation, postmortem care and, 409
Oropharyngeal airways, 366
Ostomy management, 285-290
  bacterial infections, 286-287
  fungal infections, 286
  home care considerations, 288
  infection prevention, 288, 290
  ostomy care, 285-286
  other common complications, 287-288
Oxygen administration
  description, 364
  follow up assessment, 365
  home care considerations, 365
  preparation, 365
  procedure, 365
  specific infection risks, 364-365
Oxygenation, wound care and, 275
Paracentesis, 233-234
  description, 233
  follow up assessment, 234
  procedure, 234
  procedure preparation, 234
  specific infection risks and infection prevention strategies, 233

Parasites, 62
Parinfluenza virus infection, type and duration of precautions, 104
Partial thickness wounds, 275
Parvovirus B19, type and duration of precautions, 104
Pasteur, Louis, 139
Pathogenicity, 64
Patient care equipment,
   contact precautions, 90
   standard precautions, 86
Patient placement
   airborne precautions, 89
   contact precautions, 89
   droplet precautions, 89
   standard precautions, 87
Patient transport
   airborne precautions, 89
   contact precautions, 90
   droplet precautions, 89
Pediculosis, type and duration of precautions, 104
Pelvic inflammatory disease, as reportable disease in some states, 49
Percutaneous central venous catheters, neonatal, 404-405
Percutaneous exposure
   follow up, 132-136
   zidovudine treatment, 132, 136-137
Peritoneal dialysis, 351-357
   catheter site infections, 352
   defined, 351
   dialysis catheter procedures, 353-356
      catheter placement, 354
      catheter safety, 354
      equipment, 354
      incision and catheter care procedure, 355-356
      patient preparation, 353-354
   exchange, 352
   infection prevention, 356
   patient education, 356-357
   peritonitis, 352-353
   specific infection risks, 352
Peritonitis, 352-353
   diagnosis and treatment, 353
   signs and symptoms, 353
Personal protective equipment (PPE)
   Bloodborne Pathogens Standards, 12-13
   gowns as, 165
   guidelines for use of, 94, 112
   minimum for, 117
   patient concerns related to, 112

Pertussis
   case classification, 36
   clinical description, 36
   comments on, 36
   HCW work exclusion for, 130
   laboratory criteria for diagnosis, 36
   mode of transmission, 67
   type and duration of precautions, 104, 110
Phagocytic dysfunctions, 205
Pharyngitis, type and duration of precautions, 108
Phenolic, dilution, properties and cost, 146
Pinworm infection, type and duration of precautions, 104
Plague
   case classification, 36
   clinical description, 36
   comments on, 36
   laboratory criteria for diagnosis case classification, 36
   mode of transmission, 68
   type and duration of precautions, 104
Plain soap, 75-78
   guidelines for use of and procedures, 76-77
Plasmodium, 33
   in Malaria, 33
Pleurodynia, type and duration of precautions, 104
Pneumococcal, type and duration of precautions, 105
Pneumocystis carinii, type and duration of precautions, 105
Pneumonia, 363
   type and duration of precautions, 104, 107, 108
Pneumonic plague, type and duration of precautions, 104
Pneumothorax, chest tubes and, 224
Polio
   mode of transmission, 68
   vaccine, 120
Poliomyelitis
   case classification, 37
   clinical description, 37
   comments on, 37
   HCW immunization against, 118
   laboratory criteria for diagnosis case classification, 37
   type and duration of precautions, 105
Polymorphonuclear neutrophils (PMNs), 70

Portals of entry, 65, 66
Portals of exit, 65, 66
Post-exposure plans, Bloodborne
    Pathogens Standards, 13
Postmortem care, 409-414
   home care considerations, 413-414
   infection prevention, 413
   procedure, 412
   procedure description, 409-410
   procedure preparation, 410, 412
   special populations, 413
   specific infection risks, 410
Povidone-iodine, 163
Pressurized steam, sterilization and,
    145
Proteus, in environment, 156
Pseudomonas
   contamination of surface equip-
     ment, 57
   dialysis and, 352
   in environment, 152-157
   mode of transmission, 67
   as transient organisms, 75
   urinary tract infection, 242
Pseudomonas aeruginosa, wounds and,
    274
Pseudomonas cepacia, type and dura-
    tion of precautions, 105
Pseudomonas Staphylococci, in envi-
    ronment, 152
Psittacosis
   case classification, 37
   clinical description, 37
   comments on, 37
   laboratory criteria for diagnosis, 37
   type and duration of precautions,
    105
Purified protein derivative (PPD), 123
   follow up, 123, 127
   HIV positive and, 123
   initial employee screening and test-
    ing, 123
   interval screening, 123
   standard for frequency of risk as-
    sessment and testing, 124-125
   summary of interpretation of tuber-
    culosis skin test, 126-127

Q fever
   as reportable disease in some
    states, 49
   type and duration of precautions,
    105
Quaternary ammonium compounds, di-
    lution, properties and cost, 146
Rabies
   case classification, 38

Rabies—cont'd
   clinical description, 38
   comments on, 38
   laboratory criteria for diagnosis, 38
   mode of transmission, 68
   type and duration of precautions,
    105
Rat-bite fever
   type and duration of precautions,
    106, 107
Regulated waste, Bloodborne Patho-
    gens Standards, 13
Reichelderfer, M., 53
Reichert, M., 53
Relapsing fever
   as reportable disease in some
    states, 49
   type and duration of precautions,
    106
Reportable diseases, 19-49; *see* specific
    diseases
   infectious diseases reportable in
    some states, 49
*Report of the committee on infectious
   diseases: the red book, The,*
    52-53
Reservoirs, 65-66
Resident organisms, 74-75
Respiratory care
   background on, 363-364
   endotracheal suctioning, 366-380
   infection prevention strategies, 381-
    385
     interruption of device-related
      transmission, 381-382
     interruption of person-to-person
      transmission, 382, 385
     nosocomial pneumonia, 383
   infection risks, 364
   nosocomial infections, 363
   oxygen administration, 364-366
   special respiratory equipment, 380-
    381
     manual ventilation (resuscitation)
      bags, 380-381
     ventilators and filters, 381
     ventilator tubing, 380
Respiratory infection
   failure to diagnose and infectious
    process, 57-58
   temporary isolation precautions
    for, 92
   type and duration of precautions,
    106
Respiratory isolation rooms, warning
    signs and, 14

Respiratory protection
  airborne precautions of, 89
  CDC guidelines for prevention of
    tuberculosis transmission,
    16-17
  OSHA guidelines for prevention
    of tuberculosis transmission,
    11, 14
Respiratory syncytial virus infection,
  363
  type and duration of precautions,
    106
Respiratory system
  bypassing defense mechanism of,
    61-63
  mechanical body defense, 60
Resuscitation bags, 83
Resuscitation equipment, standard precautions, 87
Reye's syndrome
  as reportable disease in some
    states, 49
  type and duration of precautions, 106
Rheumatic fever
  case classification, 39
  clinical description, 39
  comments on, 39
  laboratory criteria for diagnosis, 39
  type and duration of precautions,
    106
Rhizopus
  in environment, 152
Richettsial fevers, type and duration of
  precautions, 106
Rickettsiae, 62
Rickettsialpox, type and duration of
  precautions, 106
Ringworm, type and duration of precautions, 106
Ritter's disease
  type and duration of precautions,
    106, 107
Rocky Mountain spotted fever
  case classification, 39
  clinical description, 39
  comments on, 39
  laboratory criteria for diagnosis, 39
  mode of transmission, 68
  type and duration of precautions,
    106
Roseola infantum, type and duration of
  precautions, 106
Rotavirus, type and duration of precautions, 100
Respiratory syncytial virus, mode of
  transmission, 67

Rubella
  case classification, 40
  clinical description, 40
  comments on, 40
  HCW immunization against, 118
  HCW work exclusion for, 130
  laboratory criteria for diagnosis, 40
  mode of transmission, 67
  type and duration of precautions,
    107
Rubeola
  HCW work exclusion for, 130
  temporary isolation precautions
    for, 91
  type and duration of precautions,
    102
Rutala, W. A., 53
Salmonella, 41
  in environment, 154, 156-158
  flexible endoscopy, 346
  mode of transmission, 68
  as transient organisms, 75
Salmonella sp., type and duration of
  precautions, 100
Salmonella typhi, type and duration of
  precautions, 109
Salmonellosis
  case classification, 41
  clinical description, 41
  comments on, 41
  laboratory criteria for diagnosis, 41
  type and duration of precautions,
    107
Scabies
  HCW work exclusion for, 129
  type and duration of precautions,
    107
Scalded skin syndrome
  type and duration of precautions,
    107
Scarlet fever
  as reportable disease in some
    states, 49
  type and duration of precautions,
    108
Schistosomiasis, type and duration of
  precautions, 107
Second degree burns, characteristics of,
  293
Semicritical medical equipment, 148
Semipermeable membrane dressings,
  278, 279-280
  frequency of dressing changes, 280
  indications for use, 280
Serratia
  in environment, 153, 155-157

Severe combined immunodeficiency
disease, 205
Shigella, 41
mode of transmission, 68
as transient organisms, 75
Shigella sp., type and duration of precautions, 100
Shigellosis
case classification, 41
clinical description, 41
comments on, 41
HCW work exclusion for, 129
laboratory criteria for diagnosis, 41
Skin
cleansing/scrub preparation, 170-171
equipment, 171
procedure, 171
lesions, HCW work exclusion for,
130
as mechanical defense mechanism,
59, 60
resident and transient organisms,
74-75
shaving
equipment for, 171-172
procedure for wet shave, 172
Skin infection, temporary isolation precautions for, 92
Soap
antimicrobial, 75-78
guidelines for use of and
procedures, 76-77
plain, 75-78
Specimen collection
blood, 182-186, 189
cerebral spinal fluid, 196-197
key steps to, 181-182
self-protection of HCW, 182
sputum, 190, 193-195
stool, 190-192
urine, 187-190
wound, 196, 200
Specimen containers, 182
Spills, home care isolation precautions
for, 113
Spirillum minus disease
type and duration of precautions,
106, 107
Sporotrichosis, type and duration of
precautions, 107
Sputum specimens
children, 195
cultures, 195
defined, 190
elderly patients, 195

Sputum specimens—cont'd
infants, 195
neutropenic patients, 195
step-by-step guide for collection,
193-194
surgical patients, 195
tracheostomy, 195
Standard precautions, 84-87
gloves, 85
gown, 86
hand washing, 85
linen, 86
mask, eye protection and face
shield, 86
needle disposal, 87
patient-care equipment, 86
patient placement, 87
resuscitation equipment, 87
Standards for surveillance, prevention
and control of infection, by
JCAHO, 9
Standards for the Operating Room, 176
Staphylococcal disease
as reportable disease in some
states, 49
type and duration of precautions, 99,
107
Staphylococcus
ambu bags and, 380
in environment, 154, 158
gastrointestinal procedures, 342
mode of transmission, 67
Staphylococcus aureus
blood specimens, 183
burn wounds, 294
carriers, 62
circulatory access devices, 359
dialysis and, 352
in environment, 154, 157
HCW work exclusion for, 130
methicillin-resistant, 58
mode of transmission, 68
as resident organism, 75
temporary isolation precautions
for, 93
type and duration of precautions,
105, 107
wounds and, 274
Staphylococcus epidermidis
blood specimens, 183
circulatory access devices, 359
dialysis and, 352
State departments of health, as infection control resource, 52
Sterile drapes, 174-175

Sterile fields
  considerations for, 174
  equipment, 173-174
  establishing and maintaining, 173-175
  preparation, 173
  procedure, 174-175
Sterile urine specimens, 187-190
Sterilization
  defined, 145
  reference books on, 53
  type of object, and method of, 141-
    144
*Sterilization technology for the health
  care facility* (Reichert &
  Young), 53
Stool specimens, 190-192
  children and infants, 190
  cultures, 190
  ileostomy and colostomy, 190
  step-by-step guide for collection,
    191-192
Straight catheterization
  follow up assessment, 261
  home care considerations, 269-270
  procedure for inserting, 244-260
  risks, 243
  tips for preventing infection, 270,
    272
Streptobacillus moniliformis disease
    type and duration of precautions,
    106, 107
Streptococcal disease
    type and duration of precautions,
    107, 108
Streptococcal throat, HCW work exclu-
    sion for, 131
Streptococcus, 75
  mode of transmission, 67
  type and duration of precautions, 105
Strongyloidiasis, type and duration of
    precautions, 108
Surgical asepsis, 162-176
  environmental considerations, 173-
    175
    establishing and maintaining ster-
      ile field, 173-175
    operating room considerations,
      173
  monitoring and evaluating, 175-176
  patient considerations, 169-172
    skin cleansing/scrub preparation,
      169-172
    skin shaving/depilatory prepara-
      tion, 171-172
    wound covering, 172

Surgical asepsis—cont'd
  staff considerations, 162-169
    gloving, closed technique, 167-
      169
    gowning, 165-167
    removing soiled gown and
      gloves, 169-170
    surgical hand scrub, 163-165
  standards for practice, 176
Surgical hand scrub, 163-165
  equipment, 163
  preparation, 163
  procedure, 163-165
  purposes of, 163
Surgical patients, sputum specimens
    and, 195
Surgical procedures, 224-240
  bone marrow biopsy, 236-237
  chest tubes, 224-231
  endoscopy, 237, 239
  factors affecting patient, 238
  guidelines for soap use and, 77
  paracentesis, 233-234
  thoracentesis, 235
  tracheostomy care, 231-233
Susceptible hosts, 65, 66, 69
Syphilis
  case classification, 41-42, 44
  clinical description, 41-42, 44
  comments on, 41-42, 44
  laboratory criteria for diagnosis, 41-
    42, 44
  type and duration of precautions, 108
Taenia solum, type and duration of pre-
    cautions, 108
Tapeworm disease, type and duration
    of precautions, 108
Tetanus/Diphtheria toxoid vaccine, 120
Tetanus
  case classification, 45
  clinical description, 45
  comments on, 45
  HCW immunization against, 118
  laboratory criteria for diagnosis case
    classification, 45
  type and duration of precautions,
    108
Thermometers, method of disinfecting,
    143
Third degree burns, characteristics of,
    293
Thoracentesis
  description, 235
  follow up assessment, 235
  preparation, 235

Thoracentesis—cont'd
  procedure, 235
  specific infection risks and infection
     prevention, 235
Tinea, type and duration of precau-
    tions, 108
Toxic shock syndrome
  case classification, 45
  clinical description, 45
  comments on, 45
  laboratory criteria for diagnosis, 45
  as reportable disease in some
     states, 49
  type and duration of precautions,
     107, 109
Toxoplasmosis
  as reportable disease in some
     states, 49
  type and duration of precautions,
     108
Tracheostomy care, 231-233, 366
  description, 231
  follow up assessment, 233
  home care considerations, 233
  preparation, 232
  procedure, 232
  specific infection risks and preven-
     tion strategies, 231
  sputum specimens and 195
Trachoma
  as reportable disease in some
     states, 49
  type and duration of precautions,
     109
Transient organisms, 75
Transmission-based precautions
  airborne precautions
    patient placement, 88
    patient transport, 88
    respiratory protection, 88
  contact precautions
    environmental control, 90
    gloves and hand washing, 89
    gowns, 90
    patient care equipment, 90
    patient placement, 89
    patient transport, 90
  droplet precautions, 88-89
    masking, 89
    patient placement, 89
    patient transport, 89
Trench mouth, type and duration of
    precautions, 109
Treponema pallidum, 41, 42, 43, 44
Trichinella spiralis, 46

Trichinosis
  case classification, 46
  clinical description, 46
  comments on, 46
  laboratory criteria for diagnosis, 46
  type and duration of precautions,
     109
Trichomoniasis, type and duration of
    precautions, 109
Trichuriasis, type and duration of pre-
    cautions, 109
Tuberculin testing, 116, 119, 123-127
  CDC standard for frequency of risk
     assessment and testing, 124-
     125
  initial employee screening and test-
     ing, 123
  interval PPD screening, 123
  live vaccines and, 119
  PPD follow up, 123, 127
  summary of interpretation of tu-
     berculosis skin test,
     126-127
Tuberculosis
  case classification, 46
  CDC control program guidelines
    cough-inducing procedures, 17
    engineering recommendations, 16
    HCW counseling and screen-
      ing, 17
    HCW TB education, 17
    implementation, 15-16
    initial and periodic risk assess-
      ment, 15
    respiratory protection, 16-17
    written TB infection control
      plan, 15
  clinical description, 46
  comments on, 46
  HCW work exclusion for, 131
  high-efficiency particulate air respi-
     rators, 11
  infectious, 64
  laboratory criteria for diagnosis case
     classification, 46
  mode of transmission, 67, 68
  multidrug-resistant, 3, 58
  OSHA guidelines for preventing
     transmission, 11, 14
  respiratory precautions, 69
  respiratory protection, 88
  type and duration of precautions,
     103, 109
Tularemia
  case classification, 47

Tularemia—cont'd
  clinical description, 47
  comments on, 47
  laboratory criteria for diagnosis, 47
  type and duration of precautions,
    109
Two-stopcock system for vein catheter-
    ization, 399-401
Typhoid fever
  case classification, 47
  clinical description, 47
  comments on, 47
  laboratory criteria for diagnosis, 47
  mode of transmission, 68
  type and duration of precautions,
    109
Typhus
  as reportable disease in some
    states, 49
  tickborne, type and duration of pre-
    cautions, 106
  type and duration of precautions,
    109
Umbilical artery, 398-401
Universal Blood and Body Fluid Pre-
    cautions, overview of, 83
Universal precautions, Bloodborne
    Pathogens Standards, 12
Urinary tract infection (UTI), 241
  temporary isolation precautions
    for, 93
  type and duration of precautions,
    109
Urine specimens, 187-190
  children and infants, 189
  clean-voided (midstream), 189
  cultures, 189-190
  indwelling catheters, 189
  sterile specimen, 187-189
  step-by-step guide for collection,
    187-188
Vaccine
  administrative requirements for,
    119
  hepatitis B, 121
  inactivated, 119
  influenza, 121
  live, 119
  measles/mumps/rubella, 122
  polio, 120
  tetanus/diphtheria toxoid, 120
  tuberculin testing and, 119
  use of by HCW, 118
Vancomycin-resistance, preventing
    spread of, 90

Varicella
  temporary isolation precautions
    for, 91
  type and duration of precautions,
    109
Varicella-zoster, type and duration of
    precautions, 110
Vector, as mode of transmission, 68
Vehicle, as mode of transmission, 68
Vein catheterization, neonatal, 398-401
Venous blood samples, 185
Ventilators, 381
Ventilator tubing, 380
Vibrio cholerae, 25
Vibrio parahamolyticus, type and dura-
    tion of precautions, 100
Vibrios, in environment, 157
Vibriosis, as reportable disease in some
    states, 49
Vincent's angina, type and duration of
    precautions, 109
Viral disease, type and duration of pre-
    cautions, 109
Virulence, 64
Viruses, 62
Waste disposal
  home care isolation precautions for,
    113
  procedure, 151
  procedure preparation, 151
  regulated, 13
  specific infection risks and preven-
    tion strategies, 151
Water-borne infection, as reportable
    disease in some states, 49
Whipworm disease, type and duration
    of precautions, 109
White blood cells, 70
Whooping cough
  type and duration of precautions,
    104, 110
Work exclusions, for health care work-
    ers, 127-131
Work practice controls, 116-117
  Bloodborne Pathogens Standards, 12
Wound care
  assessment and management guide-
    lines, 276
  clean technique for chronic, 281
  history of, 273
  home care considerations, 285
  physiology of wound healing, 274-
    275
    partial thickness vs. full thickness
      wounds, 275

Wound care—cont'd
  semipermeable membrane dressings,
      278, 279-280
  specific infection risks, 275-277
    aging, 277
    nutrition, 275, 277
    oxygenation, 275
    systemic disease, 277
  sterile technique for full thickness
      wound care, 282-283
  topical wound dressings, 277-281
    gauze, 278, 279
    hydrocolloids, 278, 280-281
    hydrogels, 279, 281
    summary of, 278
  wound cleansing, 283-285
    wound irrigation (clean tech-
        nique), 284-285
Wound covering
  procedure, 172
  types of, 172
Wound gels, procedure preparation, 282
Wound infection
  temporary isolation precautions
      for, 93
  type and duration of precautions, 110

Wound specimens, 197, 200
  aspiration cultures, 197
  step-by-step guide for collection,
      198-199
  swab cultures, 197, 200
  tissue biopsies, 197
Yellow fever
  case classification, 48
  clinical description, 48
  comments on, 48
  laboratory criteria for diag-
      nosis, 48
  mode of transmission, 68
Yersinia enterocolitica, type and dura-
    tion of precautions, 100, 110
Yersinia pestis, 36
Young, J., 53
Zidovudine treatment
  dosage schedule for, 137
  side effects of, 137
Zoster, type and duration of precau-
    tions, 110
Zygomycetes, in environment, 154
Zygomycosis, type and duration of pre-
    cautions, 110